PSYCHIATRY

THE STATE OF THE ART

Volume 5
Child and Adolescent Psychiatry,
Mental Retardation, and
Geriatric Psychiatry

PSYCHIATRY
THE STATE OF THE ART

PSYCHIATRY

THE STATE OF THE ART

Volume 5
Child and Adolescent Psychiatry,
Mental Retardation, and
Geriatric Psychiatry

Edited by

P. PICHOT
Académie de Paris
Université René Descartes
Paris, France

and

P. BERNER, R. WOLF, and K. THAU
University of Vienna
Vienna, Austria

PLENUM PRESS • NEW YORK AND LONDON

Library of Congress Cataloging in Publication Data

World Congress of Psychiatry (7th: 1983: Vienna, Austria)
  Child and adolescent psychiatry, mental retardation, and geriatric psychiatry.

  (Psychiatry, the state of the art; v. 5)
  "Proceedings of the VII World Congress of Psychiatry, held July 11–16, 1983, in Vienna, Austria"—T.p. verso.
  Includes bibliographies and indexes.
  1. Psychiatry—Congresses. 2. Child psychiatry—Congresses. 3. Adolescent psychiatry—Congresses. 4. Mental retardation—Congresses. 5. Geriatric psychiatry—Congresses. I. Pichot, Pierre. II. Title. III. Series. [DNLM: 1. Adolescent Psychiatry—congresses. 2. Child Psychiatry—congresses. 3. Geriatric Psychiatry—congresses. 4. Mental Disorders—congresses. 5. Mental Retardation—congresses. W1 WO5385 7th 1983c/WM 100 W9238 1983c]
  RC327.W63   1983b   616.89   85-6376
  ISBN 978-1-4615-9369-0   ISBN 978-1-4615-9367-6 (eBook)
  DOI 10.1007/978-1-4615-9367-6

Proceedings of the VII World Congress of Psychiatry,
held July 11–16, 1983, in Vienna, Austria

© 1985 Plenum Press, New York
Softcover reprint of the hardcover 1st edition   1985
A Division of Plenum Publishing Corporation
233 Spring Street, New York, N.Y. 10013

PREFACE

The purpose of the World Psychiatric Association is to coordinate the activities of its Member Societies on a world-wide scale and to advance enquiry into the etiology, pathology, and treatment of mental illness. To further this purpose, the Association organizes mono- or multithematic Regional Symposia in different parts of the world twice a year, and World Congresses dealing with all individual fields of psychiatry once every five or six years. Between these meetings the continuation of the Association's scientific work is assured through the activities of its specialty sections, each covering an important field of psychiatry.

The programs of the World Congresses reflect on the one hand the intention to present the coordinating functions of the Association and on the other to open a broad platform for a free exchange of views. Thus, the VII World Congress of Psychiatry, held in Vienna from July 11 to 16, 1983, was composed of two types of scientific events - those structured by the Association and those left to the initiative of the participants. The first type comprised Plenary Sessions, planned by the Scientific Program Committee, and Section Symposia, organized by the WPA sections; the second embraced Free Symposia, free papers, video sessions, and poster presentations prepared by the participants. Altogether, 10 Plenary Sessions, 52 Section Symposia, and 105 Free Symposia took place, and 78 free papers and poster sessions and 10 video sessions were held.

The editors of the Proceedings of the VII World Congress of Psychiatry were immediately faced with two major problems, namely how to deal with such a great number of presentations and how to present them to the reader. The only way to solve the first difficulty was to restrict the Proceedings to Plenary Sessions and Symposia. The second obstacle was surmounted by grouping the Plenary Sessions and Symposia according to their scientific content, which meant waiving the chronological order of the Congress. In order to achieve reasonable uniformity in the lengths of the volumes, it was not possible to devote each of the eight books comprising the Proceedings to a single theme. Nevertheless, we hope that the final arrangement will enable colleagues interested in only certain subjects to restrict their purchases to the particular volume or volumes of their choice. The Proceedings in their entirety, however, represent a complete and comprehensive spectrum of the current areas of concern in psychiatry - the state of the art.

We are greatly indebted to our colleagues Rainer Wolf and Kenneth Thau. Their untiring efforts made the publication of these Proceedings possible.

Peter Berner

Secretary General, WPA
  at the time of the VII
  World Congress of Psychiatry
President, Organizing Committee
  VII World Congress of
  Psychiatry
Chief Editor, Congress Proceedings

ACKNOWLEDGMENTS

First and foremost, we should like to express our sincere appreciation to all colleagues whose scientific contributions comprise the content of these Proceedings.

We should also like to thank the immediate administrators of the VII World Congress of Psychiatry (Congress Team International), as well as the staff of the Vienna Secretariat of the World Psychiatric Association, for their collaboration in the compilation of this publication.

We should finally like to explain that, for technical reasons connected with the actual printing process, it has not been possible in every instance to eliminate minor typing errors.

Various reasons also prevented the compilation of all chapters in exact conformity with the presentations as contained in Plenary and Symposium Sessions.

Despite these problems, we hope that our aim to structure the content of the individual volumes as clearly as possible has met with an adequate measure of success.

INTRODUCTORY REMARKS

   The World Psychiatric Association was born out of the Organizing
Committee of the World Congress of Psychiatry. The first World Congress, held in Paris in 1950, was an event of the utmost importance.
For the first time, psychiatrists of the whole world met to exchange
their ideas and experiences and to promote the progress of our specialty. It later became obvious that such large congresses, convening
every five or six years, needed to be complemented by a more permanent
organization and by more frequent meetings smaller in scope and of a
more specialized nature. The national psychiatric societies decided
on the creation of a World Association which could assume all the responsibilities connected with such a complex task. I had the honor to
be elected President of this Association at the VI World Congress in
Honolulu and to hold this responsibility for six years until the advent
of the Vienna Congress.

   Whatever the importance of the various functions of the WPA, the
organization of these World Congresses has remained its major task.
It has become fashionable to criticize World Congresses because they
attract too many participants, because the scientific presentations
are not always of the highest quality, and because the multiplicity of
the subjects discussed in simultaneous sessions obliges the participants to limit attendance to only part of the entire program. Some of
the criticisms may be justified, but the fact remains that such congresses fulfill an important function. The majority of the psychiatrists of the world are not highly specialized research workers but
practitioners. Many of them live in countries where they are relatively isolated and where there is little opportunity for scientific
interchange. The World Congresses, by presenting not only the latest
technical discoveries but also general surveys through leading specialists in the different fields of psychiatry, allow every participant to keep abreast of the state of the art. There is no better
opportunity to become acquainted with developing trends, and personal
experience of this type cannot be replaced by the reading of scientific
journals. Of course, the value of such Congresses depends on the care
with which the program is prepared. The readers of these Proceedings
will have the opportunity to convince themselves that the Austrian
Organizing Committee, under the chairmanship of Prof. Peter Berner,

Secretary General of the WPA at the time of the Congress, has attained this goal, and that the scientific quality of the papers presented and now printed is worthy of the tradition of our World Congresses of Psychiatry.

Pierre Pichot

President, WPA
  at the time of the VII
  World Congress of Psychiatry
President, Scientific Committee

CONTENTS

MENTAL RETARDATION

GERIATRIC PSYCHIATRY

DEMENTIA IN LATE LIFE

RECENT ADVANCES IN PSYCHOPHYSIOLOGICAL
DISORDERS OF OLD AGE

NEUROTRANSMITTERS IN THE DEMENTIAS OF
OLD AGE AND THEIR IMPLICATIONS FOR TREATMENT

DEMENTIAS AS MULTI-STAGE PROCESSES

MENTAL DETERIORATION IN THE AGED – ASPECTS OF RECOGNITION, DIAGNOSIS, AND MANAGEMENT

PSYCHOPHARMACOLOGY IN LATE LIFE

SERVICES TO THE ELDERLY –
EVALUATION OF EFFECTIVENESS

DAY-HOSPITAL CARE FOR THE ELDERLY

SOME CRITICAL COMMENTS ON THE PROBLEM OF CLASSIFICATION AND NOMENCLATURE IN CHILD AND ADOLESCENT NEUROPSYCHIATRY

W. Spiel
Department of Child and Adolescent Neuropsychiatry
University of Vienna Medical School
Währinger Gürtel 74-76, A-1090 Wien

As we all know, child and adolescent psychiatry was the first of all medical disciplines to abandon the concept of mono-etiologic and/or substrate-related diagnoses of disease entities in favor of a diagnostic approach which focusses on the individual's life history and takes into account developmental processes occurring in a given environment and their deviations from normal. As a consequence, research has centered on the pathology of differentiating, developing and re-integrating processes affecting the maturing nervous system and psychic make-up of children and adolescents.

Thus, child neuropsychiatry was the first of the medical or rather medico-psychological disciplines to accept the principle of multi-etiologic causation and development-oriented interpretation of diseases and their symptoms: As a result, the "time factor" and "phase-specificity" assumed fundamental significance.

Labels commonly attached to a case, which were borrowed from re-educational, depth psychological and sociopsychiatric parlance, such as "neglect", "life crisis", "maladjustment", etc., have gradually disappeared from scientific publications because of their poorly defined meaning.

Historically, the diagnoses made by child and adolescent psychiatrists have thus been derived from a multi-component approach, an approach which is gaining increasing importance in other medical disciplines, e.g. in internal medicine, immunology, dermatology, etc. In keeping with this approach such terms as "multi-factor", "multicausal" and "multidimensional" have been coined to describe etiologic constellations and tri-axial or multi-axial documentation systems have been devised for better comparability of the data elicited.

1

Important as this development has been, we would be remiss if we were not to admit that any diagnostic system will restrain cognitive and conceptualizing processes needed for pinpointing the true nature and causation of diseases and disorders. In fact, the more narrowly defined a system is, the more pronounced will its restraining effect be because, whatever its nature, it will invariably reflect the conceptual background of a specific philosophy. As soon as a diagnostic system is agreed upon, access to new ideas, experiences and theories is barred at least for some time, because these will automatically be fitted in a set of preconceived ideas.

It may well be that a common diagnostic system imposed upon its users will enable them to compare their cases better. But this obvious advantage is offset by a major disadvantage in that differential evaluations of etiologic factors and symptoms of a given disease process are no longer readily understood. And what's more: it is far from certain that our n-axial systems really are such a perfect match of reality that we may slavishly adhere to them for ever without any need for modification.

If, to compound matters, symptoms other than those of the past 6 months are to be neglected, as in the ICD system of adult psychiatry, the single most important principle of child and adolescent psychiatry, i.e. the individual's life history, the developmental processes, the notorious time factor, will be grossly violated.

In proposing a differently conceived diagnostic system, which is being used at the Vienna Center, I will not deny that this, as any other model, reflects a philosophy, a weltanschauung. But its ideological foundations are, I am convinced, much less restririctive than all other pragmatic listings by etiologies and syndromes. To the best of my knowledge, there is not a single current diagnostic model which would run counter to a classification system designed to cover
  (1) the somatic, i.e. the biologic and organic level;
  (2) the psychological level; and
  (3) the social and environmental level.

In the proposed diagnostic system each of these levels is analyzed in terms of (1) the individual's basic endowment, i.e. the unalterable and constitutional factors; (2) the dynamic processes which manifest themselves in the course of an individual's life history; and (3) the impact of acute fateful events. Further differentiation may well be attempted by quantitative weighting, e.g. as "slight", "moderate" and "severe". For the sake of clarity, this aspect will, however, not be discussed, but left for a later publication.

(1) The Vienna School maintains that there is no psychiatric disorder afflicting children and adolescents which would not necessitate reflection upon the physical condition, the basic somatic endowment of the individual. This endowment should, in our view, always be considered in its qualitative

aspects. We believe it is a gross mistake to neglect the basic somatopsychic make-up of a patient, as is largely done in Rutter's and the DSM-3 classifications, for except of the individual's intellectual endowment (coded in axis 3), his primary being and innate dispositions go unheeded there. But those who are involved in child and adolescent psychiatry simply cannot sidestep an individual's constitution, the a priori conditions of his life process. Just think of the "diatheses" which ahve greatly facilitated pediatric diagnoses, or of Kretschmer's and Sheldon's "constitutional types", etc. That this aspect is fundamental for any patient appraisal and that it should be reflected upon will surely be uncontested.

Other elements to be considered at the somatic level include processes which bring about pathoplastic changes in the course of development, i.e. accelerating, retarding, dysharmonizing and deviational processes as well as processes causing discontinuities in development, in one word: variants of development. It cannot be denied that every school and every center attribute these phenomena to different origins. While some stress the importance of social factors for dysharmonizing processes during puberty, others put the emphasis on the genetically preformed forces operating during maturation. In commenting on this aspect, I would like to draw your attention to the potentially endogenous origin of developmental pathology, which should always be thought of even if the abnormality manifests itself in dysharmony, in changes of the time course of events or in deviational patterns.

Finally, acute events should be considered, i.e. events of a fateful nature which acutely inferfere with the process of somatic development, such as inflammatory conditions of the central nervous system, brain injuries or other events resulting in significant impairment of life. When eliciting these life events, it is essential to record the time of their occurrence, because it is of particular significance for developmental pathology. To ignore the phase-dependence of developmental pathology secondary to fateful life events would be tantamount to depriving child and adolescent psychiatry of one of its most sturdy pillars. This is aptly illustrated by an elementary truth: Loss of hearing before the age of 3 years will inevitably result in deaf-muteness, while the same event occurring after the third year of live will largely leave the development of speech unaffected.

(2) Let me turn to the second level, i.e. the psychological level. As at the somatic level, a triple break-down should be attempted using the criteria outlined for future documentation.

The existence of a priori abnormalities, of dispositions which are "different", may well be assumed at this level, although there is still considerable controversy about what the a priori psychic dispositions are. While it is generally accepted that intelligence, extravert versus introvert response patterns and emotional make-up are predetermined, so that the need for reflecting upon an individual's basic endowment with them will be uncontested, there are other aspects, e.g. character traits, cognitive processes and the use of cerebral functions, for which a genetic basis is disputed.

Our proposal to reflect upon an individual's basic psychological endowment should, therefore, be interpreted as an attempt for fostering further discussion.

That life events leave their imprints on development processes at the psychological level, channeling, advancing or repressing them, will no doubt be generally accepted. Consequently, common concepts of depth psychology and their significance should be documented under this heading, particularly such problems as the duration of certain events, deprivation, situations of deficiency affecting the development of functions and skills, etc.

Similarly, acute fateful events imprinting themselves at the psychological level should be considered in as much as they interfere with the dynamic processes of development, differentiation, re-integration and individuation. Even though appraisals of these events are apt to vary widely depending on the training background of the examiners, an effort should be made to distinguish between life events of a more chronic nature which slant development and those which acutely interfere with an individual's life history in a fateful manner.

(3) Finally, the socialization level should be considered. We believe that, here again, a distinction of the 3 causal factors can be made:

In assessing the process of socialization, the persistently present constituents of the individual's environment should be documented in terms of the "basic endowment". These would include stable situational conditions during early childhood, e.g. persistently held social status, presence or absence of educational rapport, educational background, etc.

In terms of the chronology of an individual's socialization, the flux of the individual's life situation should be considered, This includes continuous or discontinous conditions of socialization, the broke-home situation, events drastically changing the individual's life situation, etc.

Finally, acute events affecting the individual's socialization can be traced and their significance documented, e.g. political change, flight, unemployment.

I fully appreciate that different schools will hold different views on the delineations of sublevels within the 3 levels to be considered, their interrelationships and the definitions used, just as I am aware of the fact that, depending on the examiner's position, one and the same event may be documented at 2 different levels. In addition, opinion will surely be divided on what makes up the individual's basic endowment: Qualities regarded as constitutional by some are apt to be attributed to the flux of the life situation by others. But it may well be that the very need to reflect on the 3 sublevels outlined, i.e.

Table 1. Diagnostic system

	Basic factor/ basic endowment	Development/history/ time factor	Fateful factor/ acute situation
Somatic level	constitutional variants, e.g. neuropathic, dysplastic, asthenic, etc., sequels of prenatal/ perinatal events, base-line condition	acceleration, retardation, dysharmony orthogenetic, morphologic deviations	acute event (disease), change in circumstances of life
Psychic level	intelligence, mood extravert/introvert, unstable/stable, integr./disintegr. (psychopathy, variation), etc.	acceleration, retardation, dysharmony, developmental deviation, discontinuity, behavioral or performance defect	acute event (trauma), change in circumstances of life (irritation)
Social level	social status educational background, family (complete/incomplete), persistent contributory factors	continuous/discontinuous (break), adequacy of status, deprivation, stimulation	acute event (accidental) (fateful)

(1) the individual's basic endowment,

(2) the product of an individual's life history, and

(3) the acute events in an indiviual's life,

constitutes the true merit of this documentation system. In my thinking, other documentation systems in current use with their narrowly defined compartmentalization leave little scope for answering those specific questions which we are all deeply concerned with: What is the individual's basic endowment? What should be attributed to his development? What has made him the patient facing us? And what conclusions can we draw from the answers to these questions for his treatment?

After having expounded our basic diagnostic concepts, I would like to round off the picture by describing the classification of psychodynamic processes we have come to employ. To fully appreciate it, it is necessary to recall its conceptual foundation which is central to our thinking: Development is a dynamic process in terms of disintegration, differentiation, growth and re-integration.

A sharp distinction is made by the Vienna School between:

(a) Processes in terms of experiental responses to events which have a non-persistent effect on a person's integrity, his health, function and the homeostasis of physical and psychological mechanisms;

(b) Processes which result in an unbalanced personality development: In psychodynamic terms, these are defined as situations during a person's upbringing which cause development, differentiation, disintegration and re-integration to become persistently deviant. Just think of authoritarian education as a factor underlying the development of unbalanced personalities;

(c) Classical neuroses whose operant dynamisms can only be explained by unconscious forces and defense mechanisms.

An effort is made in each and every case to differentiate between these 3 well-defined dynamic mechanisms acting on a person's evolving psychic make-up. Once an idea has been formed about them, the information elicited is fitted in the 3-level classification system, i.e. somatic, psychological, social. We are convinced that this procedure enables us to retrace psychic processes more realistically and make their effects more transparent than other models in current use.

Ladies and gentlemen, it was my pleasure and privilege to share with you a diagnostic classification system and nomenclature which has been practiced in Vienna for years, in fact, for some decades. Once again, I would like to stress that this approach to classification permits the documentation of cases in a manner which will not hinder the discussion of other scientific positions, as other documentation systems appear to do. This is expressly why we raised this problem for consideration at the present congress.

STUDIES OF RISK, VULNERABILITY AND RESILIENCE IN CHILDREN

E. James Anthony

Washington University School of Medicine
St. Louis, Missouri, U.S.A.

Children of psychotic parents (schizophrenic or manic-depressive)
are more susceptible as a group to psychiatric disorders during
childhood and to "breakdowns" with hospitalization during adolescence
and early adult life than the children of psychiatrically healthy
controls. These general findings from a 15-year prospective investigation have been revalued by inter-group and intra-group studies that
indicate the high degree of variability in the lifetime reactions of
the offspring, differences between the children of schizophrenics and
manic-depressives, differences between the children of male and
female psychotics, differences between children in relation to the
sex of the psychotic parent, differences between the siblings of
different ages relative to the onset of psychosis in the parent and
differences based on social class and ethnic factors.

In recent years, it has become evident that the differences
between the children who have a psychotic parent are determined not
only by demographic factors of age, sex, socio-cultural influences,
but also by the presence or absence of inherent strengths and weak-
nesses. Thus, there seem to be vulnerabilities and resiliences
stemming from "constitutional" and early environmental experiences,
beginning with pregnancy and birth.

These concepts of risk, vulnerability, and resilience have
opened up new avenues of approach not only in the area of psycho-
togenesis but also in child psychiatry as a whole. The children are
now deemed to be at high risk before deviant development if there is
some significant congenital handicap, if the care giver is incompe-
tent (as with teenage mothers), disturbed and disturbing (as with
psychiatrically disordered parents, addicted parents, conflicted,
divorcing parents or physically handicapped parents), or if the

environment is disadvantageous (as in conditions of ghetto upbringing, chronic unemployment and poverty, political harassment or conditions of war and mass displacement). As with all stress experiences, it is difficult to ascertain the level of insult to the individual objectivity since subjective factors tend to add a hidden quota of influences that are not at all easy to gauge. For example, it has been found in various contexts that children who are exposed to noxious circumstances or disasters can be insulated from the effects by the protective buffering provided by the trusted parent figures. In my 15-year longitudinal study of children with psychotic parents, the risks entailed varied from family to family and from child to child within the same family because of inherent differences in the children, because of different degrees of disorganization of family life, because of the unpredictable impingements of psychosis on child-rearing, because of the idiopathic nature of psychosis, and because of the constantly shifting in the sociocultural background of everyday living.

The risk factor varies with the factor of vulnerability or increased susceptibility to stressful events. Not every child in a family is equally vulnerable to trauma, nor equally vulnerable to the same trauma. Some may be specifically sensitive, for instance, to certain aspects of the psychotic impact--the affective dysphorias or incongruities, the thought disorders, the peculiarities of communication, the delusional and hallucinatory systems, the unpredictabilities in response, and, less specifically, the violence and threat of violence, the incestuous approaches, and the sheer intensity of relationships. The elements in the individual child that enhance their susceptibility to the psychotic process include suggestibility, submissiveness, a close identification with the disordered parent, and a morbid involvement in the psychotic illness.

As a result of the interplay of the risk and vulnerability factors, two parallel conditions gradually evolve:

1. A spectrum of differences in the degree of vulnerability and resilience to the different stresses stemming from psychosis and ranging from hyper vulnerability to a relative invulnerability.

2. A wide spectrum of disorder, ranging through primitivization, folie-a-deux, transient micropsychoses, reactive disorders manifested by anxiety and depression, and simple suffering that Manfred Bleuler considers the inevitable concomitant of the psychotic process in the family.

The longitudinal study of children at high risk for psychosis offers the investigator an opportunity to study the vicissitudes of developmental psychopathology. Although all children suffer from

8

living with psychosis in a parent, and about 40 to 50% show reactive disorders and maladjustments of a non-specific nature, only a small percentage, between 5 and 15% depending on the nature of the psychosis and the degree to which the second parent is also psychiatrically disturbed, will show psychotic-like disturbances.

Furthermore, the children of schizophrenic parents are significantly different from the children of manic depressive parents in a number of ways. Whereas the children of schizophrenic parents remain heavily involved in the psychotic oppression. Secondly, whereas the offspring of schizophrenics have an increasing difficulty in discriminating affects, the children of manic depressives demonstrate an increasing sensitivity in the recognition and response to affects. Thirdly, the children of manic depressives do not display evidence of thought disorder, pathological introversion and eccentric types of response compared with the children of schizophrenics. Fourthly, the mean intelligence of the children of manic depressives is higher than that of the children of schizophrenics. Fifthly, whereas the children of schizophrenic mothers are significantly more disturbed than the children of schizophrenic fathers, this difference is not present in the children of manic depressive parents.

In spite of these differences, it is generally impossible to differentiate, under blind conditions, the first adolescent "breakdowns" of the two groups, and it is not until the third or fourth "breakdown" that critical diagnostic differences make their appearance.

A small percentage of the sample (about 8-10%) manifests a remarkable resilience that has increasingly caught the interest of the investigator. This subsample has been given various labels: stress-resilient, invulnerables, superphrenics, superchildren, etc. Stress-resilience is probably the least controversial term and is coming increasingly into practice. Some of the children are resilient from infancy onward; some are vulnerable at the beginning of life and become increasingly resilient; and some are resilient during the early phase and may then become vulnerable. There is probably no such state as total or permanent invulnerability. These resilient children do not form a homogeneous subgroup. Differences are imposed by the qualities of the cultural milieu and the possession of particular talents. For example, children from the upper social classes with special endowments (that Carlsson has related to the schizophrenic diathesis) are able, in spite of horrendous experiences at the hands of psychotic parents, to demonstrate superior adjustments coupled with creative capacities. They are generally described as "outstanding" and have a consistent record of scholastic excellence and remarkable extracurricular achievements. In addition to these competences, they are highly resistant to the psychotic process, developing defenses and coping skills that are precocious. Thus, they become almost clinically objective in their attitude to the parental illness, distance themselves from disorganizing and disturbing behaviors, and yet are often able to respond compassionately and helpfully to the parent's condition. Another group of children lack talent and high intelligence but show the same resistance to the abnormal process by responding to disintegrating effects by re-integrating the environment. They are often able to take control of the household and substitute for much of the parent's activities, at the same time maintaining a level of equanimity and superior adjustment. But, as Manfred Bleuler pointed out, all these children, who live under the shadow of psychosis however successfully, have doubts about their future and doubts about their own offspring: nor can they escape the suffering inherent in the situation. In fact, suffering is the badge of this tribe of children who have "lost" their parents through psychosis and are consequently less able to recapture any sustained period of happiness.

Conclusions

The earlier ad hoc studies of children of psychotic parents have given place to current investigations based on a risk-vulnerability-resilience model, that takes into account the recent work on stress, on trauma, on crisis and on disaster, projected against the background of the "epigenetic landscape" postulated by Waddington and Piaget. In this prospective perspective, one is better able to follow the course of life determined by the varying proportion of influences exerted by nature and nurture, make use of the risk paradigm, and monitor the striking vicissitudes of development under the influence of psychosis. It also becomes possible to understand detailed intraindividual and intragroup phenomena that may be lost in gross intergroup analyses. Out of this kind of approach, a new data-based developmental psychopathology is being born that should scientifically buttress the future growth of Child Psychiatry.

PROBLEMS IN NOMENCLATURE AND CLASSIFICATION OF MBD

Kiyoshi Makita

Department of Psychiatry and Behavioral Science
Tokai University School of Medicine
Isehara, Kanagawa 259-11, Japan

Perhaps there is no other clinical entity in the field of child psychiatry or pediatric neurology which evolved through so many changes in its designation than MBD. I do not have any intention of reciting those names here since it would be a waste of time. Instead, I want you to give just a blink on a listing of them below:

1. The hyperactive child syndrome.
2. The hyperkinetic syndrome.
3. Minimal cerebral dysfunction.
4. Minimal brain damage.
5. Minimal brain injury.
6. The brain-damaged child.
7. The brain-injured child.
8. The perceptually handicapped child.
9. The perceptually disabled child.
10. The dysfunctioning child.
11. The dyslexic child.
12. The clumsy child.
13. Chronic brain syndrome.
14. The Strauss syndrome.
15. The Prechtl choreiform syndrome.
16. Specific learning disabilities.
17. Learning disorders.
18. Maturational lag syndrome.
19. Central nervous system dysfunctions.
20. Attention deficit disorder.

If you would read the list a bit carefully, you will find that the connotations, or types of combination of the leading symptoms of each imply some delicate difference along with the difference in nomenclature. First of all, here we see a mixture of descriptive designations and of etiological, or assumptive pathogenic designations; in other words, a hodge-podge of everything.

An integration of such names resulted in the term MINIMAL BRAIN DYSFUNCTION, discarding the peripheral differences which seemed to be minor and keeping the greatest common measure, or more explicitly, by putting everything into a bigger lump encompassing all. This challenge was met by Swaiman, Peters and others trying to delineate between the hyperkinetic type and the learning disability type, but they had to settle with a mixed type in between for the formidable overlapping cases, or instead, as somebody said in trying to express the situation, they were left with a few circles and their overlappings.

Once the standard concept of MBD was established, it became necessary to compare what we call MBD now with what were called learning disabilities in the past for instance, and then to compare it with what are currently considered learning disabilities. These comparisons will definitely bring out the differences between the three, and you will re-recognize that what used to be called learning disabilities are not the same as what we term learning disability now; so that it is not adequate to consider the "learning disabilities" of the past as being synonymous with contemporary MBD.

And then, the more or less unified term of MBD is being challenged by the term ADD, i.e., ATTENTION DEFICIT DISORDER with the advent of DSM-III, which, again, is different from either MBD or MCD as it is sometimes referred to on the continent. The utmost difference between the two designations, or the two concepts lies in the fact that while MBD is derived from the pathogenetic point of view, ADD is a concept stemming entirely from the clinical and descriptive points of view, so that it is nonsense to argue which is better or which is worse, not to say which is right or which is wrong. Another difference lies in their connotation. While MBD apparently excludes psychogenous factors as the etiological element, ADD does not openly exclude the intervention of emotional factors as a pathogenic possibility, as far as the guidelines in DSM-III are concerned. So, in speaking of ADD according to the DSM-III, it is considered that some psychogenous factors may come into play to influence the precipitation of hyperkinesis, if my understanding of the latter is correct. In other words, the by-product of the MBD concept, which was the possible exoneration of the parents, was not sustained for very long.

The attitude of the biologically-oriented scientists is also becoming more flexible. While Millichap, J., was excluding emotional disturbances or environmental and socioeconomical factors in his writing in 1975, he is stressing the importance of multifacettedness in establishing the concept of MBD as well as in establishing policies of treatment in 1983. I personally agree with multifacetted, multidimensional and multifactorial thinking; of course, with the premise that the primary role of the constitution of MBD is allocated to somatogenous handicaps or impairments.

I cannot help but feel as if I am wandering in a corner of a maze struggling to find the way out and I believe many of my international colleagues may be feeling the same. I think it is true that the arrival of ADD made things more complicated, although I do not have the slightest intention to lay any blame on it. But even in the days of MBD alone, we had enough problems causing headaches. The foremost difficulty which plagues us is how we can set the appropriate diagnostic criteria for diagnosing MBD. The criteria we have employed so far is far too vague and ambiguous. Hyperkinesis is the primary feature of this disturbance. About 10 major symptoms including hyperactivity, short attention span, distractibility, impulsiveness, uncoordination, perceptual impairment, disorders of memory and concept formation, neurologic and EEG abnormalities, speech and language problems, and specific learning disabilities have been considered as the most common diagnostic criteria, but nobody ever declared that you have to have all of those features for making a diagnosis of MBD. It is well known that just a few of them will suffice. In my experience, I have found that there is some difference in the pattern of clustering of those findings, in one way or other, and many other foremost experts in the field may have found the same. And then, there also is the empirical fact that none of the cases have a full-fledged combination of the so-called "soft neurologic signs", so that the problem is to what extent and number those signs have to be witnessed in order to be called MBD and this matter has rarely been discussed so far. In fact, it cannot be overlooked that there are cases in which the above-mentioned clinical features are found but without any of the neurologic signs.

Another point of controversy is to what extent the lower limit the "normal intellectual zone" should be expanded in diagnosing MBD. Primarily, mental retardation was to be theoretically excluded in the criteria of the concept of MBD. Soon however, we were to learn that in reality, the value of measured intelligence very often came out lower than the assumed normal potential of the child just because of the aforementioned features such as hyperactivity, that is, short attention span, distractibility, etc. Consequently, it became necessary to set a standard as to what extent the "normal IQ" has to be compromised, taking the influence of the clinical, behavioral features into consideration. It was just an year ago at the IACAPAP Congress in Dublin that I was informed of the proposal by a German expert of adopting a standard of 70 in measured IQ as the limit in considering cases as MCD which he and his colleagues were utlizing. And I think this may be an appropriate discretion which I am ready to accept.

Another point of argument is that regarding the reading of EEG. Very often, some slight abnormalities may serve to impress the evaluator of a possibility of organic intervention. However, it is quite problematic to differentiate the extent to which EEG abnormalities should be considered as justification for a diagnosis of MBD. Millichap reported that among the so-diagnosed MBD cases, what he experienced could be divided into 4 groups of 12% with normal EEG, 62% with dysrhythmia, 19% with dysrhythmia characterized by sharp and slow waves of moderate severity, and 7% with spike and waves, or spike or sharp wave abnormalities indicative of seizure activity. These results seem to suggest that the severity of the clinical manifestations do not always concur with the severity of abnormalities in EEG readings. Although the designation of MBD is pathogenic in nature, I consider that the inclusion of paroxysmal grades of EEG does not deserve to be crowned with the adjective of "minimal". So, in a situation where the grade of EEG abnormality is to be utilized as a factor in making a diagnosis of MBD, I do not think that the inclusion of EEG readings implying seizure activity is appropriate or justifiable. In other words, we have here the problem of establishing standard criteria with regard to the maximum severity of dysrythmia which can be qualified as a determinant in making a diagnosis of MBD.

Just like these few that I have picked up, there are so many factors which remain unclear quantitatively as well as qualitatively. So, what we are dealing with at the moment may be no more than MBD SUSPECTS with the potential of being real cases of MBD, more or less, if such an entity ever exists. As such, the urgent need called for is the establishment of more dependable and precise diagnostic criteria. But for this purpose, a review and analysis of the current concept of MBD and its classification into a few subgroups of individual clinical features on the basis of differences which were lost in the process of integration into the present concept of MBD needs to be undertaken. I think the audience here is well aware that there is for instance MBD with hyperkinesis and without hyperkinesis, and that to consider learning disabilities as being a synonymous entity with hyperkinetic MBD is not adequate. From such clinical experience, it can be deduced that the quantitative overlapping from the standpoint of pathogenicity may be quite extensive. However, if you regard the situation at the clinical, descriptive level, the overlapping area may become much smaller and in some specific situations, it may not be going too far to say that the overlapping may become almost negligible.

As it is, meaningful comparative studies on MBD are not possible working with such ambiguous specimens as we are. The advent of some breakthrough technology which could pinpoint the existence and the function of biological involvement would go a long way in solving our problem. However it would probably be some time until such highly developed technology becomes a reality, and even such progressive techniques would probably not be able to produce significant results if the target specimen is not clearly defined.

This is the reason why I am so strongly stressing the need of a new subclassification in the framework of what we now call MBD. The approaches have to be multifactorial and multiaxillar. For instance, a comparative study may be very meaningful in trying to elucidate the determinant responsible for the divergence of the cases into the hyperkinetic and the learning disability types. Of course, better-defined comparative studies dependent on clinical observations may be necessary. Perhaps, morphological studies will not be easy given the contemporary levels of technology. But, then again, it seems to me

14

that challenges from the functional level might stand the best chance at this stage.

With the advent of the etiological hypothesis which was closely related to the progress of neurophysiological and neurochemical advances, psychopharmacological research on MBD is becoming extremely active. More so since the target symptoms are relatively easy to grasp and subsequently, the therapeutic effects can also be easily observed in this disorder. Central stimulants are catching the limelight among the improving measures today, and it is well known that methylphenidate in particular is producing quite effective results. Furthermore, it has also come to be known that a marked tendency of slowing is observed on EEG records in methylphenidate responders along with the fact that the evaluation of auditory evoked potential revealed that it was on the hypoarousal level.

In order to make pharmacotherapy for MBD more effective as well as safer, an international project is under way between a Bulgarian scientist and my staff aiming at the predictive differenciation of methylphenidate responders and non-responders from the standpoints of types of clinical manifestations, results of psychological tests (the Bender gestalt test in particular), and meticulous examination of EEG and evoked potential. This study has just been launched and still being at the stage of preparatory research, is not ready to be reported here. But still, even from our meager experience with two or three cases, some interesting findings seem to be found in the correlation between the electrophysiological changes caused by methylphenidate and the clinical symptoms. Examination of concentration levels in the blood is also planned as part of this study. But let me limit myself to introducing this preliminary data to you, since it is much too premature to bear speaking of at this point, a fact which the research associates are all well aware of.

CONCLUSION

1) The overlapping and non-overlapping specific features covered in the old nomenclature, which vanished in the process of integration into the concept of MBD, need to be reviewed and new subtypes have to be considered. The diagnostic criteria presently employed is too loosely defined, which results in our dealing with what are in reality no more than "MBD Suspects".

2) Quantitative standards for the positive signs to be justifiably called MBD is necessary in terms of soft neurologic signs, grades of intellectual potentials, EEG readings, etc.

3) Multifacetted, multifactorial and multidimensional challenges to delineate between the individual sub-classifications in MBD must be encouraged and nourished. There, for the first time, we should find ourselves standing at the true starting point from which to embark on the road toward the further understanding of MBD.

REFERENCES

Millichap, J.G., 1975, "The Hyperactive Child with Brain Dysfunction," Year Book Medical Publishers, Inc., Chicago.

Millichap, J.G., 1982, "The Hyperactive Child," Triangle, Sandoz.

Peters, J.E. et al, 1973, "The Physicians' Handbook Screening for M.B.D.," Ciba Medical Horizons.

Sakuta, T., 1982, MBD in Japan - its clinical situation (in Japanese), Psychiatria et Neurologia Paediatrica Japonica, 22-2.

Suzuki, M., 1979, "MBD," (in Japanese) Kawashima, Tokyo.

Swaiman, K.F., 1975, The practice of pediatric neurology, in: "Learning Disabilities," B.D. Wright, ed., Mosby Co., St. Louis.

ANOREXIA NERVOSA IN EARLY ADOLESCENCE

Winston Rickards

Director, Department of Psychiatry and Behavioural
Science, Royal Children's Hospital
Flemington Road, Parkville, 3052, Australia

This paper is concerned with change. Adolescence is regarded
as a period of heightened developmental vulnerability – biological,
psychological, social and cultural, where crisis can readily disrupt
continuity.

Physically, adolescence is a period of body growth and physiological changes, psychologically a period of individuation,
emancipation and striving for gender role and identity. Socially
and culturally it is a period of striving for peer group acceptance
and participation as an autonomous person in the outside world. The
transition to biological and sexual maturity is one of the dramatic
affect-arousal situations.

Adolescence is a period of maximal developmental change. The
developmental tasks of achieving identity, gender, body image and
morality are in transition.   To any given adolescent all these tasks
stem not only from innate constitutional biological patterns, but also
from powerful family, social and cultural forces.

Developmental flow is notoriously uneven with spurts and lags
which may be healthy adaptations and need not represent disorder.

Anorexia Nervosa so called,is a disorder which <u>physically</u>
disrupts body growth, promotes widespread physiological delay and
disruption to sexual and physical maturation, which <u>psychologically</u>
is characterized by disruption of processes of identity formation,
body image, gender identity, and <u>socioculturally</u> renders the
adolescence unable to compete adaptively in the social world in which
society's cultural conflicts are reflected.

17

In contrast to underdeveloped societies, in developed Western societies, dietary behaviours which we now know may represent a variety of eating disorders, are epidemic, fashionable. To vulnerable individuals are highly dangerous. To be thin is beautiful and good; not to be, may be bad. For them it is a case of starvation in the midst of plenty.

In some schools, dieting is competitive, the existence and nature of Anorexia Nervosa has become common knowledge. Some estimates suggest that in a Western metropolis, about 1 in 100 high school girls are affected.

This is not merely an adolescent subculture. Body concern has always been an anxiety. The focus has changed from preoccupation with sexuality to more global concerns. The same conflicts, a different focus.

These themes have been with us throughout history. Hippocrates gave great emphasis to the therapeutic value of diet, "excessive loss of weight and likewise fasting if taken to extremes is treacherous". Fasting and self enforced starvation throughout the ages has been a religious ritual but the disease theme of Anorexia Nervosa follows Richard Morton who in 1689 described the condition in his Treatise of a Nervous Consumption.

Sir William Gull in 1874 described the symptom complex Anorexia Nervosa: extreme weight loss, almost total failure of appetite without demonstrable physical cause, typically in girls between 16 and 25 years with amenorrhoea, bradycardia, constipation. He puzzled on the remarkable energy and ceaseless activity displayed by the patients despite their emaciation.

It is not unusual in medicine that cases of great pathological severity give rise to what is thought at first to be a rare pathological disease. The original description becomes a stereotype for diagnosis. This may explain the delay in fully recognizing its occurrence in males, children and persons with other medical conditions.

With this background we can survey a period of the last 30 years in which children with severe weight loss due to voluntary food refusal needed to be admitted as inpatients to the Royal Children's Hospital, the teaching Paediatric Hospital in Melbourne, Australia. The sample does not refer to children managed within the family or through Out-patient consultation or to the early infancy years, but to very sick children with body weight below the tenth percentile and no demonstrable organic cause.

In the first 10 years the diagnosis of Anorexia Nervosa of such emaciated children was critically reviewed as the condition was rare. The incidence doubled in the next decade and nearly trebled in the third decade and the incidence continues to rise.

In a personal series a total of 153 children were seen, 113 were girls and 40 were boys, representing 26% of the group. This sex ratio has been consistent over the years. The children in early adolescence – 12 to 14 years of age, who are considered today represent 67% or two-thirds of the sample.

Within these broad criteria a remarkable heterogeneity has been seen with a variable relationship to psychiatric disorder illustrating a range of biological vulnerabilities, e.g., metabolic, endocrine, hypothalamic, neuro-transmitters, psychological and social, and risk factors to which the early adolescent is so sensitive when approaching the tasks of the second separation individuation phase.

One searches for and finds children with the classical signs of Primary Anorexia Nervosa described so well by Hilde, Bruch and others However, in individual children these signs may be transitory and not remain in the clinical picture.

In this series children have presented with crises of adolescence, highly charged reactive disorders, depressive syndromes, severe anxiety, psychotic disorders, borderline psychosis. No child died or suicided or suffered serious physical sequelae.

Children showed clinical biological and psychological variations on entering puberty.

Children who sustain growth delays with associated dietary restrictions, fail to develop in height, weight and menstruation and other endocrine features. On the other hand, some children show rapid weight and height developmental spurts producing severe anxiety which the child appears to attempt to control by restricting food intake. "Stop the world, I want to get off". The awareness that they are biologically drafted and not in control of their bodies may produce massive anxiety and fear and they make efforts to control their bodies even to the extent of critical illness.

It is noteworthy that the series contains a high proportion of boys. These vulnerable boys seem unable to cope with the tasks of entry to adolescence. Conflicts over physical growth, sexual maturation, independent activity, control of sexual and aggressive feelings, emancipation by working through early object ties in his relationship to parents and family. Finally, coping with an aggressive competitive peer group culture.

Neurological, endocrinological and pharmacological research is exciting in this area and given good representation in this Vllth World Congress. My focus here is the clinical developmental framework from the psychological and sociocultural point of view of

food refusal. Not only were different children compared, but
particular attention paid to changing patterns of each child in
response both to treatment and developmental progress.

A spectrum was seen.

1.   Identity conflict with varied contributions from peer group,
      ethnic cultural and family demands.

2.   The adolescent trapped in a maze of dietary and body identity
      confusion arising from peer group pressures which now have
      become a widespread social phenomena involving all ages.

3.   Oppositional negativistic reaction to life situations.

4.   Reactions to life stresses with anxieties of a persecutory
      or depressive nature, e.g., stress of family disruption,
      changing family roles, educational stresses.   In particular
      some children vulnerable to family bereavement, develop
      frank depression.

5.   Phase specific conflicts and more severe internalized
      conflicts relating to sexual and aggressive impulses,
      impending bodily change, body image and psychological
      identity.

6.   In core pathology, anxiety conflict and confusion
      relating to hunger, appetite and bodily perception.

7.   Defences against abandonment – emptiness of the lost
      child's hunger for love and people that can love, but
      by not eating remaining infantile and hurt.

8.   The problem of control seen in conflicts around greed
      and fears of bulimia.   "To eat is to take from
      someone else".

9.   In the sickest isolated unavailable children core psychotic
      mechanisms can become dominant with denial; the perfect
      body is the instrument of the child's omnipotence.

Just as in normal adolescence there may be rapid massive fluctuation in levels of function and behavioural style so each of our
patients moved through the eight categories.

Now, in Australia, we are aware of further heterogeneity,
e.g., Nervous Bulimia and other disorders related to childhood fads
and media influence. More serious is the adolescent who controls the
inner psychosis through rigid defences seen in controlled eating
behaviour, vomiting, purging, exercising and does not present with

clinical weight variation, though his body image perception is grossly distorted.

Now in society to be labelled Anorexia Nervosa can be fashionable and exciting but very frightening to adolescents who have learned of its potential mortality and characteristics, e.g., the boy who said he felt he must be a homosexual as he had a girl's disease. Other adolescents experiment with disordered eating patterns, play chicken and imitate the severe cases described so vividly in the lay press. Cults are rampant. Self-help groups are taking on the problem of the community.

The pressures imposed by dietary advice through press and media remind us of the analogous situation of feeding in the Third World Countries where breast milk was devalued and the expensive artificial feeding mixtures were advertised with deleterious effects for African babies.

Clearly the adolescent is caught in a dilemma. The psychiatrist too is caught in the same dilemma and faced with cultural norms, has difficulties in understanding the adolescent patient. Clinically is he dealing with culturally determined appropriate behaviour – sometimes? or an illness out of proportion to that arising from socially approved behaviour – sometimes? or an illness out of control with critical, biological and psychological dangers – sometimes?

The challenge D.S.M. 111 offers psychiatrists now is to go beyond making a diagnosis based solely on signs and symptoms with weight loss, body image with fear of obesity as central issues. Future research needs to define biological vulnerabilities and psychosocial risk and protective factors, which together may produce clinical disorders in adolescence; some of these may be eating disorders, and some of these may warrant the diagnosis of Anorexia Nervosa.

Mr. Chairman, in conclusion clearly a constellation of syndromes around eating disorders is very important in adolescent psychiatry.

In the Plenary Session on Monday, Dr. Robert Spitzer lamented that when we understand a condition we lose it and it goes elsewhere. Quo vadis. Will research lead us to paediatrics, endocrinology, neurology, pharmacology, family process or what.

I have spoken on the child's behalf. I have stressed the heterogeneity of the conditions which makes outcome research imperative but hazardous. From the clinical perspective, three observations emphasize the point.

1.   The extent of weight loss need not necessarily reflect the severity of the child's illness.

2.   Weight gain in response to treatment need not ncessarily reflect corresponding improvement in the child's mental health.

3.   When eating disorders are becoming socially endemic, paradoxically the highly vulnerable child is specially at risk since hemay be lost in the crowd.

Whatever the perceived clinical problem now or in the future, a caring concerned medically safe holding environment is needed in which these adolescents can find a moratorium to accommodate, assimilate and work through the anxiety and conflicts of this sensitive period; an environment

NEUROPSYCHOLOGICAL DISORDERS IN CHILDHOOD AND SCHIZOPHRENIA

Reinhart Lempp

Department of Child and Youth Psychiatry
University of Tübingen
Osianderstr 14
D-7400 Tübingen

Over the last few years, neuropsychological disorders have been mentioned more and more frequently in the discussion of the aetiology of schizophrenia.
These disorders have been named basic deficiencies, a term describing functional disorders of cognition, which is supposed to be responsible for the intellectual insufficiency and the lack of ability of the schizophrenic patient.We have to differentiate between these disorders and the genuine syndromes of defects.

In child- and adolescent psychiatry, the term partial functional disorder and the term deficiencies are used to describe the above mentioned neuropsychological functional disorders.Moreover, we find these disorders rather independently from a psychosis that might appear during the psychic development of children.
In adult psychiatry, these facts tend to be overlooked when neuropsychological functional disorders are discussed.In general, we are mainly dealing with minimal deficiencies, but more severe disorders can also be found in children.The resulting learning deficiencies can range from minimal variations in aptitude to rather striking handicaps in some fields.

As compared to children of the same age, these children have an altered perception of their environment.As a result, their experience and relations to their environment deviate from the norm. These children are more or less handicapped in the creation of a "normal" perception of reality ("Aufbau eines Realitätsbezugs"). Due to these defined debilities of cognition, the children are labelled by their surrounding as different or abnormal.
Parents and teachers generally don't recognize the debilities as genuine functional deficiencies but as lack of interest and unwillingness to perform.Subsequently this may lead to emotional disturbances in the relationship between child and environment.

The term partial functional disorder is intended to abstain from any aetiological classification.But when analyzing background and neuropsychological status of the children, we yet may assume brain-organic (CNS-organic) functional disorders of various origins as a cause for these partial deficiencies.However, hereditary pre-disposing factors must not be disregarded.

Concerning their functional character, the basic deficiencies observed in schizophrenic psychosis might well be compared to the partional functional disorders.They apparently explain the phenomena of the mistaking perception and estimation of environmental situations by the schizophrenic patient.In asmuch as the partial functional deficiency - lasting from early childhood on - disturbes and labilizes a proper creation of the perception of reality of the child, the basic deficiencies - as found in schizophrenic psychosis - are responsible for the total loss of "normal" perception of reality.

So if we are in the position to find an explanation of the aetiology of partial functional disorder, then we can possibly also find explanations of the aetiology of schizophrenia, or at least one important factor of the aetiologa of schizophrenia.

For this purpose, a study of 50 adult schizophrenic patients was designed and carried out by KEPLER, LEMPP et al.(1979).These patients underwent a thorough past medical history similar to those in child psychiatry, whereby the mothers were available for inter-rogation.A similar past medical history was taken from the mothers of 50 randomly selected patients who had had accidents but none of whom ever had been treated as psychiatric patient.The study re-vealed that a preponderance of cumulatively injuring incidents in early brain development as well as a distinctliy higher number of disturbing psychosocial factors was found in the group of the schizophrenic patients.

Another study by LEMPP, ROTAR and SCHMIDT(1982) investigated the history of adults in psychiatric hospitals who at some time in their childhood had been examined, diagnosed and treated as inpatients in child psychiatric hospitals.
About one third of the patients had already been diagnosed, or at least suspected, as being psychotic at that time.One third of the patients had been diagnosed as only neurotic,or as being in a crisis of maturity, and one third had been admitted for only disorders of the organic development at that time.
Thorough examination of the child psychiatric case histories from all three groups, however, revealed a remarkable accumulation of organic symptoms from their past history as well as from medical examination.Disturbed emotional interrelations in the family en-vironment were also frequent findings.

Cautious interpretation of these results shows that organic factors disturbing the early brain development on one hand, and the emotionally conflicting environment on the other hand have sig-nificant implications for those adults who later develop schizo-phrenia.

Thus, we have to consider two possibly determinating factors for the aetiology of schizophrenia: neuropsychological disturbances, known as partial functional disorder, during the child's psychic development (recognized as basic deficiencies in adult psychiatry) as well as discontinous, conflicting experienced environment and relationships in childhood.The coincidence of these factors may lead to an instable perception of reality, and later cause an increased risk for subsequent schizophrenia.

There is no doubt about genetic factors being the cause of the occurence of schizophrenia.We assume these genetic factors to be identical with inborn partial functional disorders.

But then why do we find schizophrenia in adult age and adolescence only, and not in early childhood?

For the perception of reality,maturation of the psychic development and differentiation to some extent are necessary prerequisits for the appearance of schizophrenia, and therefore, schizophrenia as diagnosed in adults cannot occur in children before school age.

Moreover, the observations made on schizophrenic psychosis in late childhood and adolescence show a frequency of minor fluctuating disturbances in switching between reality and side reality in this age group.

In early childhood, instability and switching between different levels of experience are considered normal.This phenomenon may also occur in adolescence, but will usually resolve, and therefore is not attributed to schizophrenia - although its psychopathological image may completely resemble schizophrenic psychosis.For this condition we use the term puberty crisis.

As the child grows, the borders between reality and side reality become more defined and distinct.As long as the individual is able to control his shifting between different levels of reality, he is mentally healthy.Only if he looses the ability to distinguish - possibly due to an instable and undefined creation of perception of reality -, and if he is lost in his side reality, then we call this schizophrenic psychosis, and regard it as pathological.

Hence, the experiences of child psychiatry with variants in psychic and psychopathological development can give clues to the understanding and interpretating of the symptoms and psychopathology in adult schizophrenic psychosis.

TEACHING CHILD PSYCHIATRY IN THE U.S.A.

Rita R. Rogers

Harbor-UCLA Medical Center
1000 West Carson Street
Torrance, California 90509

There is no field of medicine that requires as much integration of the biopsychosocial mesh of human beings as the subspecialty of child psychiatry. In the U.S.A. the linkages between new knowledge of biological and psychological data and the constant changing social fabric are intricately woven into the tapestry of our perceptions about our child patients. One of the most challenging and rewarding aspects of teaching child psychiatry is delineating, studying and integrating the biological, psychiatric and social aspects of our child and adolescent patients. In doing this we should not sacrifice medical rigor, skill and ethos. The child psychiatric trainee has to increase his medical skill and knowledge by continuous artistic care of his patients and by thorough, scholarly research pursuits. He or she has to become the "artistic scientist"[1]. While learning child psychiatry, the trainee has to continually increase his knowledge of general psychiatry. Child psychiatrists treat the unresolved parental dilemmas which profoundly affect parents in their parenting roles. Parents and children are under the continuous impact of the present and the past which determines their anticipation and expectation of the future.

Developmental Tasks

The child psychiatric trainee is taught to view each child as a unique human being whose development is affected by the presenting symptomatology. Simultaneously the trainee has to learn to recognize the effects of development on presenting symptomatology, (Example: failure to thrive, learning disability, etc.). Peter Blos[2] stresses that the failure to recognize the presence of neuropsychological deficits represents an obstacle to healthy progression to adolescence and to the successful completion of the "second individuation".

At the same time one can begin to understand the vicissitudes of the youth's attempt to maintain self-esteem in light of the neuropsychological deficit and how ego structure, object relations and impulse control are influenced by the maturational difficulty. Focusing on neuropsychological deficits without integrating them into the family and social structure of a youngster's reality will not reveal, but will camouflage the picture. Let me use the following illustration: G., a bright, solemn 15 year old is the middle child of three boys. He is short in stature and not only much shorter than his older brother, but shorter than his younger brother of three years. Upon referral he suffered from insomnia and severe nausea and vomiting in the morning. Psychiatric assessment revealed that he harbored severe guilt feelings about destructive wishes he had towards his father. He attempted to hide these feelings from his father by being extremely helpful and compliant towards all adults, especially his father. G.'s younger brother, R., tall and handsome, suffered from a severe learning disorder and delinquent behavior. The neuropsychological deficit which he experienced was particularly shameful because his two older brothers were academically very successful. While G. judged himself from the perspective of comparing his height with that of his brothers, R's self-esteem was shattered by his poor scholastic achievements compared to those of his brothers. It is not enough to understand and focus only on the overt manifestations of the two brothers' sibling and parental relationships. We need to teach that clumsiness, poor judgment, poor visual and auditory perception and poor language skills, all increase vulnerability to school failure, echoic memory, discrimination of sounds, speech, recognition aspects of auditory perception and are highly linked to acquisition of verbal skills in addition to uncoordination, poor right/left differentiation and poor visual tracking, which make it difficult to participate in sports, thus additionally handicapping such youngsters from developing compensatory sources of self-esteem and mastery.[3] In attempting to understand both of these boys with different disease entities, the future psychiatrist has to remember that they are both adolescents. The author concurs with Esman[4] that adolescence is a process rather than a developmental disturbance[5]. When a youngster goes through the process of adolescence, certain struggles become highlighted. For G. height meant masculinity which meant achievement, etc. School achievement, peer relationships and peer esteem are of particular significance in adolescence. In order to understand each of these two boys, the trainee has to learn how each of these youngsters think and how they feel, how they think about how they feel and how they feel about how they think[6].

Beyond learning the impact of a youngster's disabilities on their psychosexual stage of development and how adolescence impinges on their cognitive, emotional and social skills, the budding child psychiatrist has to learn what unresolved struggles each of these youngsters reawakens in their parents. Some of these struggles might relate to the unfinished work of the parents' adolescences.

28

Hopefully the therapist of these two boys has no remnants of his sibling and parental struggles (or at least knows and understands them). The most difficult perspective to convey to the trainee is that the external realities of these two brothers have to be viewed from the threshold of the milieu in which they live (their family, their sociocultural and socioeconomic niche) not from the perspective of the trainees' sociocultural milieu. This is indeed a difficult task in teaching. It demands continuous attention to help the trainee recognize his uniqueness as a psychiatrist and therapist. Only when the psychiatric trainee has learned to recognize and respect that within himself can he differentiate his needs from those of his patients.

Child Psychiatric Disease Entities

History taking and evaluation of emotional illness in children is a multidimensional task. It also demands continuous attention and differentiation of the manifest from latent content. The child psychiatrist has to learn to compare and synthesize the parents' views and feelings about the child and his illness with those of the child and with those of himself (the child psychiatrist). He further needs to compare the parents' views of themselves in their parenting role with those of the child and with his professional view. With extreme skill and finesse the child psychiatrist will learn to recognize and assess the mutual vulnerabilities[7] which exist between children's symptomatology and unresolved, unhealed parental conflicts. The trainee will learn that through each encounter with the parents he will gain a glimpse of parental conflict in relation to this particular child and the specific meaning which this child's illness evokes in the parent.

Psychotic illness in early, middle or late childhood or adolescence can exacerbate severe parental conflict. When taking a history from the parents of a psychotic youngster, the trainee has to be exquisitely atuned to the profound emotional hurt which arises in parents when they realize that their child is emotionally ill. When one talks to parents about their child rearing techniques, one has to remember their hurt. Iatrogenic concepts like schizophrenogenic mother, etc., have increased parental guilt and hurt. One must focus on the torment of the parent and empathize with his or her suffering.

The trainee must also follow the latest scholarly literature (such as the current knowledge about anorexia nervosa, etc.) to learn that anorexia nervosa and depression share a vulnerability towards norepinephrine regulation[8]. One has to learn also about the differentiating and common features of bulimia and obesity. According to Maloney and Klykylo, the three conditions (anorexia nervos, bulimia and obesity) despite their disparate presentations, are similar in that they result from the conjunction of multiple causative factors characterized by intense, although heterogenous emotional issues combined with equally intense social and somatic concerns. Treatment requires a truly biopsychosocial approach.

It is essential that the trainee learn not to make a diagnosis based solely on the cluster of symptoms. He must integrate the somatic, personality, familial and interpsychic and interpersonal features into a conglomerate which permits not only correct diagnosis and treatment but also adequate prognostic evaluation. Parents need to plan realistically for their offsprings chances of independence versus dependence. Let me use the following example for illustration: R. was referred by her mother at the age of 11 because of bulimia. She went on stuffing binges and then attempted to control her weight by vomiting. R. was found to be a very fragmented, disturbed girl who experienced her entire environment and herself as chaotic and fragmented. R. suffered from incipient schizophrenia. Bulimia was only the presenting symptom. Unfortunately R. was treated for her bulimia. Adequate planning for hospitalization, followed by day treatment and then by half-way house was not recommended until after the family had exhausted their financial and emotional reservoir with unsuccessful outpatient psychotherapy. K., a bright, attractive 20 year old girl, referred by her father because of bulimia, also pre-sented with the same symptoms as R. She claimed that she started controlling her weight by gorging and then vomiting after she had heard many of her friends describe this as a successful weight control method. She had at one time, through fierce dieting, lost 30 pounds in three months and then gained 10 pounds in three days. Beyond the preoccupation with wanting to lose weight, K. was dealing with other losses. She had lost a boyfriend who had been her first sexual partner. It had happened at a time when she was amenorrheic (which was probably related to her heavy weight loss). She had confided her concern over her amenorrhea to her mother, but not her sexual experi-ences. She felt guilty about it. K's emotional turmoil was aggra-vated by a situation which neither she nor her mother knew consciously but experienced intensely. Her father had become involved in an extramarital affair. Both mother and daughter experienced a loss at a time when they could not comfort or support one another. Psycho-therapy helped to disentangle K. from the triangle at home. She also gained understanding about her rivalrous feelings towards her mother with a subsequent decrease in guilt feelings. When she was able to separate the loss of her boyfriend from the loss of her father's attention, K's symptoms of bulimia subsided. Her reaching for bulimia as a weight control measure was much influenced by the social mores of her milieu. In the U.S., bulimia, anorexia nervosa and obesity are reaching epidemic proportions (up to 25% of teenagers will demon-strate one of these eating disorders). Mortality of these disorders has decreased, but not their morbidity. Obesity is a culture-bound syndrome. So is violence, child abuse, etc.

Social Issues

The average American child will have watched 15,000 hour of television compared with 11,000 in the classroom by the time he or she has graduated from high school. The child will have witnessed 18,000 murders and countless episodes of beatings, robbery, arson and other forms of violence[10]. He is likely to learn and remember new forms of aggressive behavior. Television viewing can become particularly hazardous to children who are at high risk, those suffering from developmental disabilities, mental retardation, impulse disorders and psychosis. The child psychiatric trainee has to assess how his patients integrate television into their lives. Youngsters who experience blurring of their own boundaries[11] are more exposed to the contagion of violent behavior then others. Violent behavior is multiply determined and highly complex, but youngsters with fuzzy boundaries readily merge psychologically with other lacking clear-cut differentiation of their own personality structure[11]. Many patients become violent when they are traumatically overstimulated by intense feelings of an affectionate nature or by intense wishes for nurturance. The trainee has to learn that violence is a serious mental health problem. Unfortunately the most reliable predictor for later criminality is early childhood violence.

Lately in the U.S.A., two new areas of child psychiatry have preoccupied our attention. These are child abuse and child custody. We have to prepare our trainees for their unbiased role in these issues. For child psychiatrists it is more difficult to comply with the law of reporting parents for child abuse[12]. Each parent who abuses their child has been abused during childhood. Child psychiatrists recognize the unresolved childhood hurt in the parent and find it difficult to call in the punitive arm of the law to punish adults for the remnants of their childhood hurts. But we are obliged to protect children from child abuse and from becoming abusers.

The U.S.A., particularly California, is under the continuous impact of fads. There is a hunger and craving for easy quick answers. This facilitates the mushrooming of a large number of paraprofessionals who are not properly trained. They offer "cures" to people who crave direction and help. We also have to teach in the U.S.A., and especially California, the impact which immigration has on family relationships (paternal authority, family connectedness, male/female roles, etc.) and the impact which messages from our world have on children whose parents come from a place with a different language, customs, ethos, respect for the past, anticipation of the future,etc. The child psychiatric trainee has to learn to recognize the different emotional, sociocultural and religious realities of an immigrant family and has to learn how to interpret the new sociocultural milieu to the family. Immigration has a different impact on parents and children and frequently it creates role reversal. The children become easier adept than their parents at the new country's language.

Often they are needed by their parents as interlocutors and interpreters. A profound gap can emerge because the children attempt to fit in by exaggerated acceptance of their new environment while the parents nostalgically regress to exaggerated adherence to their old milieu and customs. Teaching child psychiatry is an enriching profesion. We teach our trainees that in learning about a child we learn all about the present and its connection to the past and to the future.

REFERENCES

1. D.P. Cantwell, Implications of Research in Child Psychiatry, in: Basic Handbook of Child Psychiatry, Vol. IV. I.N. Berlin and L.A. Stone, eds., Basic Books, New York (1979).
2. P. Blos, The Adolescent Passage, Developmental Issues. International Universities Press, New York (1979).
3. D.M. Robbins, Learning disability and neuropsychological impairment in adjudicated, unincarcerated male delinquents. J Am Acad Child Psychiatr 22:40-46 (1983).
4. A.H. Esman, Recent studies in adolescent psychiatry. J Am Acad Child Psychiatr 21:315-317 (1982).
5. A. Freud, Adolescence as a Developmental Disturbance, in: The Writings of Anna Freud, Vol. 7. International Universities Press, New York (1969).
6. E.J. Anthony, Normal adolescent development from a cognitive viewpoint. J Am Acad Child Psychiatr 21:318-327 (1982).
7. R.R. Rogers, Assessing parent-child vulnerabilities. Comprehensive Psychiatry 20:332-338 (1979).
8. R.L. Hendren, Depression in anorexia nervosa. J Am Acad Child Psychiatr 22:59-62 (1983).
9. M.J. Maloney and W.M. Klykylo, An overview of anorexia nervosa bulimia and obesity in children and adolescents. J Am Acad Child Psychiatr 22:99-107 (1983).
10. M.B. Rothenberg, The role of television in shaping the attitudes of children (Editorial) J Am Acad Child Psychiatr 22:86-87 (1983).
11. R.C. Marohn, Adolescent violence: causes and treatment. J Am Acad Child Psychiatr 21:354-360 (1983).
12. R.R. Rogers, The responsibilities of psychiatrist to society: the dual loyalties. J Med and Law (in press).

TRAINING IN CHILD PSYCHIATRY IN INDONESIA

Jan Prasetyo

Department of Psychiatry, School of Medicine
University of Indonesia
Salemba 6, Jakarta

INTRODUCTION

Child Psychiatry is a relatively young field in
Indonesia. It started to develop its services in 1969
when, due to the increase of child psychiatric patients
efforts were made to separate child from adult patients
at a psychiatric out-patient unit of a medical school
university hospital in Jakarta.
A subdivision of Child Psychiatry was first organized
and opened at the same School of Medicine in Jakarta
in 1973 when two psychiatrists returned from the United
States after a one year training in Transcultural Child
Psychiatry at the University of Hawaii. The subdivision
became more established after three other psychiatrists
trained in the same field, came back from Hawaii.
With those five as a core group, more structured services and training programs were developed.
The awareness of the growing demands for services and
manpower in Child Psychiatry, was greatly enhanced by
the National Workshop on Child and Adolescent Psychiatry
in 1976, and the First Asean Forum on Child Adolescent
Psychiatry (AFCAP) in 1977, both held in Jakarta.
Applications for training, requests for lectures and
short courses in Child Psychiatry came from medical and
non-medical professions.

THE PRESENT STATUS OF CHILD PSYCHIATRY IN THE MENTAL HEALTH CARE DELIVERY IN INDONESIA

The Mental Health Care Delivery System is actually
a subsystem within a larger comprehensive Health Care

33

delivery system. Mental health policy and care delivery are organized by a central government agency, the Directorate of Mental Health, which is subordinated to the Directorate General of Medical Care under the Ministry of Health. Mental Health services are primarily delivered through : State Mental Hospitals, District General Hospitals, University Hospitals, Community Health Centers, Private Mental Hospitals.

There eixts 29 State Mental Hospitals (two others are under construction, in provincial capitals where no mental health facility existed before), 10 Private Mental Hospitals, 10 Departments of Psychiatry at University/ General Hospitals, and about 250 Community Health Centers in the Country. The integration of Mental Health services in those Community Health Centers, at present is estimated to a 5% coverage.
Of all those facilities mentioned, only very few provide special services for children. Three are located in Jakarta, and one in Surabaya.

At present there are about 150 psychiatrists in the country, serving a population of approximately 150 million (1980 cencus).
Significant progress has been achieved in the development of mental health care in the country during the past two decades. The progress has accumulated such momentum that the supply for manpower is felth to be greatly lacking. It is obvious that the training of psychiatrists is strongly related to the fulfillment of those needs. At present this concerns especially the number of psychiatrists who have completed, or who are expected to complete their training in the near future.
Although it is recognized that problems of children and adolescents are increasingly pressing, especially in big cities, priority is given to the training of general psychiatrists rather than child psychiatrists and the construction of general psychiatric facilities rather than child facilities. It is still subservient to the macro-scope of mental health care delivery in the country.

THE PRESENT STATUS OF CHILD PSYCHIATRY IN THE TRAINING OF GENERAL PSYCHIATRISTS

Residency training and specialist certification used to be the jurisdiction of the professional associations and the Departments of Medical Schools. Since 1980 this responsibility has been formally taken over by the government through the Ministry of Education and

Culture. Design and approval of the training program, accreditation of training facilities and staff, and the issuance of certificates, are in the hands of a government body, the Faculty of Post Graduate Training. Presently for Psychiatry, only Departments of Psychiatry of the State Universities are authorized to give specialty training designated towards certification in Psychiatry. These Departments are from the State Universities in Jakarta, Surabaya, Bandung, Yogyakarta, Medan and Semarang. Together they have a capacity of twenty new enrollments a year, with up till now, an annual output of approximately fifteen psychiatrists a year.*

A so called Study Program Catalogue, compiled and issued by the Ministry determines the curriculum and minimum content of the training program, binding for centers designated to give training in that specialty. This is meant to insure an essential uniformity and basic quality standards in the medical specialty training throughout the country.
In Psychiatry, although particular centers are sometimes able to exceed the catalogue requirements in certain subjects, they may not quite meet the requirement in others for shortage of facilities, material, and competent teaching staff to cover these subjects.
Child Psychiatry is now formally included in the Study Program Catalogue, as a basic requirement in the training of general psychiatrists. Training Centers that do not have facilities for this purpose are obliged to develop such ones in the near future. In the meantime, visiting lecturers and consultants will cover the needs, by giving short courses in Child Psychiatry.

Although the primary priority has been for the training of general psychiatrists, the need for well-trained child psychiatrists who will devote more of their time dealing with problems of children, and who would further develop training programs and service facilities in each respective home base, is also a pressing reality.
At present, priority and greater chance for additional training in Child Psychiatry will be for faculty staff, who will later develop and establish their own units in their Departments.

---

* Of All those who have entered training since 1975, 75% are from the Ministry of Health, 13% from the Army, 10% from the Ministry of Education and Culture/Faculty Staff, and 2% are from other institutions.

To serve those needs, we have developed three types of training programs in Child Psychiatry :
Type 1, the intensification of a six months' rotation period in Child Psychiatry within the residency training in General Psychiatry ;
Type 2, the intensification of a six weeks' rotation period in Child Psychiatry for last year residents in Pediatrics ;
Type 3, the additional one and a half year training in Child Psychiatry, after completion of a residency training in General Psychiatry.

OBJECTIVES, CURRICULUM AND METHODS

Type 1

Before entering their rotation in Child Psychiatry in their third year of residency, second year residents are given thirteen hours' lectures about normal development, the diagnostic process in child psychiatry, principles of psychiatric examination of children, and principles of the psychiatric treatment of children.
The objectives of this type of training is to provide the resident with :
1. essential knowledge about the diagnostic assessment, treatment planning and management of children, parents and families ;
2. basic competence to apply it in their future work as general psychiatrists ;
3. competence to teach Child Psychiatry principles to medical/paramedical staff of his team, in his role as coordinator of mental health services in the mental hospital where he will be placed.

During this training period, the resident spends three months at the in-patients ward, where he is active ly involved in patient care roles, mostly with the severely disturbed children. Another three months is spent at the out-patient clinic, where he is trained to manage the child patient and his family on an out-patient basis besides assisting staff in consultation work.
Three case presentations with case write-ups is required for case conferences held once a week.
Seminars are given throughout the six months' period, three times weekly, focusing on normal child development (emphasizing on the cognitive and psychosocial development), psychiatric interviewing and examination of children and their parents, childhood psychopathology, and treatment modalities (emphasizing on behavior modification, parental counseling, drug therapy, family

therapy and play therapy).
At the end of the period, a written and oral examination with live-cases, is given.
Obligatory basic readings are, Anna Freud's Concept of Development Lines, Erikson's Eight Ages of Man and The Epigenesis of the Life Cycle, Phillips's The Origins of Intellect (Piaget's Theory), Simmons's Psychiatric Examination of Children, Harrison & Mcdermott's Childhood Psychopathology and Treatment in Child Psychiatry, Minuchin's Families and Family Therapies, and the DSM III.

Type 2

The general objectives of this type of training, is to provide the pediatrician with a basic understanding about Child Psychiatry, to enhance the awareness of the importance of the involvement of pediatricians in the mental health care of children, and thus, the importance of a Child Psychiatry-Pediatric Liaison.

During this period, special seminars besides individual supervision and bedside teaching, are given to the resident, with the following more specific objectives:

1. to understand the difference between Child and Adult Psychiatry ;
2. to understand normal development of children, focusing on the cognitive and psychosocial development ;
3. to understand techniques of interviewing and examination of children and their parents;
4. to understand common childhood psychopathologies frequently encountered in pediatric work ;
5. to understand about the diagnostic process, treatment planning and management in Child Psychiatry ;
6. to know about treatment modalities in Child Psychiatry.

Clinical work is limited to out-patient care, with two case assignments. One case presentation with a case write up is required at the end of this period.
Obligatory readings are limited to, McDermott & Finch's Psychiatry for the Pediatrician, Simmons's Psychiatric Examination of Children, and the Quick Reference to the DMS III as a diagnostic guide.

Type 3

In this program Fellow is given the opportunity to extend his knowledge in Child Psychiatry, and to gain competence in :
1. diagnostic and therapeutic work with children, their parents and families ;
2. consultative and collaborative work with allied professions related to child welfare ;
3. the management of service facilities for problem children and their families ;
4. the teaching of Child Psychiatry.

During the first twelve months, seminars are given three times a week, focusing in-depth on the theories of child development, childhood psychopathology, psychiatric examination of children, family theories, and treatments in Child Psychiatry (emphasizing on behavior modification, psychopharmacology, parental counselling, family therapy, group therapy, and play therapy). Throughout the whole training course, the Fellow is actively involved in the daily activities of patient care at the in-patient ward as well as at the out-patient clinic, including the administrative routines/management of the unit.

During the last six months, seminars are given about Community Psychiatry, Liaison Psychiatry and Cultural Psychiatry. To gain experience in liaison work the Fellow will spend one to two months in non psychiatric facilities i.e. the subdivisions of Child Neurology and Social Pediatrics of the Department of Pediatric ; a normal Public School, a School for the mild mentally retarded ; a detention home, under the Police Department. A written report about his work at each of those facilities has to be submitted at the end of this period.

At the end of the training, a written and oral examination with live cases is given. The final evaluation is based on : the impression of the Fellow's cognitive ability and clinical performance, his skill in liaison work, the impression of his professional and ethical attitudes, and the approved submitted reports and case write ups.

Certification is the jurisdiction of the Department of Psychiatry where the training program is carried out. Up till the present time, only the Department of Psychiatry at the School of Medicine, University of Indonesia in Jakarta is accredited for this type of training in Child Psychiatry.

Obligatory basic readings are extended to a variety of
readings in addition to the ones obligatory in Type 1,
i.e. Anna Freud's Normality and Pathology in Childhood,
Erikson's Childhood and Society, and Identity Youth and
Crisis, Harrison & McDermott's New Directions in Child-
Hood Psychopathology, Ackerman's Psychodynamics of
Family Life, Werner's Cross-Cultural Child Development
Moustaka's Children in Play Therapy, Shelden Rose's
Treating Children in Groups, Stewarts Agras's Principles
and Clinical Application of Behavior Modification.

BASIC CONCEPTS ON HYPERKINESIS IN CHILDREN

Rafael Velasco

Member of the Child and Adolescent Psychiatry Section,
World Psychiatric Association
Mexico

In the World Health Organization's International Classification of Diseases we find this definition (ICD-)*:

314. "Hyperkinetic Syndrome of Childhood". The criteria for the diagnosis uses as fundamental data distractibility, desinhibition, hyperactivity, impulsiveness, marked mood fluctuations and aggressiveness.

The American Psychiatric Association (A.P.A.), on its part, characterizes this same syndrome in its DSM 111** in the following manner:

314.01 "Attention Deficit Disorder with Hyperactivity". The criteria for the diagnosis is based on three fundamental data and three secondary ones. The first are: inattention, impulsiveness and hyperactivity; the second are: the disturbance begins before seven years of age, it lasts al least six months and the certainty that the cause it not schizophrenia, an affective disorder nor some degree of mental deficiency.

Both descriptions refer to the so-called Minimal Brain Dysfunction Syndrome, name which for some years has designated the disturbance suffered by certain children who exhibit a constellation of

---

*Mental Disorders: Glossary and Guide to Their Classification in Accordance With The Ninth Revision of the International Classification of Diseases, World Health Organization, Geneva, 1978.
**Diagnostic and Statistical Manual of Mental Disorders, Third Edtion.

41

signs and symptoms relative to behavior and learning. The procedures which permit the verification of such signs and symptoms are composed of physical and psychiatric exploration, the application of psychological tests and neurological and electroencephalographic examinations. But we ought to say that the recognition of this clinical picture was only recently translated into its inclusion in the aforementioned classifications. Formerly it was not considered necessary to designate specifically a syndrome which was previously named in very diverse manners: "brain damage syndrome", "minimal brain damage", "brain dysfunction", "hyperkinesia", "hyperactive child", etc. Even today a certain controversy exists about the legitimacy of giving it a place in nosography. A good example of researchers who harbor serious doubts is Herbert E. Rie who begins a recent publication with this paragraph (Rie, H., 1980):

"Absence of verifiable facts about a group of vexing problems seems inevitably to result in the adoption of strongly held views that tend to be indefensible. For a time the amount of controversy, of contradiction, of conceptual confusion, of questionable interpretation of observations and tangentially relevant references in the literature on minimal brain dysfunction suggested that verifiable facts were scarce indeed."

To us, from the position of the clinician dedicated to tasks of diagnosis and treatment of child psychopathological disturbances, it seems that Dr. Rie's conclusion would be reasonable, only if the "verifiable facts" were those which confirmed the "organicity" of the syndrome. But if, putting etiology apart, we study thoroughly the symptomatological manifestations which have been described in an enormous number of clinical observations and careful investigations and we assign to the signs and symptoms the value (which they undoubtedly have) of "verifiable facts", one cannot come to a conclusion other than that of the experts who request a place for the brain dysfunction syndrome in modern nomenclature. It is not a question of a "new" pathological entity, product of occured changes in man and his habitat in the course of history, rather of a condition which probably has existed always but, until this century, was not approached sistematically.

The accumulated clinical experience, repeated observations and scientific research done in diverse fields permit us to assert that the minimal brain dysfunction syndrome exists, even though we are not in a position to affirm that we know its etiopathogenesis sufficiently no in a reliable manner. Thus, in our intention to clarify where possible the meaning of brain dysfunction and its clinical manifestations, we begin by accepting a conceptual framework structured with the following elements:

a) A set of signs and symptoms can be identified which are related with what is known as the "minimal brain dysfunction syndrome", perhaps subclassifiable in types reflecting the influence of diverse secondary factors.

b) This syndrome, as any other in the pathological field, is multifactorial and exists in degrees.

c) It deals with a diagnosticable condition in which, according to the evidence obtained up to now, the organic factors seem to be essential, without leaving aside the environmental and social factors which exercise an important influence on interacting with the former.

d) As a consequence of the preceding, the syndrome is character- ized because the affected child manifests, necessarily, alterations in behavior, subjectivity and the organism and its functions.

According to our experience and to what we can conclude from a more or less extensive revision of the relevant work of many other authors, the diagnosis of the syndrome is justified when the follow- ing data are unmistakably present:

1. Hyperactivity, with the characteristics previously described as pertaining to the syndrome, and not a mere occasional, temporal or situational expression of a preponderantly emotional problem. It translates into the incapacity of the child to organize, regulate and control his motor behavior.

2. Impulsiveness, which is frequently expressed in the form of aggressiveness and unpredictable behavior, owing to changes in humor.

3. Delay in the development of specific abilities, which is translated principally into learning problems. A prominent datum related to this delay is inattention.

4. Incapacity to understand and carry out orders ("pathologi- cal disobedience"), in terms we shall describe further on.

5. Symptomatology present before seven years of age.

6. Variable behavior disturbances, provided that they can be identified as a consequence of hyperactivity and impulsiveness: very obstructed interpersonal relations, expressions of low tolerance to frustration, temerity (incapacity to evaluate danger adequately), etc.

7. Absence (definite) of different psychopathological disturb- ances which could "explain" the symptomatology: psychosis, well defined mental retardation, affective disorders.

The symptom which some lines above we called "pathological dis- obedience" merits a descriptive effort, given that in my opinion, it has not been considered with proper attention (Velasco F., 1980). Diverse clinicians have for some time referred to the incapacity of understanding verbal orders which the child suffering from brain dysfunction has. A simple observational fact is that hyperkinetic children are disobedient, but their attitude toward rules and limi- tations establised by adults who have authority over them is not that of one who disobeys knowing he has committed a misdeed which he will try to hide, but that of one who has not understood the prohibition and its significance nor much less the need to respect it. The child commits the same misdeed over and over without attempting to hide it and without understanding why he is being punished. In fact, he is surprised when someone calls his attention to it, considering that he is being treated unjustly. Regarding the behavior of these children in relation to their disobedience, mothers often express it thusly: "My child isn't capable of obeying... I've tried, even telling him things in the opposite way, but I don't get good results"; "After an explanation and a threat, I scarcely turn around, and he's doing just what I forbid him to do"; "With my child blows and punishment produce nothing, he simply doesn't register what I forbid him to do". These are statements gathered in daily practice, exactly as uttered; they show an explainable confusion for their child's very peculiar form of disobedience. It should be noted that it is not even a true disobedience in that one can hardly be said to have disobeyed an order which he has not understood. At any rate, if the interviewer looks for this datum using adequate questions, he will be surprised at the frequency with which he will find it accompanying the syndrome which concerns us. This is so much the case, that its presence together with true hyperkinesis and inattention ought to leave few doubts about a presumptive diagnosis.

Whether we are right or not in suggesting that the discrepancies in the conceptualization of this picture are due, at bottom, to different etiological approaches, the data we have brought to mind should lead us to reiterate that the brain dysfunction syndrome represents a real entity. But what are these data which from a clinical approach allow us to surmise that the responsible factors are principally "organic" ones?. Various have been mentioned; we will highlight the following ones:

1. The syndrome's antecedents, which situate the first symptoms very early in the child's life.
2. The quality of the symptoms, particularly manifestations provoking learning difficulties. Inattention, visomotor problems and evident difficulties the affected child has in organizing percepts are better explained by a dysfunction in certain areas of the brain.
3. The nature of hyperkinesis, clinically differentiable from other forms of hyperactivity in which emotional factors are predominant.
4. The incidence of numerous neurological signs, coincident with severe behavior disturbances.
5. The frequency of electroencephalographic abnormalities, significantly greater than that occurring in other childhood behavior disturbances.
6. The therapeutic effect produced by psychostimulants, distinct from the responses obtained in other clinical pictures or in normal children.

Regarding the last point, the affirmation of some authors in the sense that there are no notable differences in the response to stimulants between children suffering diverse disturbances and even healthy ones (Barkley, 1976; Sroufe, 1975; Rapoport, 1977) are very surprising to us. Precisely because our many years of experience indicates totally the opposite and because we agree on that with an enormous number of authors, we accept as one more support for the syndrome's existence the "paradoxical" response which occurs with stimulants. For these reasons, the comment of Gittelman-Klein (1978) seems very apt to us: "... if hyperkinesis is a myth, it is a myth which responds favorably to treatment with stimulants". It is obvious that the "paradoxical" term only serves to point out to us the disconcerting fact that a child responds to psychostimulants by reducing his physical activity, his aggression and his irritability. When we know with complete certainty the action mechanism of these psychopharmacals in the brain of a hyperkinetic child, it will be seen that there is no such paradoxical effect. Yet the term has been useful to point out the distinctness of the response in brain dysfunction cases.

All proposals in terms of "organicity" as the only explanation of the etiology of this picture should be rejected as incomplete and inoperative. Stimuli which can damage the organism to the degree of producing a pathological state are of a physical, psychological and social nature. The physical stimuli can break the organism's equilibrium in their chemical or antigenic properties, or in the physical ones themselves. The response is, therefore, of a physiological order and constitutes a compensatory measure to reestablish the lost equilibrium. But although the stimuli are more or less specific, the response of the organism is expressed at three levels: psychic, physical and social. In other words, a physical stimulus, as is the case of a functional brain disorder arising from a structural change (it is so at the molecular level), evokes organic responses as well as psychological and social ones. And the adaptive capacity of the child is conditioned by his own innate characteristics, by the reaction of persons having an effect on his development and by his life experiences. It does not make sense, then, to say that such and such an abnormal state "has an organic origen" or else that it is "of emotional etiology". What we want to express is that in the case of the so-called brain dysfunction syndrome, the nature of the behavioral disturbances seems to be related principally with structural changes, without which the symptoms, which could be present through the action of other stimuli, would be distinct in their qualitative manifestations. And we accept that it is a matter of inference, of a formulation still at the level of a hypothesis, but with many possibilities of verification. This position concurs with that of Rutter in 1977: "... it is highly probable that in addition to those children with brain paralysis and obvious neuropathological conditions, many others exists with some degree of damage or dysfunction in the brain".

REFERENCES

Barkley, R. A., 1976, Predicting the response of hyperkinetic children to stimulant drugs: a review, J. Abnorm. Child Psychol., 4:327.

Gittelman-Klein, R., 1978, Spectrum of action of psychostimulants and neuroleptics in childhood psychopharmacology, Adv. Biol. Psychiat., Karger, Basel, 2:23.

Rapoport, J. L., 1977, Dextroamphetamine: cognitive and behavioral effects in normal prepubertal boys, World Cong. Psychiat.

Rie, H. and Rie, E., 1980, "Handbook of Minimal Brain Dysfunctions", John Wiley and Sons, New York.

Rutter, M., 1977, Brain damage syndromes in childhood: concepts and findings, J. Child. Psychol. Psychiat., 18:1.

Sroufe, L. A., 1975, Drug treatment of children with behavior problems, Horowitz Rev. Child Devel. Res., 4, University of Chicago Press, Chicago.

Velasco, F., 1980, "El Niño Hiperquinético. Los Síndromes de Disfunción Cerebral", Trillas, México.

EARLY CHILDHOOD AUTISM AND ASPERGER'S SYNDROME

Lorna Wing

Medical Research Council Social Psychiatry Unit
Institute of Psychiatry
London, UK

In 1943 an American child psychiatrist, Leo Kanner, published his first paper on the cluster of behavioural problems he called early infantile autism (now more often known as early childhood autism). He described 11 young children all showing a similar clinical picture.

The following year, Hans Asperger (1944) an Austrian child psychiatrist published his first paper on the behaviour pattern he referred to as autistic psychopathy. His cases comprised about 200 adolescents and young adults. Later, they came to know of each other's work, but both authors were convinced that the two syndromes were different. Kanner's writing became world famous, but Asperger's although equally interesting and relevant to child and adult psychiatry, was, until recently, little known outside Austria and Germany.

In this paper, the features which each of these workers considered to be crucial to diagnosis will be compared and contrasted.

The central feature of Kanner's syndrome is the social aloofness and indifference, which is present at least for the first part of childhood (Kanner & Eisenberg, 1956). Asperger stressed that this was not found in his group but, nevertheless, the essence of the condition he described is an abnormality of social inter- action. Sometimes this takes the form of naive, one- sided, inappropriate approaches and at others a kind of superior detachment from ordinary human affairs.

Kanner and Eisenberg emphasized the diagnostic importance of resistance to change, shown by attachment to objects and repetitive stereotyped routines, such as insistence on following exactly the same route to particular destinations. Those with Asperger's syndrome tend to be unhappy when separated from their own familiar environment and, typically, are absorbed in circumscribed interests to the exclusion of all else. Examples of such interests are railway time tables, the movements of the planets, or the daily weather forecasts.

Language impairments affecting comprehension and expression are characteristic of Kanner's syndrome. About half of affected children have no speech and the rest have problems such as immediate and delayed echolalia, idiosyncratic use of words or phrases (Kanner, 1946) and reversal of pronouns. In contrast, Asperger emphasized that those in his group often spoke before they could walk, and developed large vocabularies and a good grasp of grammar. He referred to them as having 'highly sophisticated language skills'. However he also reported that some reversed pronouns in their early years, and that they tended to use speech in a concrete, pedantic way, with occasional curious misinterpretations of meaning. Asperger's suggestion that they had sophisticated language skills perhaps arose from his subjects' familiarity with long obscure words, - but, despite this, they often lack understanding of some basic verbal concepts such as 'either' or 'because'.

Whatever their level of language, members of both groups are impaired in non-verbal and motivational aspects of communication. In Kanner's children, facial expression, gesture, mime, vocal intonation and use of eye contact to convey meaning are severely limited. In Asperger's syndrome these are also limited or else abnormal in form. For instance, a recent study (D. Tantam, unpublished work) has shown that such people make eye contact with a disconcerting, fixed stare while speaking to others. This is in marked contrast to the normal alternation of making and breaking eye contact during conversation. Those with either of the syndromes have difficulty in recognizing and imitating the more subtle facial expressions, such as puzzlement, scorn or distaste.

Perhaps the most striking abnormality shown by both groups is the lack of pleasure in taking part in interpersonal communication for its own sake. People with Kanner's or Asperger's syndrome approach others to gratify their own needs or to talk about their circumscribed interests, not because they enjoy sharing ideas and emotions.

Limitation of development of imaginative play occurs in both conditions (Wing et al 1977, Wing & Gould, 1979, Wing 1981). The majority of those with Kanner's syndrome have no pretend play, but a minority have a kind of pseudo-imaginative activity in which the child repeats the same theme over and over again, regardless of suggestions from other children. One form of this is acting out, in a stereotyped way, the role of a character from television. In Asperger's syndrome also imaginative play may be absent, but in this group the narrow, repetitive pseudo-pretend play is more common than in Kanner's. Some children develop their own imaginary world, such as the young man described by Bosch (1962) who spent much time inventing the geography of an imaginary planet in pedantic detail.

Motor skills present a curious paradox in Kanner's syndrome. The more severely handicapped children, especially those who have little or no speech, can appear graceful in spontaneous movement and agile in climbing and balancing. But the more verbal Kanner's children tend to be clumsy and fearful of any activity needing good balance (DeMyer 1976). Those with Asperger's syndrome are typically poorly co-ordinated, with noticeably peculiar gait and posture. This is one of the reasons why they are often teased and bullied by other children if they attend normal school. On the other hand, the flapping movements of the limbs seen in Kanner's syndrome are much less common in Asperger's group.

Both Kanner (1943) and Asperger (1944) originally believed that children with their syndromes were of normal or superior intelligence. Over the course of time it has become clear that the majority of Kanner's group are mentally retarded, at least half being in the severe or profound range (Lotter, 1966, Wing & Gould, 1979). Asperger also noted that his syndrome could occur in people who, despite their special interests, were mildly retarded. In the present author's series of 34 cases, one in five had an intelligence quotient below 70 (Wing, 1981).

Kanner emphasized the early onset of his syndrome. He described it as present from birth, or beginning within the first 2 or 3 years of life. Asperger wrote that his condition was never recognized in infancy and often not before the third year of life. Recent work on infant behaviour has shown how early normal babies develop social awareness and interest in communication (Trevarthen, 1974). Careful and appropriate questioning of parents of a child with Asperger's syndrome often reveals that he lacked active involvement in social interaction from early infancy, even if he passively accepted social approaches (Wing, 1981).

When the diagnostic features of the two syndromes are examined, it seems reasonable to suggest that they are just different manifestations of the same underlying problems, and that the conditions are on the same continuum of pathology. Kanner described younger, more severely handicapped children, while Asperger described a less handicapped group. The contrast was heightened by the fact that Asperger saw his cases when they had grown out of some of the more marked social and behavioural problems of early childhood. This view is supported by the fact that some children who begin life as classically autistic gradually change over the years and grow up to show the behaviour pattern described by Asperger.

The relationship between the two conditions is demonstrated by the clinical pictures in 17 year old male triplets recently seen by Burgoine and Wing (1983). The most appropriate diagnosis for them is Asperger's syndrome, but all three have some features of Kanner's autism. The triplet with the most traumatic birth history has the lowest IQ and the most autistic features. The brother with the easiest birth and the highest intelligence has the fewest such features. The third triplet is half way between his two brothers for all these variables.

The evidence suggests that a variety of physical, organic factors, including genetic traits, can lead to either of these syndromes. The gross causes operate indirectly on behaviour by impairing physiological and hence psychological functions. Results of psychological tests support this view. In both conditions there are usually marked discrepancies between different skills, with comprehension of speech and non-verbal communication being most affected.

An epidemiological study was carried out in the Camberwell area of London in order to investigate the problem of sub-classification of the abnormal behaviour patterns found in early childhood psychosis, including the syndromes discussed here. As a result, the following formulation was developed (Wing, 1981).

Among children with unusual types of language, social interaction and cognition there is a group who have in common marked impairments of two-way social interaction, verbal and non-verbal communication and imaginative development. These impairments are very significantly clustered together and are accompanied by repetitive, stereotyped behaviour which can be simple or complex, self directed or object directed, or verbal in form. The impairments can be present in varying degrees of severity and can be associated with any level of intelligence (as measured mainly on visuo-spatial and rote memory tests) varying from profoundly retarded to normal or superior, but heavily weighted towards the lower end. Kanner's syndrome is one small sub-group and Asperger's is another. Other workers have selected and named sub-groups from the same pool of subjects. The particular clusters of behavioural items defined as syndromes by all these workers depended upon the types of cases referred to them, rather than a systematic examination of the whole range of clinical material.

As Anthony (1958) pointed out, the named syndromes overlap so much that diagnosing them is of little help in practice. A more soundly based system of classification awaits an increase in knowledge of brain physiology and pathology, and of how these relate to psychological function and overt behaviour. It is very likely that many different sub-groups with different aetiologies will eventually be identified. In the meantime, it is of practical value to recognize the existence of the whole group of people with the triad of impairments of two-way social interaction, communication and imagination. All children with these problems need a similar type of structured and organized education and management, and most of them will require sheltered work and living accommodation as adults. In this context, a simple classification based on levels of verbal, visuo-spatial and social ability (Gould, 1982) is of considerably more help than diagnosing the eponymous syndromes. Nevertheless we have reason to be grateful to both Kanner and Asperger for their particularly detailed descriptions, since these have formed the basis of our present recognition of a strange but fascinating group of children and adults who need very specialised understanding and help.

REFERENCES

Anthony, E. J., 1958, An experimental approach to the
    psychopathology of childhood autism. Brit. J.
    Med. Psychol. 21:211.
Asperger, H., 1944, Die Autistischen psychopathen im
    kindesalter. Archiv. Psychiat. Nervenkr. 117:76.
Bosch, G., 1962, Infantile Autism (trans. D. Jordan and
    I. Jordan), Springer-Verlag, New York, 1970.
Burgoine, E., and Wing, L., 1983, Identical triplets
    with Asperger's syndrome. Brit. J. Psychiat.
    In Press.
DeMyer, M., 1976, Motor, perceptual-motor and intell-
    ectual disabilities of autistic children, in
    Early childhood autism (2nd ed.) L. Wing, ed.,
    Pergamon, Oxford.
Gould, J. A., 1982, Social Communication and Imagination
    in Children with Cognitive and Language Impairments.
    Ph. D. Thesis, London.
Kanner, L., 1943, Autistic disturbances of affective
    contact. Nerv. Child, 2:217.
Kanner, L., 1946, Irrelevant and metaphorical language
    in early infantile autism. Am. J. Psychiat. 103:242.
Kanner, L., and Eisenberg, L., 1956, Early infantile
    autism: 1943-1955. Am. J. Orthopsychiat. 26:55.
Lotter, V., 1966, Epidemiology of autistic conditions
    in young children. I. Prevalence. Soc. Psychiat.
    1:124.
Trevarthen, C., 1974, Conversations with a two-month old.
    New Scient. 62:230.
Wing, L., 1981, Asperger's syndrome: a clinical account.
    Psychol. Med. 11:115.
Wing, L., 1981, Language social and cognitive impairments
    in autism and severe mental retardation. J. Aut.
    Dev. Disord. 11:31.
Wing, L., and Gould, J., 1979, Severe impairments of
    social interaction and associated abnormalities
    in children: Epidemiology and classification.
    J. Aut. Dev. Disord. 9:11.
Wing, L., Gould, J., Yeates, S.R., and Brierley, L. M.,
    1977, Symbolic play in severely mentally retarded
    and in autistic children. J. Child Psychol. Psychiat.
    18:167.

EFFECTS OF BRAIN INJURY IN CHILDREN

Steven White

Maudsley Hospital
London SE5
U.K.

INTRODUCTION

Some residual impairment in the learning and remembering of new material is one of the commonest and most consistent sequelae of closed head injury. However, little attention has been paid to the analysis of memory dysfunction in head injured children and this paper reports a study of such deficits.

PATIENT SAMPLE

There were 105 children, 75 boys and 30 girls, ranging in age from 4 to 16 years, with a mean of 10 years and a standard deviation of just under 3 years. Thirty five of the patients had been injured in road traffic accidents, 47 as the result of a fall and 23 had received a blunt blow to the head.

Some 70% of the children had had a period of coma following the head injury. The duration of post-traumatic amnesia (PTA) was assessed clinically by the neurosurgeons. In 38% of cases PTA duration was less than or equal to one hour, in 13% in excess of one hour but less than 24 hours, whilst in 11% it was greater than 24 hours. Overall, the median PTA duration was 3 hours. In a further 13% cases, PTA was absent and there had been no loss of consciousness. However, admission to hospital had been made since a recorded head injury had been followed by the development of symptoms such as drowsiness, vomiting, nausea or lethargy. For 23% of the sample it had not proved possible to make a formal assessment of PTA duration. The majority of these children were at the younger end of the age range. In many instances it was clear that PTA had been brief - of seconds or minutes duration.

Accordingly, overall some 75% of the sample had sustained head injuries which would be regarded clinically as mild.

As a measure of general intelligence, the English Picture Vocabulary Test (EPVT) was administered. This is a test of listening vocabulary which correlates well with more extensive test inventories such as the Wechsler Intelligence Scale for Children. The head-injured group achieved a mean standardized score of 99.5, with a standard deviation of 15.3.

One third of the sample had sustained a skull fracture, which was linear in 19 cases and depressed in 16. For one aspect of the study, it was of interest to relate memory performance to the site of the primary skull impact sustained in the head injury. In the skull fracture group this was taken as the fracture site. For the remainder the basis of classification was the recorded location of soft-tissue injury of the scalp together with eye witness accounts of the accident itself where available. In this way, it was possible to determine the site of impact in 93 patients: in 40 cases this had been to the right side of the skull, in 38 to the left side, while in 15 it had been bilateral.

13 of the children had had seizures at some stage after the injury.

The interval at which children completed the memory test after head injury covered a wide range, from just under 24 hours to 7 years in one case. However, the majority were tested relatively soon after injury, 40% within 24 hours and 70% within one week, with a median interval of just under 3 days.

CONTROL GROUP

This was a sample of 60 children admitted to hospital for a variety of orthopaedic complaints, matched for age, EPVT scores and sex distribution with the head-injured group.

MEMORY TEST

The material used was a set of 8 line drawings of common objects, comprising 4 pairs of items from 4 different taxonomic categories: animals, transport, furniture and clothing. The pictures were presented serially and subjects then recalled all the items they could remember in any order they wished. There were 4 such presentation-recall trials, followed by 2 delayed recall tests at 5 and 15 minutes after original learning.

RESULTS AND DISCUSSION

Test scores were treated statistically by analysis of variance. The head-injured children showed overall poorer performance than the controls ($p < 0.001$), recalling fewer items from the outset and their scores remaining consistently inferior. However, in the two delayed recall tests there was no evidence for markedly accelerated forgetting by the head-injured children of what they had learned.

TABLE 1.   Mean number of items recalled by head-injured and control groups

	Trial 1	Trial 2	Trial 3	Trial 4	+5 min.	+15 min.
Head-injured	5.7	6.4	6.5	6.7	6.7	6.6
Controls	6.3	7.1	7.1	7.2	7.1	7.2

Further analysis showed that the head-injured children recalled both fewer categories (animals, transport etc.) and fewer items per category than the controls, so that both category retrieval and retrieval of items from within categories seem to be equally affected by head injury. Serial position curves for both groups were similar in form and showed both primacy and recency effects. There was, therefore, no indication that the poorer recall performance of the head-injured group is attributable to a selective deficit in recalling items from particular list positions.

To simplify interpretation of the effects of laterality of skull impact on memory, only data for those children (98) who showed right hand preference were considered. Such children who had sustained impacts to the left side of the skull showed a quantitatively small but quite consistent tendency toward poorer recall than those with right sided impacts, the difference attaining statistical significance on the 15 minute delayed recall test ($p < 0.05$).

TABLE 2. Mean number of items recalled by
left and right impact subgroups

	Mean Trials 1-4	+5 min.	+15 min.
Left impact (n=38)	6.4	6.5	6.4
Right impact (n=40)	6.7	6.8	6.8

The pictures used in the memory test were readily encodable in verbal form and it seems reasonable to classify it as a verbal memory task. If it is accepted that the cerebral hemisphere ipsi lateral to the skull impact is the site of maximal injury, then this pattern of impairment is consistent with the view that lateralization of verbal function similar to that in adults is present also in children.

It is interesting that while there was some indication of a laterality of trauma effect for verbal memory, there was no corresponding trend for vocabulary performance. The left and right sided impact groups did not differ in their scores on the EFVT. This is in agreement with the suggestion made by the late Dr. John McFie (1974) of a dissociation between verbal memory processes and other verbal functions, with respect to the effects of cerebral lesions. His conclusion was that while verbal memory shows a differential sensitivity to laterality of lesion at all ages other verbal processes do not.

There was some indication that the presence of an initial period of PTA is a pre-requisite of a subsequent significant memory impairment. Accordingly, the PTA absent subjects did not differ from the controls, whereas the other PTA subgroups performed at a significantly poorer level. This is consistent with Miller's (1966) contention that PTA is "the signature of a significant closed head injury." However, when PTA has been present, a subsequent impairment of memory is evident whether the PTA is relatively short (less than one hour) or more prolonged (greater than one hour), with no significant correlation between memory impairment and PTA duration.

Nor was there a significant effect of age at injury on the severity of memory dysfunction after head trauma. It is of interest here to recall Teuber's (1970) suggestion, based on a synthesis of the animal and human literature, that while elementary sensory and motor functions may be relatively spared with earlier as compared with later cerebral lesions, more complex aspects of performance (such as memory) may be equally vulnerable to damage occurring at whatever age. Also, sparing of function may apply only to localized cortical damage and not to diffuse cerebral injury of the kind which may follow closed head injury.

No relation was apparent between memory performance and the interval between head injury and the time at which the child was tested. While several interpretations of this finding are possible, it may indicate that some degree of permanent impairment of memory function can follow head injuries which are considered clinically to be quite mild. There is support for this view in the early work of Conkey (1938) who found that, although some other aspects of cognitive function may gradually return to normal after head injury, learning and memory processes may not do so.

No significant relationship was found between memory performance and the presence of a skull fracture, whether linear or depressed, or of post-traumatic seizures. Nor was there any interaction between the sex of the child and the influence on memory scores of any of the clinical variables considered.

In conclusion, the study suggests that a significant residual impairment of memory may follow head injuries in children which would be regarded clinically as minor and that the degree of dysfunction may be related to the site of skull impact.

REFERENCES

Conkey, R.C., 1938, Psychological changes associated with head injuries, Archives of Psychology, No.232

McFie, J. 1974, Brain injury in childhood and language development, in: "Minimal Cerebral Dysfunction", M. Bax and R. MacKeith, eds., Heinemann Medical Books, London.

Miller, H., 1966, Mental after-effects of head injury, Proceedings of the Royal Society of Medicine, 59: 257

Teuber, H-L., 1970, Mental retardation after early trauma to the brain: some issues in search of facts, in: "Physical Trauma as an Aetiological Agent in Mental Retardation," C.R. Angle and E.A. Bering, eds., U.S. Department of Health, Education and Welfare, National Institute of Neurological Diseases and Stroke, Bethesda, Maryland.

CHILDHOOD HYPERKINESIS: SYMPTOM OR SYNDROME, DISCRIMINATING

THROUGH THE USE OF L-DOPA AS A THERAPEUTIC AGENT

Mauricio Knobel

Full Professor of Psychiatry, State University of
Campinas (UNICAMP)
UNICAMP, Campinas, São Paulo, Brazil

Childhood hyperkinesis is still a deem question in Child Psychiatry. We must try to clarify our diagnostic criteria, and have a "syndromic approach"in child psychiatry (3). As Ross and Ross remind us, the World Health Organization has selected the term "Hyperkinetic Syndrome" to describe the symptom constellation we all know we are talking about, and which the American Psychiatric Association in its classification of 1968 called "Hyperkinetic Reaction of Childhood" (7), which was changed to "Attention Deficit Disorder with Hyperactivity" in its DSM-III of 1980 (1). Therefore the concept of the existence of a "syndrome" is predominant, even though we cannot yet reach more uniform criteria.

We then studied hyperkinetic and non-hyperkinetic symptoms in children with problems of behavior and difficulties in relationships but with a normal I.Q. We specially observed hyperkinetic behavior. Thus, this is our first conclusion and definition we want to put forward: The term hyperactive or hyperkinetic refers to a related type of hyperactivity; that is, the child, even though disorganized, shows an interpersonal relatedness, which can be easily differentiated from the unrelated type of hyperactivity, which is seen in some schizophrenic children.

After making a breakdown in our large symptom list, some behavioral items presented an internal consistency that enabled us to select those behaviroal assessments that were highly discriminative of "hyperkinesis" and "hypokineses," and then we arrived at a conclusion in regard to the first one. We were able to state that the hyperkinetic child shows the following characteristic symptoms: 1) is not sullen, seclusive or lonely, 2) does not withdraw, 3) is hyperactive in a "related" manner, 4) is unable to postpone gratification, makes excessive demands and has poor capacity to sustain an effort 5) is not moody, and 6) is aggressive, fighting, bullying, cruel and destructive (6).

The above-mentioned symptomatology, selected for internal consistency, followed a pattern described by Guttman (2). Therefore, the Guttman scalogram analysis was possible, and we launched on a second type of treatment of our data. The six behavioral assessments provided a scale which discriminated reliably among children we studied, with satisfactory reproducibility (0.90), with a random pattern of errors, and with a satisfactory distribution of frequencies within the items.

Another breakdown of the symptoms allowed us to establish an operational definition which we called the "Infantile Hyperkinetic Syndrome." This syndrome is characterized by at least 7 of the following hyperkinetic symptoms, and no more than 2 of the hypokinetic symptoms. The hyperkinetic series consists of: 1) hyperactivity, 2) low frustration tolerance, 3) aggressiveness (including destructive, bullying and cruel behavior), 4) impulsiveness, 5) looking for companionship, 6) inability to postpone gratification (including making excessive demands and poor capacity to sustain an effort), 7) poor school performance (with normal I.Q.), 8) poor peer relationships, and 9) hostility (including rebelliousness, resenting authority and stubborness). The hypokinetic or withdrawal series is made up of: 1) feelings of depression, 2) sullenness (including seclusiveness and loneliness), 3) indifference (including being apathetic or passive), 4) moodiness, and 5) withdrawal. We show this scheme in Figure I (6).

We were also able to establish, empirically, criteria for differentiating whether the condition was of a predominantly organic or psychogenic etiology. (4)

The idea of using L-Dopa came out from experimental work and the relatedness of stimulants to the dopaminergic system. This appeared as a possible treatment procedure, according to the ideas of my co-worker Prof. Karniol, and with another co-worker, Prof. Strauss, we performed a clinical experience (5). According to our studies, we could agree that a dopaminergic imbalance could be the substrate of hyperactivity in children and that the therapeutic action of stimulants, at least partially, might be given by their ability to activate dopaminergic pathways in the brain (5). Considering that in animals the administration of small doses of L-Dopa produces a depressant effect, and that the opposite happens when larger doses are used, it is possible to consider the result of the stimulation of predominantly presynaptic receptors when small doses of L-Dopa are used and the stimulation of postsynaptic receptors with larger doses. "We hypothesized the same results in the hyperactive child, with small doses of L-Dopa producing quietness and an increase

Operational Definition of Hyperkinesis*

Hyperkinetic Series	Hypokinetic Series
1.Hyperactive.	1.Depressed.
2.Low frustration tolerance.	2.Sullen(incl.sec- clusive or lonely)
3.Aggressive(incl. destructive,bully ing and cruel behavior).	3.Indifferent (incl. apathetic or passive).
4.Impulsive.	4)Moody.
5.Looks for companionship.	5) Withdraws.
6.Inability to post pone(incl.making excessive demands and poor capacity to sustain effort)	
7.Poor school performance.	
8.Poor peer relationship.	
9.Hostile (incl. rebelliousness, resenting author- ity and stubborn)	

* A child who presents seven of the nine hyperkinetic symptoms and no more than two of the hypokinetic symptoms could be considered for diagnostic purposes a hyperkinetic child.

Figure 1

in the symptomatology or even psychotic breakdowns with larger doses." (p. 28)(5).

Encouraged by our findings, I studied a larger group of children presenting the "Infantile Hyperkinetic Syndrome," according to the previously described criteria (Fig. I)(6). Children from 5 to 10 years of age were selected, with the whole "Syndrome" in its highest presentation, disregarding those with evidence of organicity, and only accepting those which we may call of "psychogenic etiology." We may be able to change the physiological dysfunction, according to what I now call "Karniol's hypothesis."

Thus we were able to select the first 25 children with the above described condition ranging from 5 years and 2 months of age to 10 years old. Sixteen were boys and 9 were girls. Each item (Fig. I) was rated on a 0 to 4 intensity-frequency grade, 0 being not present, 1 seen rarely, 2 present regularly, 3 frequent, and 4 constant and intense. The maximum score would then be 36. The treated children showed that the total score ranged from 28 to 32, when they were selected.

	L-DOPA	BROMAZEPAN
Boys	9	7
Girls	5	4
Total	14	11

Figure 2 Treatment

We used L-Dopa and Bromazepan blindly. The prescription was made by the researcher in the form of "one tablet," "two tablets," etc. To measure the effects of treatment, evaluations were made weekly. When no improvement was seen, the dose was doubled every 2 weeks. Thus, L-Dopa was used in doses of 500 to 2,000 mgrs. a day, according to the case, the average dose of L-Dopa being 1,500 mgrs., and of Bromazepan being 12 mgrs. a day. The whole study took two months, and children were seen up until 6 months afterwards, without drug treatment. 9 boys and 5 girls were treated with L-Dopa and 7 boys and 4 girls with Bromazepan (Fig. II).

We divided the treated children into "improved" (mother and teacher's information and a score below 18 on our rating scale), and "with no changes" (mother and teacher's information and very little modification in the pre-research score).

	IMPROVED	NO-CHANGE
Boys	7	2
Girls	4	1
Total	11	3

Figure 3 Results with L-Dopa

62

	IMPROVED	NO—CHANGE
Boys	2	5
Girls	1	3
Total	3	8

Figure 4   Results with Bromazepan

The results of those treated with L-Dopa showed that 7 boys and 4 girls (total of 11) showed "improvement," while 2 boys and 1 girl (total of 3) did not change (Fig. III).   This data, treated with the Wilcoxon Sign Test (8), showed a statistically significant difference at a $p. < 0.02$, which proves that the drug used is undoubtedly efficient in the treatment of the "Syndrome" which we are now considering.

The results of those treated with bromazepan show "improvement" in 2 boys and 1 girl, and "no-change" in 5 boys and 3 girls.   That means that out of the 11 children, only 3 improved (Fig. IV).

After the 8 weeks of treatment, and after verifying the results, we tried a cross-over verification.   We treated the "no-changed" cases with the opposite drug.   The 3 with "no-change" with L-Dopa

	IMPROVED	NO—CHANGE
Boys	1	1
Girls	0	1
Total	1	2

Figure 5   Cross over of non-changed with L-Dopa

	IMPROVED	NO-CHANGE
Boys	3	2
Girls	2	1
Total	5	3

Figure 6 Cross over of non-changed with bromazepan

were then treated for one month with bromazepan and we saw that only one boy "improved," while the other boy and the girls continued in the "no-change" category. This is statistically non significant (Fig. V). The "not-changed" with bromazepan, when treated with L-Dopa, also for one month but with increased dosage, as with the previously described children, every week, showed us that 5 children (3 boys and 2 girls) "improved," while the other 3 (2 boys and 1 girls) were "not changed" (Fig. VI). Further research is necessary.

REFERENCES

1. American Psychiatric Association, "Diagnostic and Statistical Manual of Mental Disorders-DSM-III," 3rd. ed., The American Psychiat. Assoc., Washington, D.C. (1980)
2. Guttman, L., The basis for scalogram analysis, in: "Measurement and Prediction," S.A. Stoufer, ed., Princeton Univ. Press, Princeton, N.J. (1950)
3. Knobel, M., A syndromic approach to "acting-out" children, Dis. Nerv. System 20:80 (1959).
4. Knobel, M., Diagnosis and treatment of psychiatric problems in children, J. Neuropsychiat. 1:82 (1959).
5. Knobel, M., Karniol, I.G., and Strauss, L., L-Dopa and treatment of hyperactive children, Acta Paedopsychiat. 47:27 (1981).
6. Knobel, M., Wolman, M., and Mason, E., Hyperkinesis and organicity in children, Arch. General Psych. 1:310 (1959).
7. Ross, D.M., and Ross, S.A., "Hyperactivity: Research, Theory, Action," John Wiley & Sons, New York (1976).
8. Wilcoxon, F., "Some Rapid Approximate Statistical Procedures," American Cyanamyd Co., Stanford (1949).

A CHILDHOOD VARIANT OF MANIC-DEPRESSIVE ILLNESS

Richard E. Davis

Family and Child Psychiatric Clinic of Johnson County
Overland Park, Kansas U.S.A.

Use of a clinical diagnosis such as Manic-Depressive Illness or Bipolar Disorder implies that the words used in the name describe the entity to some degree. Manic-Depressive Illness of Childhood, (1) Juvenile Manic-Depressive Illness, (2), etc. all such names lead the clinician to expect either mania, depression, or classical manic-depressive cyclic behavior at some point in the illness.

Manic episodes in manic-depressive illness are described in DSM II (3) as "characterized by excessive elation, irritability, talkativeness, flight of ideas, and accelerated speech and motor activity." (See P. 36, DSM II.) DSM III (4) is more specific, but similar in its description. (See P. 208.)

Depressive episodes in manic-depressive illness are described in DSM II "by severely depressed mood and by mental and motor retardation progressing occasionally to stupor. Uneasiness, apprehension, perplexity and agitation may also be present." (See DSM II, P. 31.) DSM III gives a similar description. (P. 213.)

Manic-depressive Illness (Bipolar Disorder, Mixed) with both manic and depressive episodes, is described in DSM III (P. 217.) as a "current (or most recent) episode involves the full symptomatic picture of both manic and major depressive episodes (P. 208 and P. 213.) intermixed or rapidly alternating every few days."

Table 1

DSM-II	DSM-III
296.1 Manic-Depressive Illness, Manic Type.	296.4x BiPolar Disorder, Manic.
296.2 Manic-Depressive Illness, Depressed.	296.5x Bipolar Disorder Depressed.
296.3 Manic-Depressive Illness, Circular Type.	296.6x Bipolar Disorder, Mixed.

The descriptions for mania and depression contained in both DSM II and III are not appropriate for the group of children I call Manic-Depressive (now Bipolar) Variant Syndrome Children. These children are neither manic nor depressed by these descriptions. I will describe them and review briefly the criteria necessary to make the diagnosis Manic-Depressive (Bipolar) Variant Syndrome of Childhood. It should be noted that there are infrequent cases of classical mania, depression, and manic-depressive symptomology in persons under 18 years. These persons can be properly diagnosed as having childhood or adolescent Bipolar Disorder (Manic-Depressive Illness), if other criteria are met.

HISTORICAL PERSPECTIVE

In 1956 and again in 1959, two reports of successful lithium treatment of affectively disturbed adolescents appeared. (5,6) In 1969, Annell in Sweden published her initial accounts of treating "Manic-Depressed" children with lithium carbonate. (7) Soon followed by scattered reports -- mostly clinical trials of lithium in hostile or "Manic-Depressive" adolescents and children -- a beginning literature has accrued and was reviewed by Youngerman and Canino in 1978. (8) A further review of articles on file at the Lithium Information Center at the University of Wisconsin through January, 1980, uncovered an additional 20 reports listing 122 more cases. (9)

A number of contemporary studies support the concept that violence and abuse committed against children tend to lead these children toward violence or abuse as parents. (10) But whether there might be constitutional, biological, or genetic factors predisposing children toward committing violence as children, is less well studied. Yet Shafii, Whittinghill, and Healy reported in the December, 1979, issue of the American Journal of Psychiatry that "75% of the 944 child psychiatry emergencies (were) of violence against young people and by young people . . ." (11)

Youngerman and Canino, DeLong, Feinstein and Wolpert, Brumbach and Weinberg, Schou, and several others have initiated work or published reports which focus around childhood aggression, violence, and dysphoric mood - behaviors which often have dissipated remarkably when adequate levels of lithium carbonate were obtained. (8,1,2,3, 4,13,14,15,16) In May, 1979, in the American Journal of Psychiatry, I proposed that a specific pre-adult affective syndrome existed, the Manic-Depressive Variant Syndrome of Childhood, for more specific diagnostic and research clarity. (12) This syndrome specifies five major essential criteria, and five minor criteria (one or more of which must be met) for making a diagnosis of this syndrome.

MANIC-DEPRESSIVE VARIANT SYNDROME

Table 2

FIVE MAJOR CRITERIA

1. Affective Storms.
2. Family history of severe affective or manic-depressive behavior or alcoholism.
3. Hyperactivity.
4. Chronically disturbed interpersonal relationships.
5. Absence of psychotic thought disorder.

FIVE MINOR CRITERIA

1. "Soft" neurologic signs.
2. Sleep disturbances.
3. Abnormal EEG.
4. Findings of minimal brain dysfunction.
5. Enuresis.

All of the above are self-explanatory with the exception of "Affective Storms". An affective storm has been described as a "loss of emotional control of major disruptive force in a child or a person under eighteen years of age, which either has no identifiable precipitating factor, or whose precipating factor is grossly inadequate to explain the degree of emotional outburst." (12) These outbursts are in excess in intensity of the common emotional lability seen in children properly diagnosed as having minimal brain dysfunction. These storms are transient, irregular in occurrence, and occur over minutes or hours at most, never over days or weeks. They may appear to be of psychotic magnitude during the time of the outburst, but they are not accompanied by thought process disintegration between such episodes. They include either verbal or physical abuse or both. Such children are temporarily violent and out of self-control.

Children with Affective Storms do not want these violent behaviors and they often feel ashamed of them afterwards. They are not the result of purposeful decisions, but rather would seem to represent lowered thresholds for coping with frustration, the resulting loss of temper compounding rather than resolving the situation which precipitates the Affective Storm.

From the above noted studies, it appears these are children and adolescents who from their earliest years -- following remarkably minor frustrations or provocations -- suffer severe temper tantrums and temporary loss of affective control, and that further, selected children in this group respond remarkably well to Lithium in terms of developing adequate self-control mechanisms without either significant sedation or tranquilization. Although parental or family psychopathology may or may not be present in significant degree, many such young persons are from families without previous violent or abusive parental practices, even though such parents may eventually be provoked to it after continual onslaughts from the child over the years. Siblings in these families have not exhibited such aggressive outbursts nor have there been episodes of abusive parenting with these siblings. The violence prone child and their families are puzzled at best, are often devastated at worst by these continuous episodes of what I have labeled "Affective Storms," violent childhood behaviors precipitated by remarkably minor frustrations.

On further examination there is frequently a history of similar affective disruptions in the biological family tree, or of manic-depressive illness, alcoholism, or significant depression. Such children inevitably have serious peer, sibling, and school conflicts as a result of their unpredictable and destructive behavior. Yet these children often detest their recurrent Affective Storms and neither they nor their families can explain them. These children are not psychotic in their daily functioning or in their thought processes between such episodes.

Their symptoms begin in infancy or early childhood and per- sist despite repeated efforts to modify or treat the child or family with various psychotherapies and pharmacologic agents. Otherwise these families have the usual mixture of family strengths and problems, many with important psychodynamic factors needing attention -- but because of the continual turmoil and focus on the violent child, they are often left unattended.

It is my clinical impression that M-D (Bipolar) Variant Syndrome children most often represent behavioral expressions of a genetically transmitted CNS metabolic entity neurogenetically related to, but not identical with Bipolar Disorder (Manic-Depressive Illness) as described in DSM III. A biological cousin, if you will. It is possible some or all of these children will demonstrate as adults Bipolar (M-D) Disorder behavior, but many properly diagnosed adult M-D's did not have major Affective Storms as a part of their childhood. As such, the term Manic-Depressive (Bipolar) "Variant" syndrome seems to me more appropriate than Manic-Depressive Illness or Bipolar Disorder of Childhood (or adolescence).

68

I have now diagnosed and treated fifteen young people between ages eleven and seventeen who fit the criteria for the MDV Syndrome. Therapeutic success -- where success is defined as a dramatic decrease or disappearance of the stubbornly persistent Affective Storms - has been uniform, which I must say is both pleasing and disconcerting, disconcerting in that "nothing is 'always' in medicine." (17)

"Uniform" success refers specifically to child behavioral symptomology, particularly Affective Storms, not to the therapeutic results of treating family and parental psychopathology which has not always been possible with an equal unanimity of success in these frequently disturbed families.

Please note: The intent here is not to encourage practitioners to begin the administration of Lithium to children with "temper tantrums," nor to administer it to children indiscriminately, since Lithium in those under twelve has not been recommended for such use by the Federal Drug Administration, nor conversely has it been disapproved. It would be grossly inappropriate, indiscriminate, and unjustified to administer Lithium casually to adolescents or children without appropriate clinical knowledge and experience with Lithium, full awareness of potential risks and emphasis on unknown and possible long range factors in Lithium use in children and adolescents, and without all of these factors being shared with both the child and parents. Only when previous exhaustive medical, neurological, and psychiatric evaluation and previous comprehensive treatment efforts have been unproductive, do I currently offer Lithium therapy as an alternative to these severely distraught people. And in these carefully selected MDV Syndrome young people, the positive therapeutic response to Lithium Carbonate has been dramatic.

Whether Lithium may be related non-discriminately to excessive destructive aggression, as aspirin is related to excessive body temperature, is not yet know. The success of Lithium in the MDV Syndrome raises several questions: is Lithium a specific therapeutic for a given, or a set of given, biochemical aberrations of the central nervous system? Or is it a general defusor of excessive anger and affect?

The first double-blind study of Lithium in "Manic-Depressive Children" was conducted by Robert DeLong, M.D. at Harvard. (1) This initial double-blind, controlled study of four patients confirms the clinical impression held by many of us that Lithium is indeed a significant modifier of temper outbursts and mood disturbance in children and adolescents.

I must also add a note about an alternate treatment I have recently undertaken with youth who fit the M-D (Bipolar) Variant Syndrome. I have now treated five persons under eighteen years of age suffering the M-D (Bipolar) Variant Syndrome with Imipramine HCl (Tofranil), using a single nighttime dosage based on age and weight. Again, remarkable improvement, meaning lessened intensity and frequency of Affective Storms along with improved sleep and decreased moodiness, has occurred. That treatment program is continuing.

The pioneer clinical work indicating the need for detailed studies in a specifically defined clinical group (MDV (Bipolar) Syndrome) has been done. Using such diagnostic criteria, carefully controlled double-blind cross-over studies can be undertaken for further diagnostic and therapeutic clarity.

CONCLUSION

Children who fit the Manic-Depressive (Bipolar) Variant Syndrome criteria, and their families have led tragic, conflicted, unrelenting lives of emotional turmoil. Combined with education, appropriate psychotherapeutic help, and Lithium therapy (and more recently Imipramine HCl), all their lives frequently change dramatically for the better. Lithium or Imipramine alone for these people are inadequate therapy since most physicians still believe in treating people, not diseases. Yet these medications do seem to offer a remarkable respite from the destructive outbursts which have plagued these children's early life years. These children do not fit standard descriptions for manic or depressed people. Controlled studies of target populations fitting the MDV Syndrome criteria are now possible and justifiable because of the impressive clinical responses to certain defined medications.

REFERENCES

(1) DeLong, R., "Lithium Carbonate Treatment of Select Behavior Disorders in Children Suggesting Manic-Depressive Illness." J. Ped. 93:689-694, 1978.

(2) Feinstein, S.C., & Wolpert, E.A., "Juvenile Manic-Depressive Illness." J. Amer. Acad. Child Psych. Vol. 12, No. 1, Jan., 1973.

(3) Diagnostic and Statistical Manual of Mental Disorders. Second Edition (DSM II). APA.

(4) Diagnostic and Statistical Manual of Mental Disorders. Third Edition (DSM III). APA.

(5) Gershon, S.; Trautner, E.M., "The Treatment of Shock-Dependency by Pharmacological Agents." Med. J. Australia, 1:783-787, 1956.

(6) Van Krevelen, D.A.: Van Voorst, J., "Lithium in the Treatment of a Cryptogenetic Psychosis in a Juvenile." A. Kinderpsychiatry, 26:148-152, 1959.

(7) Annell, A., "Manic-Depressive Illness in Children and Effects of RX with Lithium Carbonate," ACTA Paedopsychiatrica, 1969, 36:292-361.

(8) Youngerman, J., & Canino, I., "Lithium Carbonate Use In Children and Adolescents." Arch. of General Psych., Feb., 1978, 35:216-224.

(9) Lithium Information Center, Department of Psychiatry, University of Wisconsin Center for Health Sciences, 600 Highland Avenue, Madison, Wisconsin 53792.

(10) "Violence and the Violent Individual." Ed: Hayes, J.R.,: Robert, T.K.; Solway, K.S. SP Medical & Scientific Books, Chapter 23, N.Y.

(11) Shafii, Wittinghill, & Healy. American Journal of Psychiatry, Dec., '79.

(12) Davis, R.E. "Manic-Depressive Variant Syndrome - A Preliminary Report." American Journal of Psychiatry. 136:702-706, May, 1979.

(13) Brumbach, R.A. & Weinberg, W.A., "Mania in Childhood." Amer. J. Dis. Child, 131:1122-1126, 1977.

(14) Schou, M., "Lithium in Psychiatric Therapy and Prophylaxis: A Review with Special Regard to its Use in Children." Edited by A. Annell, Stockholm, Proc. 4th VEP Congress, 1971, pp. 479-87.

(15) Jefferson, J.W.; Greist, J.H., "Primer of Lithium Therapy." Baltimore, Wilham and Wilkins, 1977.

(16) Lena, B., "Handbook of Lithium Therapy." Edited by F.N. Johnson, Lancaster MTP Press, 1980.

(17) Delp, M., Personal Communication During Student Clerkship in Medicine, 1953, University of Kansas Medical Center.

EPILEPSY AND PSYCHOSIS IN CHILDHOOD

Flora de la Barra Mac Donald

University of Chile, Medical Faculty, East Division
Las Condes Clinic
Santiago, Chile

INTRODUCTION

One of the possible ways of making progress in the study of schizophrenic syndrome, is to search for an ethiology and compare evolution among different subgroups of patients. Several authors, whether relying on negative bleulerian symptoms, positive schneiderian symptoms, E.E.G.s, or brain tomographies, have not been able to show differences in prognosis between functional and chronic organic psychosis in adults. The relationship between epilepsy and schizophrenic syndrome is still being intensively studied, with controversial findings, complicated by anticonvulsant use, in adult patients (2,7,9,10,11,12).

Childhood psychoses are a rare pathology, therefore it is difficult to collect a great number of cases for analysis. A further difficulty is that follow up studies in literature include cases of autism, desintegrative psychosis and schizophrenia, which are now known to constitute different clinical and prognostic entities (13). Several researchers state that schizophrenia starting in childhood is later related to severe and chronic evolution (8). Diagnosis of schizophrenia is infrequent before puberty, and in adolescence, it may also present problems. Many times, differential diagnosis with sub acute organic confusional states and with some chronic organic psychosis is very difficult.

Otherwise, it is known that epileptic children present a high prevalence of varied psychiatric disorders (5,6). The only study on the relationship between epilepsy and psychosis in children, reffers to autism (4). E.E.G. interpretation is an unreliable aid in children, due to the existence of an increasing proportion of

73

abnormalities in normal children, emotional disorders, developmental disorders and psychotic children.

MATERIAL AND METHOD

Our study was made at the child psychiatry outpatient Unit of a pediatric hospital in Santiago, Chile. The unit is situated together with the child neurology unit, and assists arround 2000 new patients each year. We do not have an inpatient unit. We included all cases who were diagnosed as schizophrenia-like psychosis between 1975 and 1979, and have followed them up to now. 14 patients had been referred before to psychiatry, either for emotional or developmental disorders.

The sample consisted of 16 boys and 9 girls, whose ages at onset of psychosis were from 6 to 16 years (most between 10 and 14). 14 (56%) were referred by pediatricians and 11 (44%) by neurologists. 14 had abnormal personal history. Both schizophrenia and epilepsy appeared in family history. 4 patients had an I.Q. under 70.

Diagnosis was rated independently by two psychiatrists, who used Bleuler's criteria for syndromatic diagnosis, therefore, all patients have at least one major sign and one or more accessory signs. At the end of follow up, diagnosis was crossvalidated by an English psychiatrist who used Schneider's criteria. Differential diagnosis with autism and desintegrative psychoses was made according to I.C.D.9. These syndromes were excluded, as acute confusional psychoses. Associated symptoms were frequent and severe. Schizophrenia-like psychoses predominated, paranoid bouts being the most frequent (Tables 1 and 2).

Table 1. Psychotic Phenomenology in 25 Patients

a) Major signs

Flat affect	= 23
Autistic withdrawal	= 16
Thought disturbance	= 8

b) Accesory signs

False perceptions	= 19
Delusive phenomena	= 18
Catatonic signs	= 21
Hebephrenic signs	= 21
Language disorder	= 6

c) Associated symptoms during psychotic bouts

Sleep disturbance	= 14
Suicidal attempts	= 7
Sexual disturbance	= 8
Psychomotor agitation	= 11
Agression	= 14
Lowering of school achievement	= 16

Table 2. Syndromatic Diagnosis of Bouts in 25 Patients

1st Bout		2nd Bout	3rd Bout	4th Bout
Schizophreniform	= 21			
Paranoid	= 13	Paranoid = 2	Paranoid = 1	
Simple	= 4	Paranoid = 1	Paranoid = 1	Paranoid=1
Catatonic	= 2			
Hebephrenic	= 2			
Schizoaffective	= 4	Schizoaffective=1		

Classification according to I.C.D.9 criteria

Even though clinical description corresponded strictly in all 25 cases to a schizophrenic syndrome, an heterogeneous picture appears when they are classified according to I.C.D. 9 categories. Epileptic psychoses turn out to be quite complex regarding contributing factors and associated diagnoses (Table 3).

Table 3. Diagnostic Classification (I.C.D.9) in 25 Children with Schizophrenia like Psychoses

Diagnosis of psychosis	Other diagnoses	Contributing factors
Organic chronic psychotic state (294.8) = 12	Epilepsy(345)=7	Paranoid hallucinatory state induced by drugs (292.1) = 1
	Epilepsy(345)=4 + M.R. (317)	Pathological drug intoxication (292.1) = 1 Induced psychosis = 1 (297.3)
Schizophrenic psychoses (295) = 10		
Induced psychosis (297.3) = 1		
Sub acute organic confusional state (293.1) = 2		

Relationship with epilepsy

10 patients had primary generalized epileptic seizures before psychosis. 8 of them had new seizures after the psychotic bout = primary generalized, secondary generalized or partial complex type. One additional patient had generalized seizures for the first time 2 years after psychosis, making a total of 11 (44%) epileptic patients. Intervals between seizures and psychosis are shorter than described in adults = 4,9 years.

E.E.G. Abnormality

All patients had several E.E.G.s which show a great degree of general abnormality specially focal alterations, which persist in time in a large proportion of cases. Association between left predominance and schizophrenia-like psychosis corresponds with literature, but the only right focus is not a schizoaffective psychosis (Table 4).

Table 4. E.E.G. Abnormality in 25 Children with Schizophrenia-Like Psychoses

```
Abnormal               = 24 (96%)
Focci                  = 18 (72%) both slow + spike waves, left
                                   focci predominate
Temporal spike focci = 3 psychomotor epilepsies
                       3 generalized epilepsies
                       4 other diagnoses
```

Relationship with Temporal Lobe Epilepsy

During the complete evolution, 10 patients had temporal spike focci. 6 of them were epileptic patients, but only three of them had clinical symptoms ascribed to the temporal lobe. The other three had generalized epilepsy. Nevertheless, 4 patients with other diagnoses, also had temporal spike focci. Therefore, only in three patients, the diagnosis of temporal lobe epilepsy could be made both on clinical and electroencephalographic grounds.

This high incidence of neurologic involvement is probably due to referral bias (8 out of 11 epilepsies and 9 out of 15 brain damage patients were referred by neurologists). It is possible that prevalence of epilepsy in Chile might be higher than in other countries (3).

Medication

18 patients were treated with anticonvulsants plus neuroleptics. 6 received only neuroleptics; and one, anticonvulsant plus benzodiazepine. In two cases, it seemed possible that neuroleptics could have triggered seizures. In one patient, it was certain that anticonvulsants triggered psychosis, and it was possible in 4 additional cases. In yet another, onset of psychosis was related to stimulant medication.

Follow up since the first bout is diverse, fluctuating from 2 to 10 years.

Outcome of Psychosis (Table 5)

We considered remission, a complete dissapearance of productive symptoms, during at least three months. It was not possible to measure intellectual deterioration. 5 patients continue having emotional or conduct disorders, although free from psychosis, and one has a schizophrenic defect.

Table 5. Outcome of Psychosis in 25 Children

Remits after 1st.bout	= 16	Abandons during 3rd. bout	= 1
Remits after 2nd.bout	= 2	Becomes chronic	= 1
Abandons during 1st.bout	= 4	Is having a 4th. bout	= 1

Duration of Bouts in 25 Children

1 - 3 months	= 13	5 years	= 1
4 - 11 months	= 7	10 years	= 1
1 - 2 years	= 5	Abandon 1st. bout	= 1
		still in evolution	= 1

Educational Outcome

A number of children are behind their age group at school, or drop out of school entirely, but it is not greater than the usual proportion of children belonging to low socioeconomic class in Chile

Outcome of psychosis is, as far as follow up goes, better than reported for child psychoses, and for adolescent and adult schizophrenia (1,13) but, our sample is not comparable with child psychoses, due to inclusion criteria. Comparison with adult schizophrenia is doubful, as it is known than only 1% have their onset before puberty.

5 Epilepsies show an unfavourable outcome. Evolution of psychosis and epilepsy can be paralell or divergent, in the same proportion. When we compare evolution of E.E.G. vs evolution of psychosis, it is concordant only in half of the cases. If we compare evolution of psychosis, epilepsies and E.E.G., we find all possible combinations, except that E.E.G. improvement is less in epileptic patients, as could be expected. There is no statistically significant difference between psychosis outcome in patients with or without seizures. There is no statistical difference between patients with or without brain damage evidence, either regarding outcome of psychosis or number of bouts.

SUMMARY

We have followed for several years, 25 children and adolescents selected initially for sharing a clinical description of schizophrenia-like psychosis,both according to Bleuler's and Schneider's criteria. When assessment included neurologic,personal and psychometric variables, we found that the children could be divided into sub groups: 11 patients have epilepsy, and 15 gather evidences for brain damage, frequently associated. No predictive factors could be identified for outcome of psychosis or of epilepsy. The initial hope that this prospective assessment and ethiologic search might cast light on the study of child psychoses, has not been completely fulfilled but, the patients themselves provide cummulative information of great clinical value. Nevertheless, further studies in children with psychoses and epilepsy are needed.

REFERENCES

1. Bleuler,Eugen (1967). TRATADO DE PSIQUIATRIA, Espasa Calpe E., Madrid.
2. Bruens,J.H.(1975). Psychosis in Epilepsy. En HANDBOOK OF CLINICAL NEUROLOGY, P.J. Venken Springer Verlag. Berlin,Vol.15, Capítulo 32,593,610.
3. Chiofalo,N.,Lirschbaum,A.,Fuentes,A.,Cordero,M.L. and Madsen,G. Prevalence of Epilepsy in Children of Melipilla,Chile.Epilepsia, 20 June, 1979.
4. Corbett,J. Childhood Psychosis.Relationship to Epilepsy and other neurological conditions.In J.K.Wing HANDBOOK OF PSYCHIATRY(1981) Cambridge University Press.
5. de la Barra,F. Devilat,M. Analysis of 50 children with psychiatric disturbance. I. Educational, Psychiatric and Neurologic Characteristics. Neurocirugia 36:322-329, 1978.
6. de la Barra,F.,Castillo,C. Analysis of 50 children with psychiatric disturbance. II.Causes of psychiatric disturbance. Neurocirugia 38: (1980).
7. Dongier,S. (1959-60). Statistical study of clinical and electroen cephalographic manifestations of 536 psychotic episodes occurring in 516 epileptics between seizures. EPILEPSIA 1:117-140.
8. Fish,B. Neurobiologic antecedents of schizophrenia in children. ARCH. GEN. PSYCHIATRY Vol. 34, Nov. 77.
9. Flor Henry,P.(1969). Psychosis and temporal lobe epilepsy. A controlled investigation. EPILEPSIA 10, 363-395.
10. Flor Henry,P.(1974). Psychosis, neurosis and epilepsy. Developmental and gender related effects and their ethiological contribution. BRIT. J. PSYCHIAT. 124-144-150.
11. Franks,R.(1979). Schizophrenia-like psychosis associated with anticonvulsant toxicity. AM. J. PSYCHIAT. 137, 7.
12. Jensen,Y., Larsen,J.K. (1979). Mental aspects of temporal lobe epilepsy. Follow up of 74 patients after resection of a temporal lobe. JOURNAL OF NEUROL. NEUROSURG. AND PSYCHIAT 42, 256-265.
13. King,L. and Pittman,G. (1971). A follow up of 65 adolescent schizoprenia patients. DIS. NERV. SYST. 328-334.

IDENTIFYING LITHIUM-RESPONSIVE CHILDREN

G. Robert DeLong and George W. Nieman

Pediatric Neurology Unit, Massachusetts General Hospital

Fruit Street, Boston, Ma

Our experience and that of others indicates that lithium has definite usefulness in certain behavioral and emotional disorders of childhood. In this paper we summarize our experience with lithium treatment of children over the past 8 years. This has been done on an outpatient basis. We have proceeded on the basis that long-term acceptance and continuation of treatment is an important index of efficacy. In every patient, during the course of treatment, there were periods of time when treatment was discontinued as either an open or blind trial - in other words, there was every opportunity to discontinue treatment.

We have recently reviewed our experience. A diagnosis was made, retrospectively, from the case histories by an observer who was blind to the outcome of treatment. We have used DSM III criteria, feeling as many others do that these criteria can be used in children satisfactorily for affective disorders and may be more restrictive, useful and precise than other proposed criteria.

We use the term childhood manic-depressive illness (MDI), in the belief it is justified, but others may prefer a more tentative designation.

Sixty-one patients met DSM III criteria for diagnosis of manic-depressive illness or mania, including 51 males and 10 females. The mean age at diagnosis was 9.8 years. Of these 20 are currently on treatment with lithium with benefit, with a duration of treatment ranging from 3 to 96 months, with a mean of 34 months. A further 16 patients have discontinued lithium after treatment extending over more than 10 months. The duration of treatment of this group ranged from 11 to 58 months, with a mean of 25 months.

The overall follow-up of these children ranges from 11 to 150 months, with a mean of 50 months. In all, 65% diagnosed as manic-depressive or manic were considered to have a beneficial long-term response to lithium treatment. The treatment, while not perfect, importantly normalized these children's lives and those of their families. Nineteen were considered treatment failures.

Forty-one children treated with lithium were diagnosed a posteriori as depression. Of these, only 11, or 27%, were treated with success. Seventeen children were diagnosed as conduct disorder. Of these, only 4 (23%) had a positive therapeutic result by the criterion of treatment continued more than 10 months.

Of more interest are 12 children diagnosed retrospectively, again without knowledge of the lithium response, as attention deficit disorder with hyperactivity. Not one of these had a useful result from lithium. None had even a transient positive response. When we looked carefully, lithium often had made these children worse, and was discontinued within a few days. (This by the way is a useful control for any halo or placebo effect of beginning a promising new medicine).

These results make certain points: 1.) Lithium is useful, on a long-term basis, for a group of children meeting criteria for manic-depressive illness. 2.) Lithium is not useful for ADDH. 3.) MDI in childhood is a distinct entity, quite separable from ADDH, on the basis of lithium response as well as symptoms. 4.) In fact, there may be an antagonism or reciprocal relationship between MDI and ADDH in childhood, in that lithium helps MDI and makes ADDH worse.

Three aspects of childhood MDI may be discussed:

A.) Clinical features

We will not emphasize the familiar "affective storms" or the manic and depressive extremes, which have been described previously. Two other features have interested us:

1.) Neurovegetative disorders of special types have been prominent, including encopresis, salt craving, increased fluid intake, increasing appetite, increased sweating especially at night, and sleep disturbances. A pungent body odor is reported occasionally.

2.) Increasingly evident to us is a tendency to obsessional interests or preoccupations – narrow intense interests in odd subjects such as paleontology, antiques, types of trucks, coins, the bones of the body, space ships, etc. Sometimes the obsessive interest takes a definite anti-social direction which may include stealing, or rarely fire-setting or sexual themes. These narrowly focussed interests seem to us to relate closely to rich fantasies and obsessive fascinations in some very young children, and with certain special or precocious abilities - several of our children have had precocious number ability, or hyperlexia, or feats of memory.

These features, which we are just now studying, suggest that many of the MDI children have not a simple attention deficit but an aberrant, strongly focussed distortion of attentional mechanisms. Again, it can be seen as the inverse of ADDH.

B.) Family History: We have found a 50% incidence of bipolar manic-depressive illness in the parents' or their first order relatives and 88% incidence of major affective disorder, using Research Diagnostic Criteria. Those children with special or precocious abilities, mentioned above, have an even higher incidence of a family history of bipolar illness.

C.) Personality and cognitive characteristics: We selected 20 typical MDI children with positive family history and lithium response, and then carefully selected a comparison group of 20 children with ADDH with negative family history of affective disorder, individually matched to the MDI group for age, sex, full-scale IQ grade level, and socio-economic status. On the Personality Inventory for Children - filled out by mothers - the MDI group had very significantly greater (p < .001) abnormalities on the items psychosis, maladjustment, depression, delinquency, aggression, asocial behavior and externalization than did the matched ADDH group.

On cognitive tests, the MDI group had significantly higher scores on non-verbal visuo-spatial subtests of the WISC-R (subsumed as a simultaneity factor), and lower scores on Halstead-Reitan neuropsychological testing on auditory-verbal perception, on verbal comprehension, and on the category test - the latter considered an index of frontal lobe function.

Thus there is evidence of a cognitive skew in MDI children with absolutely high non-dominant visuo-spatial function, relatively low dominant verbal function, and low frontal lobe function.

Preliminary observations have indicated that lithium treatment in these children is associated with some improvement in verbal function, but no improvement in attentional factors.

The K-SAD (Schedule of Affective Disorders for Children) was administered to 10 children before and during lithium treatment. The results verify a highly significant improvement in irritability, anger, episodic hyperactivity, pressured speech, poor judgment, grandiosity, and elation (all with p < .001) and less striking but still significant reductions in other features. There can be little doubt that lithium indeed ameliorates a set of behaviors characteristic of manic-depression in symptomatic children. We have confirmed similar positive effects of lithium treatment in a discontinuation double-blind crossover study in 16 children.

To summarize, 1.) There is a group of children greatly helped, on a long-term clinically-meaningful basis, by lithium treatment, permitting normalization of their and their family's lives. 2.) Most of those children probably represent a childhood manifestation of manic-depressive illness, a probability supported by the symptomatology and the very high incidence of manic-depression and affective disorder in their families. 3.) These children typically have certain specific and characteristic behavioral and cognitive features. One of the most provocative is their tendency to an obsessive or narrowly focussed distortion of attention - leading sometimes to special abilities or apparent precocity - which is in some sense the opposite of children with attention deficits. This possible opposition is illustrated by the observation that lithium is not useful in attention deficit disorder and indeed often has unfavorable affects in such children.

LITHIUM RESPONSIVE CHILDREN AND ADOLESCENTS

Kenneth L. Gordon

University of Massachusetts Medical Center
Worcester, Massachusetts

The validity of the concept of affective disorders in
children has long been debated. Recent advances have been made
in the diagnosis and treatment of Major Depressions in children.
This paper is based on observations of seriously disturbed,
hospitalized children who have distinctive physiological and
behavioral states, and respond to lithium.

The patient population studied are children 15 years old and
younger, who have histories of multiple treatment failures
including previous psychiatric hospitalizations and medication
trials, psychotherapy, special school programs and legal involve-
ments. They have been previously diagnosed as Tension Discharge
Disorder, Borderline, Psychotic, Conduct Disorder and Hyperactive.
Hospitalization became necessary when they could no longer be
safely contained in the community.

The physiologic and behavioral states observed will be
referred to as "low" and "high" periods. During their "low"
periods these children experienced disturbance in sleep and
morning experience. Specifically, these children developed
overly lengthy, overly sound, dreamless sleep. Upon arising in
the morning they felt angry, irritable or tired; or had stomach
or headaches. The morning dysphoria and somatic symptoms improved
over ½ - 4 hours. Pubertal children also had decreased libido.
These children often appeared energetic, but close observation
often demonstrated psychomotor changes. Appetite and weight
changes were of no diagnostic value. During "high" periods there
was a different sleep disturbance, motor restlessness, excessive
appetite and thirst, and, in adolescents, increased sexual energy.
During this state the children took hours to fall asleep; they

had restless sleep with multiple awakenings; and, most strikingly, nightmares with violent imagry including killings and mutilations with explicit visualization of blood and crushed body pieces. Behaviorally, during their "high" periods the children appeared either euphoric or hostile. If euphoric they were mildly oblivious, pleasantly happy or silly, and non-angrily impulsive. Psychotic euphoria was not seen. If hostile, there were characteristic temper tantrums of "psychotic intensity." These tantrums were typically triggered by specific psychodynamically loaded events such as limit setting or confrontations by parental or authority figures. During the tantrums, the children appeared out of control and out of touch for periods of $\frac{1}{2}$ - 6 hours. Attempts at engaging them only aggravated the tantrum. Space, time and sedating antiphychotic agents were frequently useful in terminating these episodes. These children also had extended periods of non-violent anger, during which they sought isolation.

Other inconsistent findings in these children were dysphoric affect with crying spells and death wishes; symptomatic phobias and panic attacks; tension headaches; subjective anxiety and muscle tightness. Lying, stealing and other secretive behaviors were common. A history of enuresis was common. There was also an overrepresentation of actual abandonments in the life histories of these children. Family histories were positive for affective illnesses, alcoholism and violence. Psychodynamically, the children appeared to have deep abandonment fears with a prominent counter-dependent style.

When treated with lithium, at blood levels of 1.0 - 1.2 meq/1, these children had marked improvement in their disturbances. Sleep, dream, appetite and libido normalized. Morning experience, anxiety and depression improved. Restlessness, impulsivity and tantruming decreased. Social provocativeness, lying, stealing and other secretive behaviors also decreased. Attention and learning improved. Treatment, however, was frequently complicated by the counter-dependent stance of these youngsters.

Case Presentation

At the time of his admission, Howie was an 11 year old boy with a long history of hyperactive, distruptive and runaway behaviors. He had come to the attention of the social agencies early in his life, and had received the benefit of several years of psychiatric counselling and special school programs. However, Howie could no longer be contained in the community when he began to light fires, carry knives, be involved in street fights, and steal money.

Howie's life history is striking for a number of abandonments, and exposure to much violence. He was placed in foster care at

birth, where he remained until the age of 6 months, when he went
to live with his Mother and her Husband. Mother left Howie and
Husband three years later due to Husband's drunken abuse. Howie
did not see Mother again until he was eight. He lived with his
step-Father until five months prior to his admission. At that
time he was placed by the social agencies, into the custody of
his Mother due to step-Father's abuse.

The developmental history available revealed that Howie
achieved both verbal and motor milestones early, and was a talk-
ative and active child. Behavioral problems were first noted
during his second year, and were chronic. Peer relationships
were very inconsistent.

Howie's Mother had a history of psychiatric hospitalizations
secondary to drug abuse, a suicide attempt, and a possible
depression.

His medical history was unremarkable.

At admission, medical and neurologic evaluations were unremarkable. Of interest, however, was a positive dexamethasone
suppression test.

Following a brief period of relative quiescence, Howie
became a significant management problem for the nursing staff.
He displayed much physical activity, was distractible and hyper-
alert. His mood fluctuated rapidly: at times he was irritable
and abusive; at other times he seemed sad. He constantly
struggled with the staff about rules and limits. He could only
engage with peers for brief periods and would extend himself only
when it was to his advantage. He was involved in numerous reck-
less and dangerous activities. Because of his provocativeness,
impulsivity and overt displays of anger he frequently required
placement in a seclusion room. However, instead of calming there,
he would remain tense and angry for hours. At night, he was
afraid of the dark, and would require many hours to settle for
bed. His sleep was restless and he had numerous awakenings. He
also would talk and curse in his sleep.

When I first met Howie, he was continuously tense and
irritable, and resistant to all attempts to engage with him.
There was no evidence of a psychosis, although it was apparent
that his judgement and insite were quite impaired.

Howie told me of his fear of the dark, and that when he went
to bed he felt tense, and would think for hours before falling
to sleep. Prior to admission he had begun taking a knife and his
Teddy Bear to bed with him. He slept lightly, woke up numerous
times each night, and frequently fell out of bed. He had night-

mares in which he saw people being blown apart by gun blasts, and vividly described the gore and blood. He also had a recurrent falling dream in which he would hit the ground and bounce, instead of waking up or being hurt. Howie recalled other times when he did not have nightmares, and slept so soundly he could not be aroused.

He described frequent angry feelings that could last for hours or days, and were only helped by isolating himself. With continued contact during these angry periods, he often lost control and became violent. There was partial amnesia during these violent outbursts.

He had also been feeling as if he had too much energy, which he could not discharge. He also had been eating much more than usual for him.

A review of phobic symptomology revealed a prominent counter-phobic stance. Although afraid of the dark, and being home alone, Howie revealed his "love" of numerous dangerous activities such as hanging from bridges and cliffs, and darting in front of moving automobiles. He also "loved" thunder and lightening, fires and bombs and owned several pet snakes.

Howie was placed on lithium carbonate, with serum lithium levels controlled between 1.0 - 1.2 meq/l. The drug was tolerated well. During the second week after this level was achieved, striking objective and subjective changes were noted. Howie ceased being provocative, irritable and labile. Struggles with staff and peers ended. Howie experienced and reported a reduction in energy level and angry moods. At school there was improved attention and learning skills. Sleep and eating symptoms normalized.

Confirming this lithium response was a return to the admission behavior and physiological state when Howie was temporarily taken off of lithium, and a further remission shortly after a therapeutic lithium level was again achieved. Further possible corroborating evidence of a physiological change comes from the dexamethasone suppression test. On admission this test indicated an early release of cortisol suppressed by 1 mg. of dexamethasone; that is the test was positive. After Howie's first response to lithium, this test became negative. When the lithium was temporarily discontinued and the exacerbation of symptoms occurred, the test again became positive. A fourth test was not done.

DISCUSSION

The case presented is typical of the roughly 20 children who fit the clinical description presented, and who have shown marked improvement with lithium. For an equal number of children, the recommendation of a lithium trial has been made, but no trial attempted. This represents a significant percentage of the several hundred hospitalized children seen by us during the past few years. If it were not for the current thinking about Affective Disorders in children, Howie would merit only a Conduct Disorder diagnosis by D.S.M. III criteria, and a Tension Discharge Disorder diagnosis by G.A.P. criteria. Since his symptomology is not consistent with R.D.C. or D.S.M. III criteria for a Major Affective Illness, lithium as the appropriate psychopharmacologic intervention, might not be considered.

The relationship between this syndrome and adult Manic Depressive Illness is not entirely clear. Follow-up studies are needed and are in progress. Two children, of the six on whom there are several years of follow-up, and who are 16 years old or older, have developed adult manic, psychotic episodes that remit with increased lithium levels. It does not seem surprising that development might exert such a "phenoplastic" effect on the manifestations of disorders. A well known example is the pseudodementias in the aged, that respond to treatment of the etiologic affective illness. Likewise, it is necessary to carefully consider the diagnosis of a lithium responsive condition in children who have severe behavioral disorders. Failure to diagnose and treat the affective component of these severely disturbed children, greatly enhances the risk of severe affective morbidity and permanent character pathology.

ALTERED PROLACTIN RESPONSE IN ANOREXIA NERVOSA

K. Toifl[1], F. Waldhauser[2], and J. Spona[3]

1: Department of Neuropsychiatry in Childhood and
   Adolescence; 2: Department of Pediatrics;
3: Department of Gynecology and Obstetrics;
All: University of Vienna, A-1090 Vienna, Austria

In females amenorrhea is essential for diagnosis of anorexia
nervosa (AN)[6]. Even though AN is accompanied by a variety of endocrine disturbances such as reduced sex steroid levels [5], reduced basal serum gonadotropins[18], diminished response of gonadotropins to
luteinizing hormone, releasing hormone (LHRH)[4], alterations in growth
hormone and cortisol levels [12], low serum, triiodothyronine values and
blunted thyrotropin response to thyrotropin releasing hormone (TRH)[15],
it is generally believed that the prolactin (PRL) response to stimulation is not altered in this disorder[4]. Basal serum PRL has been reported to be normal[3,11] or slightly diminished[8], and PRL values after
TRH stimulation were found to be normal by most investigators[4,21].

PATIENTS AND METHODS

We examined serum basal PRL values and serum PRL values after
stimulation either with thyrotropin releasing hormone (TRH, 200 µg/m²)
or with insulin (4 IU/m²) in 27 female patients with AN, 12,5 to 18,3
years of age, diagnosed as anorectics according to the criteria of
Feighner (6). The patients, of whom two had primary amennorrhea, 25
secondary amenorrhea, were admitted to an inpatient ward. They had
a body weight ranging from 53 % to 88 % of their ideal body weight
(IBW).

Before any psychotropic medication, and while on a low caloric
diet (700 to 1000 kcal/day), the patients were given an insulin tolerance test (ITT) and one day later an TRH test. Nine healthy females, 28,8 to 28,3 years of age, with normal menstruation served
as controls.

The PRL response was evaluated 20, 30, 60, 90 and 120 minutes after stimulation.

RESULTS

Basal PRL values

The basal PRL values were low in anorectics but not significantly different from the controls (table 1).

PRL response after TRH stimulation

Stimulation with TRH caused a PRL increase in both patients and controls. The PRL increase in AN was significantly less than in control subjects as indicated by comparing individual PRL stimulation values (table 1).

PRL response after insulin stimulation

PRL stimulation values 60 minutes after insulin administration and later were significantly lower in anorectics than in controls (table 1).

Because PRL did not rise in some subjects of both groups after insulin administration, data were recalculated using the nonparametric Fisher's exact test. This test also confirmed the diminished PRL response to insulin in AN ($p < 0,01$).

Table 1. Prolactin response after TRH or insulin in AN (n = 27) and controls (n = 9); * $p < 0,05$, ** $p < 0,01$, *** $p < 0,005$

	Anorexia Nervosa (n = 27) $\bar{x} \pm$ SEM	Controls (n = 9) $\bar{x} \pm$ SEM
PRL value (after TRH)		
0'	6,8 ± 0,8	9,9 ± 1,3
20'	34,0 ± 4,1 *	50,40± 7,2
30'	30,9± 3,6 ***	58,7 ± 7,4
60'	20,0 ± 1,7 *	33,7 ± 7,4
90'	14,1 ± 1,3 *	21,4 ± 3,5
120'	10,0± 0,9	15,9 ± 2,1
PRL value (after Insulin)		
0'	8,9 ± 0,8	12,8 ± 2,2
20'	8,1 ± 0,7	10,4 ± 1,7
30'	12,1 ± 3,4	20,0 ± 5,9
60'	16,6 ± 4,7 *	76,3± 21,9
90'	12,7 ± 2,3 **	61,8± 15,8
120'	11,2 ± 1,4 **	31,5 ± 7,3

DISCUSSION

Basal serum PRL values in our patients with AN were low but not significantly diminished when compared to controls. This is in agreement with previous reports which found low normal[4,11] or diminished PRL values[8,10]. In other reports[14,20] elevated basal PRL values in AN were recorded. In most of these early papers no specific reference to treatment was given.

We found a reduced response of PRL to TRH in anorectics.

Isaacs et al. (11) also observed a significantly reduced PRL response to TRH in anorectics before and after weight gain. They found no correlation between PRL response and ideal body weight. In contrast, most other authors found no changes in PRL response to TRH in AN[4,21].

However, data on PRL response to stimulation are limited, and in most instances such studies were performed frequently and on few patients[13,21].

To our knowledge the ITT has never been used as a stimulant for PRL release in AN. In recent years intracellular glucopenia due to insulin has been established as a potent and relatively reliable stimulus for PRL secretion. The great majority of normal individuals respond satisfactory to insulin if it is administered in sufficient amounts[22].

An interesting aspect of this test is that in contrast to TRH, which acts directly on the lactotrophes, insulin seems to exert its influence on PRL release through the hypothalamus. Thus, this test has been considered to be more appropriate than other PRL stimulation tests for evaluating the integrity of the hypothalamic pituitary[22].

PRL secretion has been considered to be a marker of brain dopaminergic function. The PRL release from the pituitary is controlled basically by inhibitory effects of hypothalamic dopamine; therefore a change in hypothalamic dopamine content influences PRL secretion[19]. In the feedback control of the dopaminergic hypothalamic system disturbances has been suggested to exist in AN[1,16,17]. Normally, this feedback regulates the neuronal activity to a balanced system. In AN disturbances of this regulatory mechanism might cause chronically supersensitive postsynaptic DA-receptor activity. This hypothesis seems to be attractive because stimulation of dopamine receptors causes inhibition of prolactin secretion[5], and reduction of dopamine turnover. Furthermore in simple starvation the PRL response to TRH is blunted[2]. High estradol levels, observed in sexually mature women[9], are believed to cause the elevated PRL response to stimulation tests. Low estradiol values in AN may on the other hand be sufficient to explain the PRL alterations.

REFERENCES

1. V. C. Barry and H. L. Klawans, On the role of dopamine in the pathophysiology of anorexia nervosa. 38:107 (1976)

2. D. J. Becker, A. I. Vinik, B. Pimstone, and M. Paul, Prolactin responses to thyrotropine-releasing hormone in protein-caloric malnutrition. J.Clin.Endocrin.Metab. 41:782 (1975)

3. P. J. v. Beumont, M. G. Friesen, M. G. Gelder, and T. Kolakowsaka, Plasma prolactin and luteinizing hormone levels in anorexia nervosa. Psychol.Med. 4:219 (1974)

4. P. J. v. Beumont, C. G. W. George, B. L. Pimstone, and A. I. Vinik, Body weight and the pituitary response to hypothalamic releasing hormones in patients with anorexia nervosa. J.Clin.Endocrinol.Metab. 51:1283 (1976)

5. P. Dally, I. Gomez, A. J. Isaacs, "Anorexia nervosa". William Heinemann Medical Books Ltd., London (1979)

6. P. Doerr, M. Fichter, K. M. Pirke, and R. Lund, Relationship between weight gain and hypothalamus pituitary adrenal function in patients with anorexia nervosa. J.Steroid Biochem. 13:529 (1980)

7. J. P. Feighner, E. Robins, S. B. Guze, R. A. Woodruff, G. Winokur, and R. Munoz, Diagnostic criteria for use in psychiatric research. Arch.Gen.Psych. 26:57 (1972)

8. R. J. Frankel and J. S. Jenkins, Hypothalamic-pituitary function in anorexia nervosa. Acta Endocrinol. 78:209 (1975)

9. S. Franks, M. A. F. Murray, A. M. Jeguier, S. J. Steele, J. D. N. Nabarro, and M. S. Jacobs, Incidence and significance of hyperprolactinaemia in women with amenorrhaea. Clin.Endocrinol. 4:597 (1975)

10. A. G. Frantz, Prolactin. New Engl.J.Med. 298:201 (1978)

11. M. G. R. Hull, M. A. F. Murray, S. Franks, and H. S. Jacobs, Endocrinopathy of weight-recovered anorexia nervosa in women presenting with secondary amenorrhea. J.Endocrinol. 69:43 (1976)

12. A. J. Isaacs, R. D. G. Leslie, J. Gomez, and R. I. S. Bayliss, The effect of weight gain on gonadotropins and prolactin in anorexia nervosa. Acta Endocrinol. 94:145 (1980)

13. J. Landon; F. C. Geenwood, T. C. B. Stamp, and V. Wynn, The plasma sugar, free fatty acid, cortisol and growth hormone response to insulin, and the comparison of this procedure with other tests of pituitary and adrenal function, II. J.Clin.Invest. 45:437 (1966)

14. C. Macaron, J. F. Wilber, O. Green, and N. Freinkel, Studies of growth hormone (GH), thyrotropin (TSH) and prolactin (PRL) secretion in anorexia nervosa. Psychoneuroendocrinology 3:181 (1978)

15. R. S. Mecklenburg, D. L. Loriaux, R. H. Thompson, A. E. Anderson, and M. B. Lipsett, Hypothalamic dysfunction in patients with anorexia nervosa. Medicine 53:147 (1974)

16. K. Miyai, T. Yamamoto, M. Azukizawa, K. Ishibashi, and Y. Kumahara, Serum thyroid hormones and thyrotropin in anorexia nervosa. J.Clin.Endocrinol.Metab. 40:334 (1975)

17. P. Riederer, K. Toifl, and K. Jellinger, Is there a hypothalamic dopaminergic dysfunction in anorexia nervosa? In: "Biological Psychiatry", C. Perris, G. Struwe, and B. Jansson ed., Elsevier, North-Holland Biomedical Press 1059 (1981)

18. P. Riederer, K. Toifl, and P. Kruzik, Excretion of biogenic amine metabolites in anorexia nervosa. Clin.Chim.Acta 123: 27 (1982)

19. B. M. Sherman, K. A. Malmi, and R. Zamudio, LH and FSH response to gonadotropine-releasing hormone in anorexia nervosa: effect of nutritional rehabilitation. J.Clin.Endocrinol. Metab. 41:135 (1975)

20. M. O. Thorner and I. S. Login, Prolactin secretion as an index of brain dopaminergic function. Adv.Biochem.Psychopharmacol. 28:503 (1982)

21. P. Travaglini, R. Beck-Peccoz, C. Ferrari, B. Ambrosi, A. Paracchi, A. Severgnini, A. Spada, and G. Faglia, Some aspects of hypothalamic-pituitary function in patients with anorexia nervosa. Medicine 53:147 (1974)

22. R. A. Vigersky, D. L. Loriaux, A. E. Andersen, R. S. Mecklenburg, and I. L. Vaitukaitis, Delayed pituitary hormone response to LRF and TRF in patients with anorexia nervosa and with secondary amenorrhea associated with simple weight loss. J.Clin.Endocrinol.Metab. 43:893 (1976)

23. P. D. Woolf, L. A. Lee, and W. Leebaw, Hypoglycemia as a provocative test of prolactin release. Metabolism 27:869 (1978)

ARTISTIC MEDIA IN THERAPY FOR CHILDREN

WITH DEVELOPMENTAL PROBLEMS

Eva A. Frommer

Department of Child and Family Psychiatry
St Thomas' Hospital
London SE1

There are two main aspects of treatment in child psychiatric work. One is the elimination or at least the moderation of out-standing symptoms that cause distress. The other must be to stimulate and foster the development of the individual child and to influence and advise those individuals who are in his environ-ment and who relate to him so that their life together can take as normal and as healthy direction as possible.

The most obvious symptoms of psychiatric distress in child-hood are behavioural and in the last few years there has been a great deal of interest in devising behavioural modification programmes directed to extinguishing inconvenient or distressing symptoms. These programmes can be very effective and what makes them so popular apart from their identified and limited aim is that results are immediately measurable. They also require only relatively brief involvement of the therapist with the client, in contrast to the psychoanalytically directed psychotherapies that were fashionable until recently.

The latter have proved useful in removing symptoms only in a very limited number of patients, notably where psychic stress such as bereavement has precipitated the inappropriate behaviour of a morbid grief reaction for example.

Psychiatric Background to Developmental Problems

Psychiatric illness such as a depressive state may underlie behavioural symptoms at any age. In such cases a behavioural modification programme without other measures could prove disastrously inappropriate. The illness itself disrupts concentration and memory, and so there is no learned benefit for the patient.

In many children we see evidence of chronic anxiety underlying their presenting symptoms, and a careful history of life events and styles of behaviour usually reveals severe and often repeated stress. Chronic anxiety inhibits normal psychological maturation and is related to developmental problems. The behaviour of the affected child is inappropriate to his chronological age and maladaptive to the environment. Some stresses are endogenous, as in children with delayed or abnormal development of language, or articulation difficulties for example, or children with sensory or neurological deficits. Others succumb to cultural and emotional deprivation, growing up in a developmentally inadequate environment.

For such problems intervention directed only to correct the maladaptive behaviour, or the standard psychotherapeutic techniques is likely to fail, as the child's chronically anxious state has usually disabled his learning faculties. Perception, concentration and memory are disrupted or even distorted by the child's inner preoccupation. Methods of intervention are needed that can re-establish the child's capacity to perceive what is around him and stimulate him sufficiently to interest himself in what he finds in the world and also in himself. He needs to be able to build confidence in himself and his future and to meet others including his family in a positive spirit.

Artistic Media in Therapy

It is fortunate that the most powerful stimulus to learning in childhood and perhaps also in later life, is the instinct to imitate the adults in the environment. This instinct can become our greatest ally in therapy. It is particularly useful if we undertake artistic activities with him.

To become a therapist who is able to stimulate artistic activities in children it is important to be an active, creative person oneself. Colour, music, poetry, drama, movement such as eurythmy, are the vehicles through which one can stimulate reciprocal activity in most children. These media are themselves living creative forces that have pervaded human life and affected man's experience of nature throughout history. With the increasing availability of technology, there has been a tendency to lose the natural relationships and instinctive awareness of the role that colour, music and so forth play in normal life. Even worse, the division between city life and country life experiences, where despite a great deal of mechanisation nature is at least still visible, has become increasingly difficult to bridge. Direct experience of growth and development is rare for families living in deprived inner city areas.

Music in Therapy

The artistic media all carry creative energies within them.
In this city music must be the prime example that springs to mind.
A Haydn symphony, a Mozart sonata, a Beethoven quartet, are spiritual
structures with creative force both for performers and audience. I
am not speaking of reproduced music on disc or tape. Their use for
entertainment is a very different thing. Nor am I advocating a
string quartet in every child psychiatry department - though I know
of no better way of building team consciousness in a group of four
people. If music is included in the therapeutic programme of a
clinic it must be living experience to which children and therapists
contribute. It is not necessary to be very ambitious. The
instruments that are used must however produce tone of good quality.
I have found that a certain amount of courage is required before
adults, who were often told as children that they were ungifted for
music or indeed any of the other arts, will pick up a pair of beaters
and try their luck on a xylophone or glockenspiel. The Orff type
percussion instruments have proved invaluable in helping children
to listen, to hear, and to express moods and feelings for which
they had no words. On this basis more sophisticated musical
communication can be developed by therapist and child, alone or in
a group. Singing communications, once the child hears and listens
are often far more successful than speech, and the sung ring games
of childhood which are such a treasury throughout Europe can become
a truly socialising activity as the children find their way into
them with the help and encouragement of the therapists. We have
also found the songs of the traditional body image games invaluable
for children who are either unable to form a normal body image
because of neurological deficits, or, as happens more frequently
with our local deprived population, because of environmental and
emotional deprivation. No one had ever played such games with them
in infancy.

Colour in Therapy

Colour and its creative energies has been a subject for study
and work in our department for many years. This has included
careful consideration of the colours that have gone on the walls of
various rooms in our treatment unit, and their furnishings. Water
colour is a directly accessible medium for adults and children, and
we have mainly worked with this on wet or dry paper. Gradually,
skill develops and the colours enable the expression of mood, of
feeling and of experiences in the child's life with which he can
then begin to come to terms.

Stories in Therapy

The genuine folk tales such as those collected by the Grimm
brothers come out of the depths of human life experience. For the

treatment of disturbed children, these are an indispensable treasury. Almost every horror that emerges in the histories of our disturbed children can be found in such folk tales, where however there is usually a solution to the problem, that depends to some extent on human qualities of caring, of truthfulness, or perseverance against odds, and of perception of what is and what is not important. In our experience a well-chosen folk tale can become a far more successful behaviour modifier for a disturbed child than a psychologically devised programme. He can identify with the "cast" in the story, and its offer of a solution gives him hope without any direct challenge to his autonomy. The stories need to be tactfully chosen and carefully paced. The decision is always supervised by a clinician in regularly held case conferences.

Staff Training and Attitudes

Another very important aspect of the work I have been describing is the general spiritual context in which it takes place. A framework within which criteria of normality of progress and of failure can be recognised by the therapists and the patients is essential. One aspect of such a framework is a continuous process of communication both at a social and professional level among the clinic staff. Meetings at which the work and progress of the therapists as well as the children are discussed and new ideas developed must take place regularly. It is very tempting, particularly when working with artistic media though not oneself an artist, to fall into a sort of colour or music routine, with the result that the activities lose creative direction and energy. This is particularly likely with overworked staff who have become tired. We devote two days a month to art classes and other study projects for the staff. Their own further development as individuals can also be monitored in this way. The framework also depends upon awareness of the spiritual reality of man within himself, and his relationship in the world to others and to nature.

There can be undue anxiety over the perception of time as a real element in therapy and in building relationships. Our intervention must be seen within the context of the life-history of the members of the child's family, problems that have grown and developed through many years, even generations, cannot be resolved in a set short term programme. The seasonal festivals offer an indispensable opportunity for this. We mark these with appropriate celebrations and an appropriate choice of songs, games and poems so that children are not expected for example to paint snowmen in mid-summer!

Such celebrations do not need to have a specifically religious connotation although they stem from awareness of the spiritual realities in our natural world. They give rhythm, form and definition to the artistic endeavours of the whole unit and also opportunities for very necessary fun and enjoyment.

IMPORTANCE OF NEUROLEPTICS IN TREATING PSYCHIATRIC DISORDERS OF CHILDHOOD AND ADOLESCENCE

Michel Dugas

Service de Psycho-Pathologie de l' Enfant
et de l'Adolescent, Hôpital HEROLD
7, place Rhin et Dunube, 75935 Paris Cedex 19

In **adolescents** just as in adults the major indications for prescribing neuroleptics are manic episodes of manic depressive illness or of the bipolar form of affective disorders, and paranoid schizophrenia. In France, CHLORPROMAZINE and HALOPERIDOL are the most widely used neuroleptics, followed by TRIFLUOPERAZINE, FLUPENTIXOL, FLUPHENAZINE and PIPOTHIAZINE. The hebephrenic form shows little or no sensitivity to neuroleptics as side effects such as apathy and reduction of activity compound the deficiency syndrome of schizophrenia. Neuroleptics used in doses which lead to weak concentration at the synaptic level selectively block pre-synaptic dopaminergic receptors; on the contrary, when synaptic concentration is high, they block post-synaptic domapinergic receptors. The monitoring of plasma levels of the administered neuroleptic and the estimation of the total action of neuroleptics at the synaptic level using the membrane radio-receptor procedure, should permitt treatment of "minus" forms with doses which cause weak synaptic concentration and "plus" forms with doses which cause a high concentration. Hopefully, clinical results will confirm the correctness of these propositions.

Just as it does not make sense to discuss schizophrenia as a homogenous entity, it also contradicts pharmacological data to consider neuroleptics as having identical properties. Actually, they differ in : (i) their blocking power of dopaminergic receptors ; (ii) their preferential sites of fixation on the receptors of different dopaminergic systems ; (iii) their blocking action on dopaminergic, noradrenergic and serotoninergic systems, and their selective action on the dopaminergic system ; (iiii) their differential affinity for dopaminergic receptors ; (iiiii) their sedative or stimulant clinical activity.

We may also mention two other indications for using neuroleptics with adolescent which are less frequently reported - treatment of psychotic anxiety and of sub-agitated states sometimes found in anorexia nervosa (wether hyperactivity or feelings of persecution).

In children, indications for neuroleptics are less clear and certain. In a survey carried out in France in 1982 on 100 parisian child psychiatrists, who practiced in the public sector, it was found that 15 of them never prescribe neuroleptics and that 65 seldom use them in treating childhood psychosis. Main prescribers of neuroleptics in children are therefore general practioners and pediatricians (in France, sales of neuroleptics for children represent 8 % of the total sale of this drug).

Although criteria for usage and non-usage of neuroleptics in children has remained quite empirical since 1952, controlled studies have assessed neuroleptic action in this age population. These are four useful indications for neuroleptics :

1°) Childhood psychosis (pervasive developmental disorders) ;

2°) Behavioral disorders associated with mental retardation ;

3°) Attention deficit disorders ;

4°) Gilles de la TOURETTE's syndrome and its incapacitating forms. Neuroleptics act upon with-drawal hypoactivity, anxiety, other and self-oriented aggressiveness, and abnormal movements. Such action probably reflects the side effects of the neuroleptics rather than direct anti-psychotic action.

What are the disadvantages of administering neuroleptics to children and adolescents ?

Among the short-term effects, let us mention drowsiness, extrapyramidal effects (dystonia, akathisia, tremors) ; as long-term side-effects weight gain and abnormal movements. The latter may develop in the course of prolonged treatment or following treatment interruption (withdrawal emergent symptoms). Such movements are usually temporary , very infrequently, they become long lasting, as in the tardive dyskinesia of adults. But the symptomatology is different from that of tardive dyskinesia, localized dystonia, diskinesia of the extremities,

choreic and ballistic movements, myoclonia, ataxia and
"facial tics". This important question deserves to be
studied within a strict methodological framework.

**What progress can we expect frome treating psychiatric
disorders of childhood and adolescence with neuroleptics ?**
    Three conditions need to be met in order for
progress to take place :
1°) The development of studies bearing on a specific
patient population, selected according to agreed-upon
criteria, common to several different centers. The
DSM-III system is likely to give us the needed starting
point for the next few years. For each specific research,
this type of classification can be complemented by
inclusion and exclusion criteria which are adapted to a
particular goal ;
    2°) Controlled studies must integrate pharmacologi-
cal and pharmacokinetic date ; these are needed for both
children and adolescents since it is has been established that they are different for each stage of development. Results from a pharmacological study on HALOPERIDOL
in children an adolescents, conducted with P. MORSELLI
and E. ZARIFIAN, show that in children there is an
important interindividual variability in haloperidol
plasma concentrations, that there is an important age
effect on the disposition of the drug, and, more important, that the incidence of adverse effects is significantly correlated to the drug concentrations in plasma.
Possible relationships with the therapeutic effects are
less evident and further work along this line is needed.
    3°) The determination of therapeutic effects and
adverse effects must use evaluation procedures for which
the validity, sensitivity, relevance, and reliability
have been established.
    The use of neuroleptics in treating psychological
disorders of childhood and adolescence is numerically
inferior to what it is in adults. On a qualitative level,
its results are inferior to those observed in adults.
The results are comparable to those for adults in
adolescents with similar indications. In children and
adolescents, neuroleptics should neither be to fully
dismissed nor used undiscriminately. It would be desirable that those who work in the field of biological
psychiatry of children and adolescents form a worldwide
network.

MENTAL HEALTH SCREENING OF CHILDREN IN JAPAN

Kunihiko Asai

Vice-Director of
Asai Mental Hospital : Psychiatrist
38, Katoku, Togane City, Chiba Prefecture, Japan

With the use of a computerized system we have carried out two projects on Mental Health Screening of Children since 1975: "Health examination of 10,000 three-year-old children", and "Follow-up study of two cohorts of children from the age of three to their entrance of elementary school". In this paper we would like to present several interesting results and discuss the advantage of the longitudinal periodic health examination and certain desirable health-records keeping methods for study of health and mental health of children.

1) Results from a survey on use of medical services in Chiba

A survey was conducted in Chiba prefecure on the number of children of dfferent age who consulted doctors on a given day in 1978. Of the 166,490 individuals (440 per 10,000) who consulted doctors in 2014 medical institutions or doctor's offices in Chiba Prefecture, those under 12 years of age were 42,527, representing 27 percent of the toal consultations. Among them, 3.4 percent were under 1 year old, 9.5 percent between 1 and 3 years old, and 6.8 percent between 4 and 6 years old. The total of preschool children thus accounted for 20 percent and elementary school children formed 7.7 percent of all consultations.

2) Health examination of 10,000 three-year-old chidren

Health examination of 10,000 three-year-old children revealed that 14.2 percent of the three-year-olds suffer from some kind of physical and/or psychiatric ailments of varying severity requiring the attention of specialists. As shown in Table 1, those clearly diagnosed as physical disorders were 52 (0.7%) and psychiatric disorders were 90 (1.1%) the majority of which suffered from mental retardation. 2.7 percent of all chidren examined were mildly mentally retarded, 1.7 suffered from mild motor dysfunction, 2.5 percent had emotional disorders, 4.6 percent had physical ailments, and 4.1 percent were over or underweight.

3) Follow-up study of the children from the age of three to their entrance of elementary school

We made 3 year follow-up studies on two samples at 3 years of age and 6 years of age, as shown in Table 2. Of the three-year-old children, those clearly diagnosed as having physical and/or psychiatric disorders were 3.7 percent in 1976 and 3.5 percent in 1977. When we compared these results to those of follow-up health examinations three years later, we found a considerable difference between them. Those diagnosed as physical and/or psychiatric disorders increased from 3.7 percent to 4.3 percent for Sample I and from 3.5 percent to 4.1 percent for Sample II. The marked decrease of physical disorders in both samples, from 2.2 percent to 1.1 percent for Sample I and from 1.8 percent to 0.9 percent for Sample II is in striking contrast to the doubling of the prevalence rates of psychiatric disorders, from 1.5 percent to 3.0 percent in Sample I and from 1.3 percent to 3.0 percent in Sample II. While mild motor and physical problems decreased over 3 years in both samples, emotional disorders, weight problems and mild mental retardation increased dramatically in both samples.

These results may be understood by the fact that physical problems discovered by the health examinations of the 3-year-old children have been treated successfully. But the psychiatric or emotional problems have not only been handled ineffectively, they have increased with the advance of age probably due to either increased awareness on the part of the parents or increase of stress in family or kindergarten.

4) Study on the response of family to children with physical and/or psychiatric disturbance

We have followed up 113 cases of all children diagnosed as physical and/or psychiatric disturbances following the medical examination conducted by us. 60 children out of 113 cases were with psychiatric disturbances and 53 with physical problems.

Table 3 shows a marked difference in the age of discovery of physical disorders versus psychiatric disorders. 75 percent of children with physical disturbances were discovered under the age of three, in contrast to only 20 percent of children with mental disorder including mental retardation. 80 percent of the latter were found at the age of four or older. The lack of awareness regarding children's mental functioning is noteworthy.

Table 4 shows that mothers take a lead in finding their chihldren's problems with physical and psychiatric disturbance. However, the fathers account for only about 5 percent, a dismal figure, which may be an indication of their relative lack of contacts with children of these ages. In cases with physical problems, medical personnel such as specialists, home doctors and public health nurses, account for 43.5 percent. In cases with psychiatric problems, however, medical staff account for only 12.5 percent. It should be noted that 33 percent of the cases with psychiatric problems were not noticed by anyone including mother, any member of the family, or medical people, while every physical problem was accounted for by them.

How did family members regard their children's abnormality? The family members' attitude toward their children with physical problems differs greatly from those with psychiatric problems. In cases with physical problems, those who "found their children's abnormal signs in its early stage" accounted for 35.9 percent. Those who "found their children strange, not corresponding to the normal development" were 35.9 percent, and those who "felt strange without knowing why" were 34 percent. There were only a few family members who refused to acknowledge their children's abnormality and considered that their children with physical problems" could not yet acquire daily practice "or "were just a baby and too immature" or "were restless and short-tempered".

The situation was quire different in the cases with psychiatric problems. On the one hand relatively few family members discovered their children's abnormality. Those who "found their children's abnormal signs in the early stage" accounted for only 7.5 percent, those who "found their children strange, not corresponding to the normal development" were 7.5 percent. On the other hand, many family members did not acknowledge their chidren's abnormality and tried to trace their abnormality to different origins. Those who thought their children with psychiatric problems only "were slow learners" accounted for 77.5 percent, those who thought their children "could not acquire daily life skills" formed 57.5 percent. It seems that the Japanese family finds it difficult to recognize the signs of psychiatric disturbances or mental retardation in children. This difficulty seems to be reinforced by the traditional stigma against mental disorders that still prevails in Japan. Many family members refused to admit the presence of signs of psychiatric disturbances or mental retardation in their children and tend to seek other explanations for the abnormality. This results in their contrasting attitudes to the children with physical versus psychiatric problems as well as the patterns of seeking help to solve the problems.

Table 5 shows that about 57 percent of all cases with physial ailments consulted a doctor immediately, 20 percent consulted special public institutions such as Child Consultation Center or Public Health Center. For the cases with psychiatric disorders, however, 25 percent of children did not receive any help frcm anyone or any agency. Only 15 percent of them "consulted school or kindergarten teachers" and 12.5 percent consulted doctors.

Table 6 shows that only 26.4 percent of children with physical disability are attending regular elementary schools, in contrast to 71.9 percent of chldren with psychiatric problems that are in the school. 34 percent of children with physical problems are in hospital care and 39.6 percent in welfare institutions for the handicapped, as compared to only 1.7 percent of children with psychiatric problems who are cared for in hospitals and 26.7 percent in welfare institutions for long-term care. These figures clearly indicate the lack of public interest and lack of public resources for care of children with psychiatric problems in Japan, while the family and the regular school are left with the burden of providing care for them.

Discussion

In Japan the health examination system for children is now established firmly and put into practice nationwide. It is conducted for neonates, children under the age of one, one and a half, three, before entrance of elementary school, and school chidren. At present, however, health examinations are performed without uniformity or continuity. Each physician or public health officer uses his or her own methods and there is no provision for keeping he records the same child systematically for a long period of time. Furthermore, there seems to be very little attention given to psychological, mental or social aspects. We strongly advocate a comprehensive and logitudinal health examination system for all children at various ages of their development. The recent advance in computerized record-keeping technique and its availability and economy certainly will make such an important health examination system within the reach of many who are concerned and interested in the wholesome growth and development of children in Japan and elsewhere.

The marked differences observed between physical and psychiatric problems of chidren in a number of important aspects deserve special attention. The physical disorders are recognized earlier by the family and are better taken care of by specialized care programs or institutions, while psychiatric disorders or mental retardation tend to come to the attention of their parents and other family members late and receive little special care. The prevalence rates of the children with physical problems decrease to half in three years in both Samples I and II, while those of children with psychiatric problems rose in the same periods - speaking eloquently of this desparate attitude and handling by the family and society of these two categories of children's problems.

Table 1 : Type of Physical and/or Psychiatric Disorders

(Health examination of 10,000 three-year-old children)
YEAR 1978   N=7,950

	No.	%
Physically and/or Psychiatrically ill	195	2.5%
Physical Disorders	52	0.7%
Psychiatric Disorders	90	1.1%
Others	53	0.7%
Mild Mental Retardation	215	2.7%
Mild Motor Dysfunction	135	1.7%
Mild Emotional Disorders	199	2.5%
Mild Physical Ailment	366	4.6%
Weight Problems	326	4.1%
Result of First Step Screening	1,158	14.6%

Table 2 : Three Year Follow-up of Three Year Olds
           (Medical examination of 10,000 three year-old children)

	SAMPLE I			
	Three-Year-Old		School Age	
YEAR	1976		1979	
TOTAL NUMBER OF CHILDREN	544		532	
	No.	%	No.	%
Physically and/or Psychiatrically ill	21	3.9	23	4.3
Physical Disorders	12	2.2	6	1.1
Psychiatric Disorders	8	1.5	16	3.0
Others	1	0.2	1	0.2
Mild Mental Retardation	9	1.7	20	3.8
Mild Motor Dysfunction	8	1.5	4	0.8
Mild Emotional Disorders	5	0.9	7	1.3
Mild Physical Ailment	24	4.4	12	2.3
Weight Problems	23	4.2	33	6.2
Result of First Step Screening	84	15.4%	86	16.2%

	SAMPLE II			
YEAR	1977		1980	
TOTAL NUMBER OF CHILDREN	545		533	
	No.	%	No.	%
Physically and/or Psychiatrically ill	19	3.5	22	4.1
Physical Disorders	10	1.8	5	0.9
Psychiatric Disorders	7	1.3	16	3.0
Others	2	0.4	1	0.2
Mild Mental Retardation	9	1.7	19	3.6
Mild Motor Dysfunction	7	1.3	3	0.6
Mild Emotional Disorders	4	0.7	6	1.1
Mild Physical Ailment	16	2.9	16	3.0
Weight Problems	20	3.7	39	7.3
Result of First Step Screening	71	13.0%	83	15.6%

Table 3 : Time of Discovery

Subjects Age	Physical Disturbance 53		Phychiatric Disturbance 60	
0	3	5.7%	C	
1	6	11.3%	0	
2	10	18.9%	3	5.0%
3	15	28.3%	5	8.3%
4	6	11.3%	8	13.3%
5	3	5.7%	9	15.0%
6	1	1.9%	13	21.7%
7	1	1.9%	2	3.3%
unknown	8	15.1%	20	33.3%

Table 4 : Dicoverer of Children's Problems

Subjects Discoverer	Physical Disturbance 53		Psychiatric Disturbance 60	
Mother	18	34.0%	21	35.0%
Father	13	5.7%	3	5.0%
Grandparents	0		3	5.0%
School Teacher	2	3.8%	4	6.7%
Home Doctor	4	7.7%	2	3.3%
Medical Specialist	15	28.3%	2	3.3%
Public Health Nurse	4	7.7%	1	1.7%
Others	4	7.7%	2	3.3%
not noticed	0		20	33.3%

Table 5 : Help-Seeking : Consultations and Treatment

Subjects Adviser	Physical Disturbance 53		Psychiatric Disturbance 40	
Home Doctor	4	7.6%	2	5.0%
Medical Specialist	26	49.1%	3	7.5%
Child Consultation Center	6	11.3%	6	15.0%
Public Health Center	4	7.6%	2	5.0%
Social Welfare Office	1	1.9%	1	2.5%
School or Kindergarten Teacher	2	3.8%	6	15.0%
Other Families	10	18.7%	10	25.0%
None	0		10	25.0%

Table 6 : Institutional Care at School Age

Subjects Treatment	Physical Disturbance 53		Psychiatric Disturbance 60	
Child Welfare Institution	21	39.6%	16	26.7%
Hospital	18	34.0%	1	1.7%
Elementary School	14	26.4%	43	71.7%

USE OF RUTTER SCALES WITH INDO-CHINESE CHILDREN

G. Graves, L. Alexander, G. Burrows, N. Carson,
E. Chiu, R. Frieze, J. Krupinski, A. Mackenzie, E.
Morrison, Y. Stolk, E.-S. Tan and B. Tonge

Mental Health Research Institute

35 Poplar Road, Parkville, Victoria, Australia 3052

To provide the context within which this paper is set, it will be necessary to give you a very brief outline of our study of recently arrived Indo-Chinese refugees. All arrived in Victoria, Australia, in the last 6 months of 1981 and were seen by Indo-Chinese health professionals (mainly doctors) within weeks of their arrival and typically at the hostel in which they were accommodated. All Indo-Chinese refugees arriving during this period were seen as long as the family group contained at least one member who was aged between 5 and 24 years of age. Heads of household were interviewed to establish the usual demographic details and to find out about losses endured and stresses experienced in their country of origin, on the journey, in the camps and in the early days following arrival in Australia.

In all, 510 families were seen and these families included 336 children aged 5-14 and 650 adolescents aged 15-24 years. Adolescents and young adults are the subject of a separate paper which will be presented at another time by the psychiatrists involved. Of the children, 60% were male. The majority (81%) were Vietnamese, with 12% from Cambodia and 7% from Laos. Parents (or, where parents were not present, their surrogates, who were in many instances elder siblings) were asked to complete the Rutter questionnaire (Scale A2) to screen for behavioural disturbance. The Rutter questionnaires were translated into the four languages - Vietnamese, Chinese, Cambodian and Laotian. While every attempt was made to pinpoint problems through detailed explanation and exploration of the meaning of the behavioural descriptions in the Rutter parent questionnaire and through back translation, it is inevitable that some items will contain nuances of expression which render them, at least in part, non-comparable conceptually with their original form.

The survey is a longitudinal one with follow-up interviews at periods of 6, 12 and 24 months after arrival and, at these stages, the Rutter teacher questionnaires will be administered, in addition. In this paper, however, we will be dealing only with the interviews which took place shortly after arrival in this country and for this reason discussion will be limited to the Rutter parent questionnaire and the parent and child psychiatric interviews.

Eighty four children and their parents or parent surrogates were selected and 78 children were seen for a psychiatric interview using a form closely modelled on the procedure described by Rutter and Graham (1968) for the child psychiatric interview and a modified and shortened form of the parent interview, as described by Graham and Rutter (1968).

Thirty seven of the 322 children (11.5%) whose parents completed the Rutter questionnaire exceeded Rutter's cut-off point of 13 and, of these, 35 were seen for psychiatric interview. In addition, a control group of 43, whose scores on the Rutter questionnaire ranged from 0-12, were seen for psychiatric interview. These represented a stratified sample of 20% of those with zero scores, 10% of those with scores between 1 and 5, 20% of those scores between 6 and 8 and 25% of those with scores between 9 and 12. Those selected for the subsample and their parents were interviewed by one of the Australian child psychiatrists or psychologists (4 in all), usually in the migrant hostels in which they were accommodated. The Australian clinicians were accompanied by Indo-Chinese health professionals who were used, in this instance, as interpreters. Such interviews commonly took place some weeks and possibly months after the initial interview. Typically, 'parent' interviews took place with the father, the mother or an older sibling in the presence of the child whereas, if at all possible, the child was interviewed on his or her own. Interviews with the parent and the child took approximately one hour, half an hour for each.

The relation between scores on the Rutter parent questionnaire and the overall judgment of psychiatric state made on the basis of the psychiatric interview was tested by Chi Square. The association between the two was significant at the 5% level of confidence.

While there is a statistically significant association between behavioural deviance and judgments concerning psychiatric state, it was apparent that, while 72% of those whose scores on the parent questionnaire equalled or exceeded 13 were found to have some degree of abnormality, the same was true of 44% of those who did not show behavioural deviance, as indicated by the Rutter parent questionnaire.

Goldberg (1972) has developed measures by which the sensitivity and specificity of the screening instrument (in this instance, the parent questionnaire) can be calculated. The questionnaire was found to have a sensitivity of 57% and a specificity of 71%, with overall efficiency of 63%. It was apparent that it is under-predicting judgments of psychiatric abnormality. This would support the argument of the use of denial as a defence mechanism by the parents in completion of the questionnaire.

This proposition is lent added support by an analysis of the proportions at various cut off points below 13 who were detected as having some degree of abnormality at psychiatric interview. It is notable that 42% of those with zero scores were found to show either mild or definite abnormality, whilst 36% of those with scores on the parent questionnaire between 1 and 5 and about half of those with scores between 6 and 8 and 9 and 12 showed such abnormality.

A further comparison can be made between various items on the parent questionnaire and the ratings made by the clinicians following the parent and child interview. For example there are three items on the parent questionnaire..."Very restless, has difficulty staying seated for long", "Squirmy, fidgety child" and "Cannot give attention to anything for more than a few moments" which can be compared with the ratings of over-activity, fidgetiness and distractability made on the basis of the child interview. Similarly "Often worried, worries about many things" and "Tends to be fearful or afraid of new things or new situations" can be compared with observed anxiety and "Often appears miserable, unhappy, tearful or distressed" can be compared with observed mood level.

Analysis of the data reveals that, whereas parents more commonly described their children as restless and distractable than did clinicians, parents less commonly described their children as anxious or depressed than did clinicians. This would suggest that cultural and conceptual factors may be operating as important determinants in perception. What was perceived as restless behaviour by the Indo-Chinese parent was infrequently perceived as such by the Australian health professional and, similarly, what was perceived as anxiety and depression by the Australian health professional was not usually observed as such by the Indo-Chinese parent.

There are various questions which we would like to consider in relation to the data obtained from the Rutter parent questionnaires and, to facilitate this, we are using, as a comparison group, data obtained from a survey conducted in 1980 in the Westernport region of Melbourne, Australia (Mawdsley and Graves, 1980). This survey was carried out on 881 children with a similar age distribution to the Indo-Chinese refugee sample and, for 602 of these children, a Rutter parent questionnaire was obtained.

The rates of children whose scores reached or exceeded Rutter's cut-off point of 13 were very similar - 11.5% of the Indo-Chinese sample and 11.8% of the Westernport region sample.

Since in this paper we are considering the usefulness of the Rutter parent questionnaire in a cross-cultural study, it may be of interest to compare the prevalence of the checking of each of the 31 behavioural descriptions in the two studies.

The Spearman rank order correlation coefficient was of the order of 0.48 which suggests a fair level of agreement but detailed inspection of the data would suggest some interesting differences in the rank ordering of such behavioural descriptions.

Both groups of parents reported restless behaviour and irritability in their progeny but the Indo-Chinese children were more commonly described as complaining of headaches (rank 4) than were their Caucasian counterparts for whom 'headaches' ranked 20. Similarly, 'has stomach ache or vomiting' ranked 7 for the Indo-Chinese and 22 for local children. Thus, there is some support for the widely held notion that the Indo-Chinese tend to somatize their problems and to deny psychological problems (See, for example, Kleinman and Mechanic, 1981, and Lin et al., 1981). Note in this connection that, while 'often worried, worries about many things' ranked 2 in the Westernport survey, it ranked 12 for the Indo-Chinese.

It would also appear that the Indo-Chinese are less likely to report behavioural descriptions which have an anti-social connotation. Thus "is often disobedient" ranked 6 for the Indo-Chinese but was rank 1 for the Westernport sample.

As part of the parent interview, inquiries were made about all items checked in the Rutter parent questionnaire as other than zero. In particular, inquiry was directed at whether the symptom was still present or had diminished in either frequency or severity. This inquiry also elicited a certain amount of information about the possible misunderstanding or misinterpretation of the item.

Whilst the original administration of the parent questionnaire referred to the period of the last 12 months and covered some time in the country of origin, on the journey and in refugee camps, the enquiry in the psychiatric interview concerned the present time, which was not infrequently some weeks and sometimes months after they were first seen.

It was apparent that many items and, in particular, items concerning headaches and vomiting, being fearful or afraid of new things or new situations and of school resistance had diminished but the restlessness, irritability and anti-social behaviour, where reported, had persisted. Misunderstandings were few, except where asthma or attacks of wheezing had been checked. Inquiry often elicited that such symptoms had occurred with head colds or similar minor illness and bore no apparent relation to asthma.

At this point, I wish to discuss some of the more qualitative data which was gained from an analysis of the child psychiatric interview. Areas which were covered in the interview included peer relationships, anxiety, fears, depression, anger and preferred activities. In addition, they were asked to draw a dream and to draw a person.

Over 40% of the children indicated that they were lonely in Australia and, typically, this was related to missing the close relatives and friends who had remained behind in Indo-China. Such peer relationships as had been established in Australia were of a superficial kind and involved fellow refugees from the hostels or the language centres. Feelings of sadness and depression were expressed by over one-half of the children and were primarily related to the absence of loved ones. Not infrequently, such feelings were originally denied and then almost immediately contradicted.

A similar pattern of denial was evident in relation to worries and, even more strongly, in the expression of anger. The majority (66%) claimed that they had never been involved in fights, although 47% were prepared to admit to angry feelings, primarily relating to teasing by their siblings or peers. Angry feelings were rarely acted upon and more typically led to withdrawal or "bottling up". Where anger was directly expressed, it was more often expressed by verbal than by physical means.

In contrast, three quarters of the children were prepared to admit to fears. Main fears were of ghosts or dogs or related to some aspect of their experiences on the journey. Snakes were also feared.

Dreams of any kind were denied by one third of the children interviewed and, of the remainder, a further 20% denied bad dreams. Bad dreams, which were reported by 47% of children, commonly involved threat situations, many of which had obvious connections with their

113

experiences in Indo-China or during the escape. As one child said "I dream about ghosts - sitting on a tomb. Now I dream about my mother and she is crying".

It is said that "when you translate, you interpret and, when you interpret, you limit" and this would certainly accord with my own experience and with that of my colleagues. As we have tried to show, there were a number of areas in the Rutter parent questionnaire in which, for reasons linguistic, cultural and conceptual, there were important differences in the perception of Indo-Chinese parents. The most basic of all was in the lack of psychological-mindedness of Indo-Chinese parents and in their concentration on somatic problems and denial of psychological ones. It is our view that, while the Rutter parent questionnaire provided valuable information which is of use in screening for psychological disturbance, its application to an Indo-Chinese population is subject to qualification and caution. The instrument is conceptualised in Western terms and inherent in its use is the underlying assumption that what is appropriate in the West in the recognition of behavioural deviance will remain appropriate in translation to an Indo-Chinese population, whose cultural norms and perceptions are so very different from our own.

REFERENCES

Goldberg, D.P. 1972. "The Detection of Psychiatric Illness by Questionnaire." Maudsley Monograph no. 21. Oxford University Press: Oxford.

Graham, P., and Rutter, M. 1968. The Reliability and Validity of the Psychiatric Assessment of the Child: II Interview with the Parent. Brit. J. Psychiat., 114, 581-592.

Kleinman, A. and Mechanic, D. 1981. "Mental Illness and Psychosocial Aspects of Medical Problems in China", in Normal and Abnormal Behaviour in Chinese culture. Ed. by A. Kleinman and T.-Y. Lin. Vol. 2. D. Reidel Publ. Co.

Lin, K.-M., Kleinman, A. and Lin, T.-Y. 1981. "Overview of Mental Disorders in Chinese Cultures: Review of Epidemiological and Clinical Studies", in Normal and Abnormal Behaviour in Chinese Culture. Ed. by A. Kleinman and T.-Y. Lin. Vol. 2. D. Reidel Publ. Co.

Mawdsley, J.A., and Graves, G.D. 1980. "A Survey of Behaviour Problems in School Children to Aid Planning for Change in Service Delivery", in The Child in His Family: Preventive Child Psychiatry in an Age of Transition. Ed. by E. James Anthony and Colette Chiland. Vol. 6. John Wiley and Sons.

Rutter, M., and Graham, P. 1968. The Reliability and Validity of
the Assessment of the Child: I Interview with the Child.
<u>Brit. J. Psychiat.</u>, 114, 563-579.

Rutter, M., Tizard, J. and Whitmore, K. (Eds.). 1970. Education,
Health and Behaviour. Longmans: London.

THE PSYCHOPATHIC NUCLEUS IN ADOLESCENT PSYCHOPATHOLOGY

Mauricio Knobel

State University of Campinas (UNICAMP)
UNICAMP, Campinas, São Paulo, Brazil

Adolescence can be considered a stage of life during which the individual tries to establish his/her present identity and at the same time prepare him/herself for the future adult identity, through early internalization of parental objects and their relationships and also by continuous testing of reality of the social environment. All of this is achieved through the developing biophysical elements which tend to stabilize personality on a genital level, and through a basic threefold mourning process of the lost infantile body, lost infantile identity and role, and childhood parents loss, in the maturational process toward adulthood.

It is necessary to understand underline adolescence as a developmental period which, due to its special characteristics, demands a certain amount of "psychopathic" behavior, that is necessary for the process of working-through what we consider the normal adolescent mourning, as well as for becoming able to establish him/herself in an extrenely conflictive and violent society (1).

Because of biological and psychodynamic structuring, adolescence must be a period of turmoil and uneasiness, expressing itself through inner conflicts and external battles running from open defiance of society (including here the questioning of family structure and dynamics), the well known and frequently described "generation conflict," to isolation and bewilderness, or to creativeness or violent destruction.

Thus a "Normal Adolescent Syndrome" or a "normal abnormality" during adolescence can be described (3)(5). The very process of adolescence implies an amount of psychopathic-like behavior with the use of true psychopathic mechanisms. The exaggerated intensity or persistence of these phenomenae constitute <u>psychopathy</u> in the nosological sense of the term.

But the permanent use of psychopathic mechanisms during adolescence invades both normal and abnormal behavior. In this last situation psychopathy becomes an integrative part of the different pathological entities an adolescent may be presenting. We may see depressive, schizoid, or even schizophrenic adolescents with their specific pathological traits, among which, as mentioned, pyschopathy will be appearing and at times disguising <u>Psychopatic Nucleus</u> in all psychopathological syndromes, running from "Personality Disorders" through "Neuroses" and up to "Psychoses," during adolescence.

Adolescent changes are slow and no inner or outer haste will help the process because it has the characteristics of mourning, and requires time for a real working-through. The pathology of this kind of mourning relates adolescents' psychopathology to 'psychopathy,' because it leads toward acting-out, denial, impulsivity, and poor object relationships. These are the traits we shall look for when considering any kind of adolescent psychopathology in order to realize that the existing 'psychopathic nucleus' is very active in all those cases.

Within our concpet of adolescence three fundamental kinds of mourning can be observed:

1) The <u>mourning for the infantile body</u> occurs because of the characteristic biological changes of adolescence. While his/her mind is still infantile, there is a feeling of both the loss of the infantile body and the emerging changes into an adult body. The contradiction experiences causes a very real phenomenon of depersonalization which pervades adolescent's thinking and that is related to the evolution of thinking itself. This fluctuating process of depersonalization allows for acquiring psychopathic characteristics because of its exaggerated intensity or due to a developmental fixation. Symbolization fails, symbols and that which is symbolized become confused, and ideas tend to develop on a "physical," level which is what leads toward action in short circuits, one of the typical ways of thinking of the psychopath. There appears "confusion," a symptom of both normal and pathologic adolescents, and a sign of the psychopathic nucleus actively participating in dimming many psychopathologic adolescent's syndromes. This mourning leads to the phenomenon of intellectualization and to physical acting-out, both characteristic traits of psychopathy.

2) The <u>mourning for the infantile identity and role</u> stems from childhood natural dependency which has to be lost. While the child accepts his/her relative impotence and the need that other should assume certain kinds of ego functions, the own ego becomes enriched through the projection-introjection process which makes <u>identifica-</u>

tion possible. During adolescence, there is a confusion of roles: the adolescent cannot maintain infantile dependency nor assume adult independence, and he/she suffers a failure of personification. This behavior permits him/her to depersonalize other people and to treat them as objects necessary to his/her immediate gratifications. This "lack of consideration" for people and things in the real world makes all of the object relationships as frail as they are, at the same time, excessively intense. These psychopathic features also appear in diverse adolescent's pathology, denouncing the permanent activity of the psychopathic nucleus. Mourning for the infantile role turns into emotional acting-out, just as mourning for the infantile body turns into motoric acting-out. During this development, and partly by denial of mourning and by use of projective identification with his/her contemporaries and parents, the adolescent goes through periods of identity confusion. We must now remember that the above mentioned traits do appear as symptoms in more specific nosologic entities such as the "clinical picture of identity diffusion" to which Erikson called our attention (2). Thought processes begin to work according to group characteristics that normally allow for greater stability, through the support and enhancement acquired by identification with the ego of others. But when "psychopathy" takes over, this becomes one of the basic reasons for the "gang" phenomenon, where some adolescents apparently feel very safe, adopting changeable roles and sharing group behavior, responsibilities and guilt.

In the psychopath, the affective short circuit, by avoiding thinking whereby guilt can be worked-through, allows the definite ill-treatment of real and fancied objects, producing an impoverishment of the ego. This then tries to maintain itself unrealistically in an infantile situation of irresponsibility, but with apparent independence. Failing in the mourning for the infantile identity and role leads toward psychopathic handling of affection and love.

3). Mourning for the childhood parents. Impotence in dealing with physical changes, the suffering of infantile identity and role struggling with the new identity and its social expectations drives the adolescent to a process of denial of those very changes which take place simultaneously in the figures and images of the parents and the link with them. Parents obviously do not remain passive under these circumstances, for they have to work through the loss of the infantile submissive relationship of their children and the process of getting older. All of this gives rise to an interaction I call "Double Mourning." Behavior is expressed in a series of contradictions with denial of dependence and a true "show" of independence. There is no reality perception. Though contradictions show the lack of a conceptual working-through. They cause perplexity in dealing with the internalized parental object relationship and sever communication with the real outer parents, now completely displaced in the adolescent personality context.

Instead of seeking the solitude that would help work-through the loss of childhood parents, the psychopath constantly avoids it, trying to dissolve his/her personality through massive projective identifications with delinquent or marginal groups, where anxieties, of psychotic nature, can be acted-out. The psychopath perceives the outer world as frustrating and threatening. There is a real distortion of perception, a true "psychotic-like perception" which prevents the psychopathic adolescent from testing reality and forces to experience frustration as a death threat, against which defense is made through short-circuit responses, whereby the distorted perception acts as the triggering cause of overwhelming fearful affects and aggressive behavior.

Those behavioral traits related to the threefold mourning in any adolescent pathology and not only in psychopathy itself. No matter what the syndrome or personality disorder may be, these outlined traits will be found showing us that the "psychopathic nucleus" is permanently active in the psychopathological manifestations of this period of life.

If we also look at the conceptions of time and space in adolescence, we may be able to add some more knowledge of the structuring of the "psychopathic nucleus" we are talking about. A child has a phenomenological conception of the boundaries of space but lacks conception of time, which is then limitless. An adult has a sense of infinite space and of the temporality of existence. But the adolescent enters into "a crisis of temporality": space and time become intermingled and confused. Thinking shows the contradictions of immediateness or of infinite delay before any possibilities of fulfillment. Those are again traits of the underlying psychopathic structure which may appear in any psychopathological behavior disturbance during adolescence.(4)

True judgement gradually operates as a replacement, working-through the threefold mourning process hereby described, enabling the adolescent to place the infantile body, role and parents in the past, to accept the passage of time, and with it the concept of death as a natural and irreversible process of development.

The psychopathic type of behavior, on a basic schizoid personality structure, configurates defense mechanisms and object-relationships that permeate the other types of characterologic traits different adolescents may have, in health and illness.

The frail though intense link to objects and persons, the envious type of relating to the therapist and other persons, and the constant paranoid-schizoid anxiety, underlying and coloring permanently all kinds of behavior, has to be considered as a persistent frame of reference in therapy with adolescents.

This is the core of the "psychopathic nucleus," understanding by nucleus a part of the whole mental apparatus, structured in a special pathological interrelationship, which may have several and different particularities in its metapsychological functioning, which remains isolated within the Ego, but which manifests itself either smoothly and uneventfully in general, or strongly participating in . psychopathological disorders. In adolescent psychopathy, this "nucleus" has a psychopathic structure and manifests itself strongly and permanently. This understanding will certainly help a therapeutic approach, especially a psychodynamic one.

REFERENCES

1. Aberastury, A., Knobel, M., and Rosenthal, G., Mourning as a way to maturity: thinking in normal and psychopathic adolescents, in: "The Psychoanalytic Forum," J.A. Lindon, ed., International University Press, New York (1972).

2. Erikson, E.H., "Identity and the Life Cycle," International University Press, New York (1959).

3. Knobel, M., On psychotherapy of adolescence, Acta Paedopsych. 33:168 (1966).

4. Knobel, M., El pensamiento y la temporalidad en el psicoanálisis de la adolescencia, in: "Adolescencia," A. Aberastury, et al., ed., Kargieman Ed., Buenos Aires (1976).

5. Knobel, M., El sindrome de la adolescencia normal, in: "La Adolescencia Normal," A. Aberastury and M. Knobel, eds., Paidos, Buenos Aires (1981).

MINOR PSYCHIATRIC ILLNESS IN MOTHERS

OF YOUNG CHILDREN

Ian Berg, Alan Butler, Jackson Houston and Ralph McGuire*

Department of Psychiatry, University of Leeds
15 Hyde Terrace, Leeds 2
*University of Edinburgh

A survey of minor psychiatric illness in women with young children was carried out in Harrogate, a non-industrial town in the North of England. They were patients of one group practice composed of three family practitioners with 2,000 patients each. Previous surveys have mostly involved industrial and socially disadvantaged areas in Britain and a high prevalence of minor psychiatric illness has been found linked to poor living conditions and having a large number of children (Brown and Harris 1978, Goldberg and Huxley 1980). In our survey it was considered important to look at age of mother, number and spacing of her children, social factors, interpersonal difficulties, life events and contact with medical services. Disturbance of the children was also studied. Harrogate is a reasonably affluent part of the country where severe social problems are rare.

The Leeds Scales (Snaith et al 1976) and the Malaise Inventory (Rutter et al 1970) were used as screening questionnaires for disturbance in mothers. They are easy to complete and acceptable for use in the general population. There is evidence that they pick out the same disturbed individuals as does GHQ, the general health questionnaire, which has been more extensively used in Britain for community surveys (Forrest and Berg 1982).

240 women with children aged between 2 and 11 were studied. About a third were found to be suffering from mental distress (score of 7 or over in the above scales). This is a similar prevalence to that found in less affluent parts of Britain. Childhood disturbance measured using the BCL, the behavioural checklist (Richmond 1977)

123

for pre-school children and the Rutter A Scale (Rutter et al 1970) for children of school age was associated with maternal disorders.

Having isolated the mothers with problems, a randomly controlled double blind study, using a long-acting preparation of amitriptyline, lentizol (William Warner Ltd.) was carried out by the family doctor. The use of medication is traditional and acceptable in general practice and other approaches are more time-consuming and expensive.

The general practitioner interviewed women selected by the questionnaires as suffering from mental distress, clinically assessed them and completed a social scale. Quite a high percentage of women were excluded because he did not consider them sufficiently disturbed or because they were pregnant or considering pregnancy, or because they felt they should be able to cope without medication. The remainder were offered treatment in the trial following full explanation of the procedure.

13 received active drug and 12 placebo, 50 mgms of lentizol was taken each evening for three months (Houston et al 1983) the patients being seen at two weeks, one month, two months and three months. Each time they consulted their family doctor they filled in a Leeds Scale and a Malaise Inventory. The scores were unknown to him throughout the trial. Blood levels of amitriptyline and nor-triptyline at one and two months showed good compliance with treatment. The patients were interviewed one year later. It was found that the depression scores on the Leeds Scales went down significantly on amitriptyline and were still significantly improved compared with the controls after one year.

In the survey, younger mothers were more depressed and anxious than older ones. No relationship with the number and spacing of the children emerged. Although living conditions were good, minor psychiatric illness was still found to be associated with poor personal relationships and difficulty in getting out and about. Women with mental distress did not attend their doctors more than others.

It is often assumed that because symptoms of anxiety and depression found in community surveys are related to social factors, appropriate management should be some sort of counselling or psychotherapy. Women who could not be included in the drug trial, mostly because of possible pregnancy, were offered regular counselling by a specially trained Health Visitor and it was hoped to evaluate this in the same way as in the drug trial. However, insufficient women agreed to co-operate with regular Health Visitor sessions to discuss their problems, despite considerable effort to get this arranged.

It is concluded that the use of tricyclic anti-depressant medication should be considered as a first line of action in the treatment of minor psychiatric illnesses with symptoms of depression in general practice. It would appear that this approach would be reasonably acceptable to the patient, in keeping with the family doctors' usual way of dealing with distress, more economical than counselling sessions and likely to be effective in reducing the symptoms of depression.

REFERENCES

Brown, G. W. and Harris, T. 1978, Social Origins of Depression. Tavistock Publications, London

Forrest, G. and Berg, I., 1982, Leeds Scales and the GHQ in women who had recently lost a baby. British Journal of Psychiatry, 141, 429-430

Houston, J., Berg, I., Butler, A. and McGuire, R., 1983, Treating depression in general practice with amitriptyline. British Journal of Psychiatry, 142, 103-104

Rutter, M., Tizard, R. and Whitmore, R., 1970, (Eds) Education, Health and Behaviour. Longmans, London

Snaith, R. P., Bridge, G. W. K., and Hamilton, M., 1976, The Leeds Scales for the self-assessment of anxiety and depression. British Journal of Psychiatry, 128, 156-165

BRAIN DYSFUNCTION AS A CAUSE OF

READING DISABILITIES-CROSS CULTURED

Chen-chin Hsu*,**, Wei-tsuen Soong**, Seng Shen***
Shu-jane Su**, and Fang-wan Wei*

* Provincial Tao-yuan Mental Hospital; ** Children's
Mental Health Center, National Taiwan University
Hospital; *** Taipei City Psychiatric Center, Taipei
Taiwan, R.O.C.

While reading disabilities have been considered as a problem
of serious concern in Western nations, they were seen as a rarity
and even non-existence in Asian countries. Most authorities agree
that at least 5 - 10% of the Western elementary children evidence
the characteristics of reading disabilities, the Chinese primary
school teachers are unaware of the existence of such an issue.
"When the characteristics of reading disabilities are explained to
them, they remarked that only a very limited numbers of their
students fell into such a category of exceptionality. (Kuo, 1978)."
The same point was made by a Japanese psychiatrist who wrote, "...
the incidence of reading disabilities in Japan is so rare that
specialists in Japan do not get any referrals. (Makita, 1968)."

The most plausible and widely accepted explanation for the
marked discrepancy in incidence of reading disabilities between
Western and Eastern cultures was proposed by psychologists like
Rozin et al (1971), psychiatrists such as Kline (1977), and
linguists like Martin (1973). They argue that Chinese and Japanese
are easier to learn to read because the Japanese syllabary provides
consistencies between symbols and their pronunciations and the
ideographs of Chinese characters (used both in Chinese and Japanese)
offer possibilities for response to whole units that do not exist
in alphabetic writing system. The phonological basis of alphabeti-
cal orthography has been considered to be the major cognitive
barrier to initial progress in reading English. (Rozin and
Gleitman, 1977.) Morrison and Manis (1983) suggest that the major
difficulties for the beginning reader of English is the formidable
tasks of mastering sound rules in spelling that are complex and
irregular. They go on to argue that the primary cause for the

lack of reading disabilities among Chinese and Japanese children is that the units of the written languages are related simply and regularly to their pronunciations.

What is striking through all of the above mentioned theories and arguments is that no well designed study had ever been carried out to verify that reading disabilities actually are a rarity among Chinese and Japanese children. There, of course, had been no comprehensive study which elucidated the clinical pictures of reading disabled Chinese and Japanese children.

The first part of this paper intends to present evidences which indicate that reading disabilities do exist among Chinese children. The second part of this particular paper present findings of the performances of poor readers on a set of cognitive tests designed for a crosscultural study. Finally, a preliminary clinical findings of reading disabled Chinese children will be supplemented to support the view point that brain dysfunction should be considered as a cause of reading disabilities across culture.

A. Eastern children do evidence reading disabilities

A 3-year "International study of children's reading" was carried out using large samples of 5th graders from Minneapolis (U.S.A.), Sendai(Japan) and Taipei (Taiwan, R.O.C.). The methods and materials of that study have been described in detail elsewhere (Stevenson et al in cooperation with Hsu and Kitamura, 1982) and will not be reiterated here. Suffice it to say that a reading test which was reliable, culturally fair, and accurately reflecting the curricula of the 3 countries was constructed. In addition to the reading test, 10 culture fair cognitive tasks and a mathematics test were constructed. Tasks were selected either on the basis of a hypothesized differential relation to reading ability in the three languages or on the basis of prior research in which same tasks have been related to reading ability. The mentally retarded children were all excluded from the randomly selected subjects of the 3 cities. Minneapolis was selected because of the very low frequency of minority children in its population.

The results show that approximately 3.5% of the Minneapolis children, 3% of the Taipei children and 7.3% of the Sendai children failed to meet the criteria for success at grades 3, 4 and 5, and were, therefore, over two grades behind in their reading level, a common criterion for defining reading disability. Another definition of reading disability is low reading ability together with average or near-average I.Q.. An approximation of each child's I.Q. scores was obtained from a Z-score computed for each child on each of the ten cognitive tasks, standardized within each country. Percentage of children within each country who were both within the lowest 10% of the distribution of reading scores and who obtained an average Z-score higher than one standard deviation below mean for both verbal and performance tasks was determined. The percentage of subjects in the three cultures classified as reading disabled by this criterion were 6.3% in Minneapolis, 7.5% in Taipei and 5.4% in Sendai. The same study was replicated last year in another city in Taiwan about 200km south of Taipei. The result showed that 4.2% of the subjects evidenced reading disabilities according to the first criterion (Guo et al, 1982).

These findings offer no support to the belief that reading disabilities are absent or rare among Chinese and Japanese children, nor to the hypothesis that orthographic systems of Chinese and Japanese preclude the development of disability in reading.

B. Clinical manifestations of Chinese children with reading disabilities

1. Reading Chinese

A brief introduction to reading Chinese may be pertinent here for those who are unfamiliar with this particular language. Approximately 3,000 Chinese characters (單字) have to be mastered for reasonable literacy in Chinese. A character is not equivalent to a word. Most Chinese words are composed of two or more characters, e.g., two characters "銀行" stand for "bank", "症候群" mean "syndrome" and "精神分裂病" are equivalent to "schizophrenia". Major problems faced by the teachers of Chinese are to get the children to pronounce each character correctly. A phonetic spelling system called zhu-in-fu-hao (注音符號) is used to assist in the pronunciation of characters. Zhu-in-fu-hao is a set of 37 symbols, for each of which there is consistent grapheme-phoneme correspondence like the English phonetics. Pronunciation of all Chinese characters can be represented by no more than 3 of the 37 symbols. Markers indicating the 4 tones of Mandarin are further aids to pronunciation. For instance, the English phonetics m∧ pronounced in different tones represent completely different characters and meanings, i.e., the first tone 媽 (mother), the second tone 麻 ∕(numb), the third tone 馬 ∨(horse), the fourth tone 罵 ∖(scolding). Another formidable task of reading Chinese is, in many cases, the same character has to be pronounced differently in different context within the phrase/sentence and with its specific combination with other character. For instance, 行∕人 (pedestrian), 銀 行∖(bank), 一 行∖(one line), 行∕ 為 (behavior) 行∖家 (expert), 他 很 行∕(he is very good at......), etc.

Many Chinese characters are very similar in their orthographies, but have to be pronounced differently and, of course, stand for completely independent meanings. For example, 白 (white),

自(self), 日 (sun), 曰 (saying), 目(eye), 月(moon), 貝(shell), 見(look),etc.

From the above one can imagine that Chinese is not so that easy to read and comprehend as have been widely assumed. Like all other languages learning to read and comprehend Chinese do pose serious challenges to the cognitive functions of the brain. Without the help of phonetic symbols (starting from the text of the fifth graders) one may have to resort more to one's memorized vocabularies in reading each character correctly. Then the reader may have to rely more on the memory of the whole context in which a character is used to comprehend the right one of the many meanings represented by that character. This may explain partly why the Chinese 5th graders performed significantly better than their American counterparts on verbal memory and vocabulary out of the 10 cognitive tasks related to reading as reported by Stevenson and his colleagues(1982).

The clinical findings to be presented here are very preliminary in nature and were obtained during the very initial phase of an ongoing project designed to elucidate the nature and possible causes of reading disabilities among Chinese children. Examples of mistakes in writing and reading were made by 23 5th graders of two schools diagnosed as evidencing reading disabilities. For neurological assessment, each reading disabled child was assigned a case with grade appropriate reading ability matched by sex, classroom and learning potential within ± 2 points on Raven's Standard Progressive Matrices scores.

2. Mistakes in Writing

1) Typical mirror writing: Mirror writings similar to English speaking cultures. Examples are: 7→Γ, 3→Ɛ , 4→ϯ , 人 (human)→入(enter), 馬(horse)→馬 (N.M., no meaning).
2) Partial mirror writing: It is hypothesized that a Chinese character is composed of one or more basic caligraphic units. For example "人" is represented by only one basic unit, while 来(come) is composed of two "人" and another basic unit "木" (tree). Partial mirror writing is characterized by typical mirror writing of one or more basic caligraphic units of a character while the rest of the basic units are written correctly, such as, 來→來, 媽(mother) →媽 , (N.M.), 外(outside) →外(N.M.), and 版→版 (N.M.).
3) Displacement of basic caligraphic units: Basic units are displaced horizontally or vertically, e.g.,知(know)→咦 (N.M.), 昌(prosperous)→冒 (N.M.), 唱(sing)→啚 (N.M.),都(capital) →階 (N.M.), and 昏(dark)→民 (N.M.).
4) Rotation of basic caligraphic unit: A basic unit within a character is rotated by 90 degree, such as,把(hold)→把 (N.M.), 縣(county)→縣 (N.M.), and 相(phase)→柙 (N.M.).
5) Sequence reversal of characters composing a word: Examples are挫折 (frustration)→折挫 (N.M.), 皮包 (wallet) →包皮 (foreskin), 台北(Taipei) → and 北台(northern part of Taiwan).

6) Addition, omission or substitution of caligraphic units: In this category we gathered the following examples, e.g., 監 (inspect)→藍 (blue), 償 (compensate)→賞 (reward), 買 (buy)→賣 (sell), 肉 (meat)→內 (inside), 藍 (blue)→籃 (basket), 模 (model)→摸 (touch), 律→律(N.M.), etc..

7) Writing wrong character of same pronunciation: Examples are, 示 (indicate)→是 (yes), 忘 (forget)→望 (look up), 直 (straight)→只 (only), and 就 (at)→舊 (old).

3. Mistakes in reading

1) The most common mistakes made are wrong pronunciation of the 4 tones. For example 馬 (horse)→麻 (numb), 印→ (print) 因 (cause), and 採 (collect)→菜 (vegetable).

2) Pronouncing only a part of or a basic caligraphic unit of a character. Examples obtained are 便 (convenient)→更 (alter), 例 (example)→列 (itemize), 愁 (worry)→秋 (autumn), etc..

3) Pronouncing characters of similar caligraphy. The following examples were observed; 溝 (ditch)→講 (speech), 恕 (forgive)→怒 (anger), 完 (complete)→安 (easy), and 拖 (drug)→施 (give).

4) The term "Contextual error" is coined by the authors to indicate reading the wrong one of the more than one pronunciations of a character which should be read differently within specific context. The following sentence will be enough to illustrate such an error; 他在銀行 (bank) 工作，他每天走人行 道 (side walk) 上班，要在二十四行 紙 (24-line paper) 寫字，他的字很行 (good)，可以説是行家 (expert) 之一．

5) Reading erroneously one character of a word composed of two characters: Examples are 博覽 (exhibition)→博物 (general science), 獲勝 (to win)→勝利 (victory), 張燈 (to hang a lantern)→張貼 (to poster), and, 最後 (the last)→最終 (the very end.), etc..

6) Inability of identifying right one out of many characters of same pronunciation. One of our cases could not identify a character of his own name "銘" used in a sentence containing characters of same pronunciation like 明，鳴 and 名．

4. Neurological findings

Since this is a very preliminary study, the pre-, peri- and post-natal history of the cases were not obtained from the mother and the hospital. Taylor's Neurological Examination Sheet and scoring system were tried on each of the 23 cases and their controls. The average neurological scores for the reading disabled were 5.56±4.03 and 2.96±2.28 for the control, significantly higher for the former. Five out of the 23 reading disabled scored below 3 points, while 3 out of the 23 control children scored above 5 points. The tentative conclusion one makes out of the results of neurological examination, therefore, is as a group the reading disabled scored significantly higher on the Taylor's Neurological Examination designed for detecting soft-signs, but approximately 1/5 of the reading disabled children did not manifest more soft signs than the control group, while approximately 1/8 of the control children scored higher than the mean scores for the reading disabled children.

Summary

Some of the very preliminary clinical findings of reading disabled Chinese children as outlined above may well be explained by "inattentiveness", "carelessness", "lack of motivation" or "not trying hard enough". However, most of the clinical evidences such as typical mirror writing, partial mirror writing, pronouncing a part of the character, inability to differentiate the four tones, inability of identifying even one's own name out of characters with same pronunciation, etc., together with the significantly higher scores of positive soft neurological signs do indicate the possibility of brain dysfunction. Most of them also have their counterparts among the reading disabled American children. We would, therefore, intend to conclude that brain dysfunction should be considered as one of the major causes of reading disabilities accross cultures.

References

Guo Y.C.: A study of reading disabilities among the fifth graders in Tainan City. Collected Papers, Taiwan Provincial Health Administration, 1982.

Kline, C.L.: Development of dyslexia: An overview of transcultural factors. Paper presented at World Congress of Mental Health, Vancouber, B.C., August 1977.

Kuo, W.F.: A preliminary study of reading disability in the Republic of China. Collected papers, 1978, 20: 57-78, National Taiwan Normal University.

Makita, K.: The rarity of reading disability in Japanese children. American Journal of Orthopsychiatry, 1968, 38: 599-614.

Martin, S.E.: Learning to read: Why Taro finds it easy but Jonny finds it hard. Paper presented at the Second Japan-U.S. Joint Sociolinguistic Conference, Tokyo, August 1973.

Morrison, F.J. and Manis, F.R.: Cognitive processes and reading disability: a critique and proposal. In C.J. Brainerd and M. Pressley (Eds.), Advances in cognitive development. Vol.2, New York, Springer-Verlag, in press.

Rozin, P., Porits Ky, S., and Sotsky, R.: American children with reading problems can easily learn to read English represented in Chinese characters. Science, 1971, 171:1264-1267.

Rozin, P. and Gleitman, L.R.: The structure and acquisition of reading. In A.S. Reber and D. Scarborough (Eds.), Reading theory and practice. Hillsdale, N.J., Erlbaum, 1977.

Stevenson, H.W., Stigler, J.W., Lucker, G.W., Lee, S.Y. in cooperation with Hsu, C.C. and Kitamura, S.: Reading disabilities: The case of Chinese, Japanese and English. Child Development, 1982, 53, 1164-1181.

Taylor, E.: The neurological examination in children with disorders of behavior and learning. 1972, Unpublished manuscript.

THE SOCIAL-CLASS BACKGROUND OF MENTALLY RETARDED

CHILDEN: A STUDY IN MANNHEIM[*]

Brian Cooper and Birgitt Lackus

Zentralinstitut für Seelische Gesundheit
J 5, D-6800 Mannheim 1

INTRODUCTION

Reports of a number of surveys, mainly in the Eng-
lish-speaking countries, have indicated that mild and
severe grades of mental retardation differ in their social-class distributions within the general population.
While parents of mildly retarded children have been found
predominantly among the lower social classes, those of
severely retarded children are said to be proportionately
distributed over all social strata (Kushlick & Blunden,
1974).

The absence of a social-class gradient for severe
retardation has been interpreted as meaning that exposure
to the biological risk factors responsible for the primary
impairments of this group must occur independently of
socio-economic status. There have been, however, some
discrepant findings Bayley (1973), for example, reported
that 65 per cent of mildly and 47 per cent of severely
mentally retarded persons in Sheffield, U.K., belonged
to the lowest social-class category, compared with only
26 per cent of the city's population as a whole. Similarly, in a survey of mentally retarded children in Mannheim (Liepmann, 1979; Cooper et al., 1979), 76 per cent
of the families were categorized as working-class, compared with 52 per cent of the city's inhabitants and

---

[*]Abbreviated version of a paper published in Social
Psychiatry, Vol.19 (1984), No.1.

40 per cent of the West-German population as a whole.
Less expected was the finding that no fewer than 70
per cent of severely retarded children were drawn from
working-class families, so that in Mannheim, as in
Sheffield, the hypothesis of an even social-class distribution for this group of conditions could not be confirmed.

The present study can be seen as a replication of
the earlier Mannheim survey, making use of more accurate
and reliable research methods.

RESEARCH DESIGN AND METHOD

The survey sample consisted of all children of German nationality, born in the period 1962-1971, whose parents or guardians were resident in Mannheim on the census
day (1.10.78) and who because of mental handicap were
unable to attend either a normal school or a school for
'learning-handicapped' children.

Investigation of the children and their families included a standard medical examination of each child, administration of four sub-tests from a standardized test-
battery for the mentally retarded (Bondy et al., 1971),
assessment of the child's handicaps and behaviour by
means of the HBS schedule (Wing, 1981), and, finally,
assessment of family and social problems by means of a
semi-structured interview.

The medical data used in the present analysis consisted of a clinical diagnostic assessment and a weighted
score for the extent and severity of neurological impairment (NI-score). Following testing on criterion
groups of brain-damaged and normal children, an NI-score
below 20 was judged to mean no significant CNS abnormality, a score of 20-49 to mean mild or borderline impairment and a score of 50 or over to mean severe impairment.

The social-class distribution was analysed in terms
of occupational prestige and based in each instance on
the occupation of the father or chief family breadwinner
(Moore and Kleining, 1960).

THE SURVEY FINDINGS

1. Size and Representativity of the Sample

The number of children ascertained as mentally retarded was 242, corresponding to an age-specific administrative prevalence of 7.0 per 1,000. A group of 28 children, all of whom were severely or multiply handicapped, were excluded from further detailed investigation because they were in residential care at some distance from Mannheim. Of the remaining 214 children, consent was obtained from the parents or guardians to examine 208 (97.2%).

2. Social-Class Distribution of the Sample

A relative excess of mentally retarded children was again found in the lower social classes. The findings of the two Mannheim surveys, separated by a four-year interval, were insofar closely similar. The fall in administrative prevalence during the interval had not resulted in any change in class distribution.

Class-specific rates for mental retardation could not be calculated, since no population-based data on social-class distribution are available for Mannheim. The only information to hand comes from a classification of economically-active persons according to type of employment, which is not hierarchical but does enable the proportion of unskilled and semi-skilled workers to be estimated. This proportion was significantly higher among parents of the mentally retarded (74%) than among the inhabitants of Mannheim as a whole, indicating that the pronounced social-class skewing of the survey sample is a feature of families of the mentally retarded rather than simply of the local population.

3. Social Class and Type of Mental Retardation

Although the observed class gradient was steeper for families of the mildly retarded, it was also present among those of the severely retarded: indeed, no significant difference in this respect was found between the two groups.

Classification according to aetiology proved difficult, because of the incompleteness, and at times poor quality, of the anamnestic data and diagnostic information in the case records. Nevertheless, a systematic attempt was made to allocate a specific diagnosis whenever possible, and the distributions then compared for the two main social-class categories. The main difference appeared to be a relative excess, among the lower-class children, of cases of no known aetiology. When these were removed from the sample, the diagnostic distribution of the remainder was broadly similar across the social classes. Toxic and infective causes were recorded more frequently among the lower-class children and 'brain damage of unspecified cause' in the higher-status group; in view of the obvious difficulties of differential diagnosis, however, these differences are of doubtful significance.

The social-class distribution was next compared with that of the neurological impairment (NI) scores. The proportion of children with neurological deficits was lower in the working-class than in the higher social-class groups. Nevertheless, the absolute number of lower-class children with such deficits - 72 out of a total of 105 - was higher than that to be expected if the social-class distribution of neurological damage were in fact random. Thus, there appears to be an association between social class and the prevalence of neurobiological abnormalities, associated with severe mental retardation.

4. Economic and Living Conditions

The sample was next examined in relation to a number of other socio-economic indices, based on information derived from the family interviews. The social-class ratings were found to be to some extent predictive of the economic situation and living conditions of the families. Of the working class families, one-quarter were afflicted by chronic illness or disability; one-quarter had an unemployed or disabled head of household and one-third were rated as severely socially disadvantaged. Since the families in this group comprised three-quarters of the total sample, poor economic and living standards appear to be characteristic of the families of mentally retarded children in Mannheim.

No significant difference was found between the families of mildly and severely retarded children, with regard to parental levels of occupation and educational attainment. The two groups of families seem to be drawn from very similar social backgrounds. The families of the severely retarded enjoyed, however, rather better economic and living conditions than did those of the mildly retarded. It may be hypothesized that the frequency of severe mental retardation is raised among working-class families generally, because of a high birth prevalence; whereas the milder forms of retardation, which are in the main socio-culturally determined, tend to occur predominantly in those working-class families which are downwardly socially mobile, or which are burdened by an accumulation of social pathology.

5. Areas of Residence

Each family was given a rating based on the socio-economic status of its area of residence. For this purpose, the 78 statistical districts of Mannheim were divided into four groups, according to the proportion of unskilled workers among the economically-active residents. Ratios were calculated which could not be accepted as accurate prevalence estimates (the denominators used being based on the last population census, in 1970), but which do reflect relative frequencies of mental retardation among school-age children.

The spatial distribution was found to be very uneven and to vary with social characteristics of the neighbourhood. The frequencies both of mild and of severe forms of retardation were inversely related to the social status of the neighbourhood. While the trend is slightly more pronounced for the mildly retarded group, there is no significant difference between the distributions for mild and severe grades of retardation. Once again, therefore, the survey findings do not support the hypothesis that severe mental retardation is evenly distributed among the social classes.

6. Possible Sources of Bias

The findings of the present study are not in agreement with those of most research groups in other countries, who have examined the same question. This disagreement suggested that the Mannheim data might have been affected by some anomaly in the research method, or by some peculiarity of the local situation, which would reduce comparability with the other reported findings. Various possible sources of error or bias were therefore examined as systematically as possible. No single variable or combination of variables was identified, which could account for the observed social-class gradient in the prevalence of severe retardation. Mental retardation tended to be associated, as expected, with above-average family size and with a late position in the birth order; but these findings applied equally to severe and mild grades of retardation, and are in any case not peculiar to Mannheim.

CONCLUSION

It is not possible, on present evidence, to say whether or not the reported association between parental social class and the prevalence of mental retardation (both mild and severe forms) is due to an increased birth prevalence of these conditions in the lower social-class groups, and hence is linked with aetiology. Further investigation of this issue would seem justified, both nationally and with the help of international collaborative studies. Unfortunately, recent legislation on data confidentiality in West-Germany and in some other European countries now presents a major obstacle to further epidemiological research in this field and seems bound to slow down scientific progress.

Quite apart from any causal significance, the research findings have some implications for the care and education of the mentally retarded. The great majority of mentally handicapped children in Mannheim are to be found in those sections of the population which, in view of their economic situation, housing conditions and standard of education - to say nothing of the frequency among them of various forms of social pathology and deprivation - are least well-equipped to cope with the ensuing problems. There appears to be an urgent need to establish and to evaluate programmes of medico-social support for the families of mentally retarded children with special attention to those living in deprived urban areas.

Acknowledgments

This study formed part of a project, "Mentally retarded children in Mannheim", which was undertaken within Special Research Programme 116 (Psychiatric Epidemiology) of the University of Heidelberg, with financial support from the German Research Association (Deutsche Forschungsgemeinschaft).

References

Bayley, M.(1973): Mental Handicap and Commmunity Care. A study of mentally handicapped people in Sheffield. London, Routledge & Kegan Paul.

Bondy, C., R. Cohen, D. Eggert & G. Lüer (1971): Testbatterie für geistig behinderte Kinder (TBGB). Ingenkamp, K. (Hrsg.). Weinheim, Beltz.

Cooper, B., M.C. Liepmann, K.R. Marker & P.M. Schieber (1979): Definition of severe mental retardation in school-age children. Findings of an epidemiological study. Soc. Psych. 14, 197-205.

Kushlick, A. & R. Blunden (1974): The epidemiology of mental subnormality. In: Clarke, A.M. & A.D.B. Clarke (Hrsg.): Mental Deficiency - the Changing Outlook. 3rd Edition. London, Methuen.

Liepmann, M.C. (1979): Geistig behinderte Kinder und Jugendliche. Z. Kinder- und Jugendpsychiatrie, Beiheft 4. Bern, Huber.

Moore, H. & G. Kleining (1960): Das soziale Selbstbild der Gesellschaft in Deutschland. Köln. Z. Soziol. Sozialpsychol. 12, 86-119.

Wing, L. (1981): A schedule for deriving profiles of handicap in mentally retarded children. In: Cooper, B. (ed.): Assessing the Handicaps and Needs of Mentally Retarded Children. London, Academic Press.

THE IMMIGRANT CHILD IN THE SCHOOL

Joan Hart

Aldergrove Child and Family Clinic

3131 Lakeshore Blvd., West, Toronto, Ontario

Next to the family, the school is the major agent of socialization in the child's life. To the immigrant child and his family,
the school assumes even greater significance. For many children, it
represents the first institution encountered in a strange environment, one to which they must assimilate for many years. Secondly,
sucess within this institution is usually implicit within the family's
value system, as most immigrant parents cite educational opportunities as the major motivating factors in their decision to immigrate.

The stresses on the child are considerable - the need to acquire
a new language, differing expectations and customs and the inevitable dilemma of divided loyalties for his family, and his traditional heritage.

In his efforts to regain a feeling of self-worth the child is
confronted with pressures of varying degrees to conform to a new
way of living, behaving, dressing, that imply a displacement of his
original heritage. This is inconsistent with the goal of education
in a multi-cultural society, one in which the dignity of the individual is respected, with members engaged in a mutual learning process and in which the established culture is enriched with a new
diversity.

Canada has officially endorsed a policy of multi-culturalism
since 1971, (Berry et al 1977). Ethnic minorities are encouraged to
maintain their cultural diversity and at least in principle, the
melting pot philosophy is rejected.

Immigration patterns have significantly altered the character of
Toronto. Until 1945, the population of the city was primarily

white, British and Protestant. Today, the community is one of the most ethnic in Canada - one third of the population is non-British in origin (Hughes & Kallen, 1974). The impact was felt disproportionately in the suburbs, as one half of all immigrants to Canada from 1971 to 1976 (aged 5 and over) settled in these areas (Social Planning Council, 1979, V.I.).

The suburbs have been poorly prepared for such changes. Adaptation is difficult here due to the settlement pattern of highly dispersed, culturally diverse pockets of immigrants. Self help societies, extended family and kinship networks for informal support are lacking as compared to the more developed internal core of the city.

The Borough of Etobicoke has the lowest population of recent immigrants, but a high percentage of school-aged children, many with special learning and transitional needs. Population statistics from 1976 to 1981 illustrate the rapid growth here. Three ethnic groups have increased by close to or beyond 100%: Chinese, Portuguese, Indo-Pakistani. Due to recent Latin American immigrants, there has also been a large increase in Spanish-speaking citizens (Statistics Canada, 1981). Statistics are not available for West-Indian immigrants, but this group is thought to be the largest.

Population trends result in fewer households having a direct relationship with schools, as children of established residents mature. In 1976, 56% of families contained no child under 17, the highest such percentage in Metro (Social Planning Council, 1979, V.I.).

Consequently, there is limited political momentum to focus attention on problem areas.

The challenge to schools is considerable. Teachers require knowledge of different ethnic groups to avoid stereotyping, teachers must deal with their own feelings of prejudice, respond constructively to feelings students manifest, yet maintain standards of excellence, and strive to develop the full potential of each child.

The educational programmes provided by the Etobicoke Board of Education, to accomodate immigrant children will now be outlined:

1. T.E.S.L. (Teaching English as a Second Language)

This is the most extensive, frequent type of programme provided by school boards in the Metro area.

The programme is available at the elementary and high school level. Classes are self-contained with average duration of enrolment two to three years.

The sucess of this programme depends greatly upon appropriate integration into regular stream classes. However, declining enrolment in this Board has virtually eliminated this possibility at the elementary level. Smaller schools, with larger classes mean teachers are less willing to accept additional students.

2. Transition

This programme was initiated in 1975 in response to large scale immigration from the West Indies. Although a common language, familiarity with an English school system better prepares these children in comparison to those of non-English speaking backgrounds, significant discrepancies in childrens' educational history, numerous dialects, point to the need for transitional classes. Classes are on a half day basis, with integration the remainder of the day. Maximum length of stay is two years to avoid unnecessary isolation from mainstream education.

Children from other English speaking countries are also enrolled in large numbers: Phillipines, Africa, Guyana.

3. Community Liaison Workers

Elimination of independent immigration in 1980 resulted in a decline in black enrolment. The Board responded by cutting transition classes at the high school level and instead three Community Liaison positions were created. A fourth was added this year to deal with Indo-Chinese enrolment.

These workers, experienced teachers, were charged with the responsibility of dealing only with "visible minorities" (defined by skin colour). They outline their role as facilitating communication between the child and his family and the school, by interpretation of the school's expectations and assisting in the socialization process for the child. The workers are part of a Task Force on Multi-Culturalism, established in 1977, designed to promote mutual respect, tolerance and understanding.

An interesting project of this group is an annual multi-cultural camp week for students selected from different schools. The emphasis is on developing leadership skills rather than a direct focus on racial tensions.

How sucessful are these programmes in meeting the needs of the immigrant child? To determine this, interviews were conducted with teachers, principals, the community liaison workers, special education consultants, representatives of parent groups and community organizations. Observations from families in this Clinic's Day Treatment Programme (operated jointly with this School Board) are included.

In the absence of formal evaluation of these programmes, a summary of opinions and impressions will be presented.

Evaluation

Despite this Board's longstanding committment to multi-cultur-alism, the view was frequently expressed, particularly by the community workers, that in reality this is a token gesture. Committment to long term planning, and necessary evaluation of programmes is lacking. Efforts at intervention are "crisis oriented". Immigrant families are not informed of the workers' services upon en-rolment. Instead, children are referred by principals, guidance teachers, and due to their heavy work load, workers can only respond to situations already in crisis.

The mandate of the workers represents a puzzling contradiction. They are charged with the responsibility of promoting multi-cultural attitudes, yet they can only deal with "visible minorities". They can respond to needs for other children only if specifically repre-sented and are not encouraged to foster relationships with other ethnic community groups.

The Board decision not to keep statistics (a practice followed by only one other Board in the Toronto area), was widely interpreted as further evidence of administrative denial and intent to minimize problems. This practice also shields the Board from being account-able to ethnic groups whose population is increasing. For example, increase in Vietnamese immigration and national public support for this group led to the hiring of an additional community worker. Yet, no similar recognition has been awarded to swelling members of Spanish-speaking immigrants.

How does this tokenism contribute to pressures on the child? Inadequate focus on issues results in poor preparation by schools in welcoming children. One principal, upon the enrolment of a child from El Salvador, questioned "Where is that?" When minority group members increase, posing a threat to the existing equilibrium, feel-ings of prejudice intensify. Workers observe teachers react to increasing numbers, and when enrolment approaches 15-16% of the school population, begin to talk about "the problem". Complaints about students can take on ehtnic overtures "he just doesn't fit in", or "he's different". Hostility is expressed towards workers' intervention, with the view that undue attention is devoted to immi-grants. Teachers quiery, "when are you going to represent the maj-ority?"

Pressures to conformity are more intense when the student vio-lates behavioural expectations through aggression or threat of aggression. It should be emphasized this pattern does not occur exclusively with immigrant children. The diagnosis of "hyperactivity" has frequently been attached to children with a pattern of restless and aggressive behaviour, leading to enrolment in special education classes, with prescription of Ritalin strongly encouraged. Significantly, aggressive behaviour is the most frequent symptom of children referred to this Clinic by the schools.

Lack of assessment prior to enrolment results in the teacher assuming responsibility for detecting special language and learning needs. Teachers and principals must then use their own ingenuity to find access to overcrowded resources. A frequent comment was "I had to go to the top to get service for this child." Occasionally, community groups compensate by providing remedial tutoring. However, this is inadequate, as qualified teachers are not involved and the programme has limited credibility with parents.

There was virtually unanimous agreement amongst counsellors, teachers that more adequate services will not be provided until attitudes of resistence, denial and inadequate knowledge fostered by tokensim, are broken down.

This Board's tendency to respond to pressure groups perpetuates the low priority for immigrant needs. Apart from traditional parent-teacher associations, only one community organized parent group exists and it is poorly attended. Economic factors, cultural trad-itions (for West Indians particularly) of viewing education as the responsibility of the school make active parent involvement difficult. Teachers feel the Board is not aware of parents' dissatisfaction, particularly concerning limited opportunities for integration, and a misuse of vocational placements. In one elementary school with 40% black enrolment, parents resist vocational recommendation in at least 50% of cases. For parents who view this country as a land of new opportunity, this feeling is understandable. The vocational solution often reflects the school's failure to provide adequate early education, with the result that the student's poor motivation, underachievement means no alternative exists.

It is extremely important to bring parents into the educational process. The following recommendation of the Social Planning Council is strongly endorsed: "Linkage of parents means more than forming an association with the school, it means multi-lingual workers ...to work with existing ethno-cultural and family groups and develop parent orientation and education programmes." 1.

Increased numbers of community workers with a broader mandate are extremely important in fostering necessary attitudes of mutual respect and understanding.

1.   Social Planning Council of Metro Toronto, 1980, V.II, p. 199

REFERENCES

Berry, J., Kalin, R., Taylor, D.: Multi-culturalism and Ethnic
    Attitudes in Canada. Ottawa, Minister of State, for Multi-
    culturalism, 1976, 1977

Hughes, D., Kallen, E.: The Anatomy of Racism. Canadian Dimensions
    Harvest House, Montreal, 1974

Social Planning Council of Metro Toronto: Planning Agenda for the
    Eighties: Policy Report. Metro Suburbs in Transition, 1979,
    V.I; 1980, V.II

Statistics Canada: Selected Mother Tongue Groups in Metropolitan
    Toronto, 1981

SOCIOCULTURAL DETERMINANTS OF POSTNATAL DEPRESSION AND

POSTNATAL BLUES: HOW IMPORTANT ARE THEY?

John L. Cox

University Department of Psychiatry
Royal Edinburgh Hospital,
Edinburgh, EH10 5HF, Scotland

INTRODUCTION

In the 19th century Esquirol first observed that large numbers of women with "mild to moderate" puerperal psychiatric illness were cared for at home and "never recorded" and more recent prospective studies from Sweden (Nilsson and Almgren, 1970), Uganda (Cox, 1979a, 1983) and the United Kingdom (Pitt, 1968; Kumar and Robson, 1978; Cox et al., 1982) have confirmed this earlier observation and found that 10-15% of mothers are depressed following childbirth. The majority of such depressed mothers only rarely consult doctors and most do not receive adequate treatment.

Women in the United Kingdom who realised the importance of these findings have established self-help organisations such as the Association for Post-Natal Illness, whilst in Africa the puerperium is also known as a time when mental illness may occur. The trad-itional Ugandan puerperal illness "amakiro", for example, is well recognised, its most common symptom being the belief that a mother may wish to eat her baby and the cause is regarded as promiscuity during pregnancy (Roscoe, 1911; Cox, 1979b). Another traditional puerperal illness in Nigeria "Abisiwin" is not caused by faulty social relationships but by excessive "heat". Thus culture may determine not only the explanation for a puerperal mental illness but also in-fluence attitudes to a mother who is depressed at this time. In Western society, this latter predicament is poignantly illustrated by Welburn (1980) in the frontispiece to her book which shows a young mother with downcast eyes tightly holding her baby with above the quotation: "You have to go about with that big smile on your face and people saying "Aren't you lucky to have such a dear little baby" and you feel utter despair."

In the United Kingdom as well as other European countries professional interest in post-partum depression has increased substantially, and has also become linked to popular beliefs that the cause may be related to the changing role for women, the increase in medicalization of childbirth or having a hospital rather than a home delivery. Childbirth in Africa is therefore commonly regarded as being more harmonious, or "natural", than in a Western country, and postnatal depression thought less likely to occur.

The Scottish study of postnatal depression was completed in 1982 and had a similar design to the African research carried out earlier between 1972 and 1974; both studies were prospective and both used the Standardized Psychiatric Interview Schedule (SPI) of Goldberg et al. (1970). The women were followed from their first antenatal attendance to the postnatal interview about three months after delivery. The Scottish mothers (N = 103) were also interviewed during the third trimestre, and at one week after childbirth. An overall clinical assessment of psychiatric morbidity was made by the author and a total score obtained by summating the ratings of defined symptoms and observed abnormalities of the mental state. The postnatal interviewer was blind to information as to whether the mother had been depressed in pregnancy and strenuous attempts were made to ensure reliability, and in the African study the accuracy of the interpreter. A control group of non-pregnant, non-puerperal African women matched for age, marital status and parity was also interviewed. The antenatal interviews usually took place at the maternity clinic whilst the postnatal interviews were carried out at home. The obstetric and socio-cultural data were obtained from the obstetric case records.

RESULTS

38% of Scots and 19% of the Africans were primigravidae; almost all the Scottish subjects were married (96%) whilst only one half of the Africans were married with a bride price paid; one third of the Africans were co-wives. Of the Scots 15% worked outside the home whereas most of the Africans remained at home caring for children, cultivating the shamba (garden) and cooking for the family. Most of the Africans belonged to the Ganda tribe whilst almost all of the Scots were Caucasian and born in Britain.

Postnatal Depression

Of the 183 Africans who were interviewed during pregnancy and again in the puerperium 18 (10%) had a postnatal depressive illness and 11 of these 18 had a Depressive Psychosis; in 14 the depression had an onset after delivery.

The frequency of postnatal depression in the Scots was 13% and of these 13 depressed women 9 had become depressed after childbirth (Fig.1). There were in addition a further 16 women with depressive

148

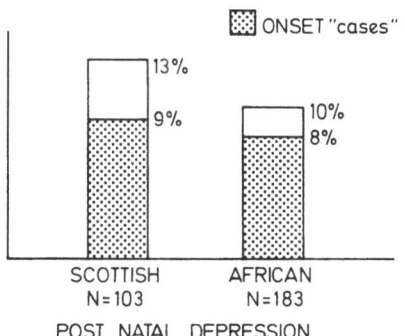

Figure 1

episodes which, though lasting more than four weeks in all but two, had improved by the time of the postnatal interview.

The depressed Africans were in general more impaired than the Scots, six could only dig or carry water on one of the preceding seven days, whilst none of the Scots had a Major Depressive Disorder and all fulfilled the Research Diagnostic Criteria for Minor Depressive Disorder (Spitzer et al., 1976) and had less severe work impairment.

Of the depressed Africans only two reported guilt or self-blame whereas 9 of the 13 depressed Scots were guilty at not managing their baby as well as they believed they should. Physical symptoms of depression were described more frequently by the Africans than by the Scots.

There was no association found in either study between postnatal depression and primiparity, an assisted delivery, and for the African mothers, a hospital rather than home delivery. Those Africans who were more educated, and therefore possibly more Westernised, were no more likely to become depressed than mothers with less education.

Antenatal Depression

As shown in Fig.2, depression during pregnancy was three times as likely to occur in the African than the Scottish subjects. Comparison with the African control group of non pregnant and non puerperal women showed that psychiatric symptoms, predominantly anxiety, were more likely to occur in childbearing women. In both Scottish and African samples, unmarried women were more likely than married women to report psychiatric symptoms during pregnancy.

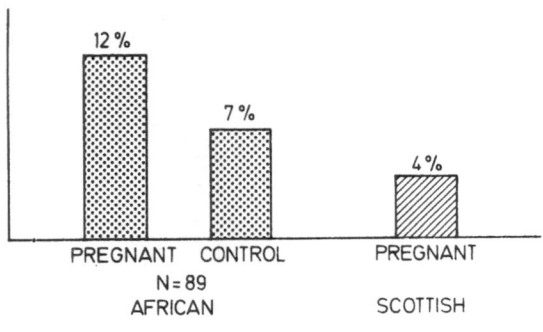

Figure 2

DISCUSSION

These results indicate that postnatal depression can readily be diagnosed in rural Africans, and was more severe than that found in the Scots. Although Field (1960) described depressed women after childbirth at a Ghanian healing shrine there are no other previous reports of postnatal depression in non-hospitalised Africans. Depressive illness in women admitted to a psychiatric unit had however been reported by Ebie (1972), Swift (1972), Collomb (1972) and Makanjuola (1982).

Our findings are somewhat similar to those of Orley and Wing (1979) who also found depression in rural Africans to be more severe than in London women. However these authors found more pathological guilt in the depressed Africans - 80% compared with only 10% in our study. The Scots readily talked about their difficulty coping with the baby and their guilt at not managing as well as they thought they should but only rarely did the Africans talk in this way. Although somatic symptoms of depression were spontaneously described by many of the depressed Africans a direct question whether or not the mother was sad usually enabled the mother to describe a low mood. Only rarely however was depression complained of spontaneously whereas the Scots more readily described this mood disturbance.

The frequency of antenatal depression in the African study was similar to the findings of Assael et al. (1972) in Uganda and also to that found in London by Kumar and Robson (1978); the finding of a much lower rate of antenatal depression in Edinburgh may be explained by differences in social and marital status between the Scottish, English and Ugandan subjects.

Thus although child-bearing in Africa confers high status, it is also a time of apprehension and anxiety; there was little "relaxed contentment" and indeed there is a sub-group of mothers who become depressed after delivery, and who also suffer considerably because of this illness. Our finding of similar rates of postnatal depression in two contrasting cultures might suggest that obstetric and socio-cultural variables are less important in the aetiology of puerperal depression than popular belief might expect and may therefore provide some indirect support for biological theories of causation.

It is therefore of interest that in the Scottish sample a quarter of women with severe postnatal blues went on to develop a depressive illness. It is also likely that postnatal blues (transitory emotionalism of the first post-partum week) are not directly caused by socio-cultural factors since the blues are known to occur in Tanzania (Harris, 1981), Jamaica (Davidson, 1972) and also amongst Japanese women (Morsbach et al., 1983) as well as in the U.S.A. (Yalom et al., 1968) and Britain (Pitt, 1973).

In Edinburgh, together with Professor R.E. Kendell and Dr. W. MacKenzie, we have recently completed a study comparing daily mood ratings for 10 days after elective Caesarian section with a control group of women who had a hysterectomy for non malignant conditions. Our preliminary findings show that depression and tears are more likely to occur on Day 5 in the Caesarian than in the control group. This finding therefore confirms earlier observations and studies are under way to determine whether hormonal changes can account for this 5th day peak of mood disturbance.

CONCLUSION

Our findings indicate that although socio-cultural factors may determine the symptom of depression and the choice of healer, the aetiology of this disorder is more likely to be linked to physiological factors, or possibly to longstanding personality characteristics.

It is likely that postnatal depression is not a "culture bound" disorder that is restricted to a Western country and it is unlikely to be caused by hospital confinement, initiated by a role conflict or provoked by a forceps delivery. The African and Scottish women were unlikely to seek help for their depression and despite the increased medical observation in the puerperium only rarely did such medical personnel recognise this disorder.

It is to be hoped that the implication of these findings for the training of medical and nursing staff in the psychological as well as the obstetric complications of the puerperium will be reconsidered. The recognition of post-partum mental illness is an important priority for Maternal and Child Health Services in any culture or country.

REFERENCES

Assael, M.I., Namboze, J.M., German, G.A. and Bennett, F.J., 1972, Psychiatric disturbances during pregnancy in a rural group of African women, Soc.Sci.Med., 6:387-395

Collomb, H., Avena, R. and Diop, B., 1972, Psychological and social factors in the pathology of childbearing, For.Psychiatry, 1:77-89

Cox, J.L., 1979a, Psychiatric morbidity and pregnancy: a controlled study of 263 semi-rural Ugandan women, Br.J.Psychiatry, 134:401-5

Cox, J.L., 1979b, Amakiro: a Ugandan puerperal psychosis? Soc. Psychiatry, 14:49-52

Cox, J.L., 1983, Postnatal depression: a comparison of African and Scottish women, Soc.Psychiatry, 18, 25-28

Cox, J.L., Connor, Y. and Kendell, R.E., 1982, Prospective study of the psychiatric disorders of childbirth, Br.J.Psychiatry, 140:111-7

Davidson, U.R.T., 1972, Postpartum mood changes in Jamaican women and discussion on its significance, Br.J.Psychiatry, 121:659-63

Ebie, J.C., 1972, Psychiatric illness in the puerperium among Nigerians, Trop.Geogr.Med., 24:253-6

Esquirol, E., 1845, "Mental maladies; a treatise on insanity". Translated by E.K. Hunt, Lea and Blanchard, Philadelphia

Field, M.J., 1960, "Search for security", Faber and Faber, London

Goldberg, D.P., Cooper, B., Eastwood, M.R. and Kedward, H.B., 1970, A standardised psychiatric interview for use in community surveys, Br.J.Prev.Soc.Med., 24:18

Harris, B., 1981, Maternity blues in East African Clinic attenders, Arch.Gen.Psychiatry, 38:1293-5

Kumar, R. and Robson, K., 1978, Neurotic disturbance during pregnancy and the puerperium, in: "Mental illness in pregnancy and the puerperium" M. Sandler, ed., Oxford University Press, London

Makanjuola, R.O.A., 1982, Psychotic disorders after childbirth in Nigerian women, Trop.Geogr.Med., 34:67-72

Morsbach, G., Sawaragi, I., Ridell, C. and Carswell, A., 1983, The recurrence of 'maternity blues' in Scottish and Japanese mothers, J.Repr.Infant Psychology, 1:29-35

Nilsson, A. and Almgren, P.E., 1970, Paranatal emotional adjustment. A prospective investigation of 165 women, Acta Psychiatr.Scand. Suppl. 220:65-141

Orley, J. and Wing, J.K., 1979, Psychiatric disorders in two African villages, Arch.Gen.Psychiatry, 36:513-20

Pitt, B., 1968, Atypical depression following childbirth, Br.J. Psychiatry, 114:1325-35

Pitt, B., 1973, Maternity Blues, Br.J.Psychiatry, 122:431-435

Roscoe, J., 1911, "The Baganda", Macmillan, London

Spitzer, R.L., Endicott, J. and Robins, E., 1978, Diagnostic criteria, in: "Biometrics Research", N.Y.State, Department of Mental Hygiene

Swift, C.R., 1972, Psychosis during the puerperium among Tanzanians. East Afr.Med.J., 49:651-7

Welburn, V., 1980, "Postnatal depression", Fontana Publications

Yalom, I., Lunde, D., Moos, R. and Hamburg, D., 1968, Postpartum blues syndrome, Arch.Gen.Psychiatry, 18:16-27

PUERPERAL PSYCHOSIS: DEFINITION AND FUTURE DIRECTIONS

Ian Brockington

The University of Birmingham
Birmingham B15 2TH

Definition is essential in science, and the study of puerperal psychosis has been hampered by the lack of a generally accepted definition. Many studies fail to distinguish between the rare psychosis of early onset, and simple 'postnatal depression' which is common during the months following childbirth. The concept of 'puerperal psychosis' originates from the observation that hitherto normal women suddenly become insane during the first few days after delivery. If we start with this fact, we can progressively tighten the definition, asking in sequence: (1) During what time period is there an excess of new episodes of psychosis ? (2) What sort of illnesses begin during this period ? (3) When do illnesses of this sort begin ? Onset is sometimes difficult to pinpoint, but the answer that is beginning to emerge is that onset is usually during the first week , and 2 weeks can probably be taken as the limit. The clinical picture includes mania, schizoaffective mania, schizophreniform psychosis and depression, but not hebephrenia or chronic paranoid schizophrenia.

Puerperal mania is in such clear contrast to normal behaviour that its definition presents few problems. In depressed patients, however, it is sometimes difficult to decide whether minor depressive or neurotic symptoms during pregnancy constitute the onset of the illness. Also any sample of puerperal depressed patients, defined purely by onset, is likely to be contaminated by patients with postnatal depression presenting unusually early, for example when the mother rejects the baby. The presence of obvious social stress could be used to exclude these patients. A systematic study of life events and difficulties in patients admitted to a mother and baby unit, compared with a community sample of recently delivered women, showed that puerperal psychosis

Table 1. Stress and puerperal psychosis
_____

Major events and difficulties were found in

21% of 80 community puerperal women
     (of whom 22 were depressed)

21% of 35 patients with puerperal psychosis

60% of 22 depressed community puerperal women

is not associated with social stress (Table 1, Martin, Brown &
Brockington, unpublished observations). It would be wise, therefore,
to exclude depressed patients with prominent psychosocial problems
such as unmarried motherhood or an unwanted baby.

I therefore propose that <u>puerperal mania</u> be defined by

1   clinical picture of mania (any subtype) or
     schizophreniform psychosis

2   onset within 2 weeks of delivery, ignoring
     depressive or neurotic symptoms during pregnancy.

<u>Puerperal depressive psychosis</u> should be defined by

1   clinical picture of depression

2   onset within 2 weeks of delivery, excluding patients
     with depressive or neurotic symptoms during pregnancy

3   absence of major stress or hostility to the baby.

(Patients not meeting this definition would be classed as
postnatal or prenatal depression).

These definitions are provisional, and it is hoped that a
clinical study of the symptoms of puerperal and postnatal
depression will provide discriminating clinical features, which
will improve the second definition. A preliminary analysis carried
out at Manchester in 1978 showed a large number of differences,
amounting to 22 of the 218 variables studied in 40 puerperal and
54 postnatal depressed women. Six variables showed differences
at the .01 level of statistical significance, and it appeared
that puerperal depressed patients had more confusion, while
postnatal depressed patients had more obsessional symptoms, sadness
and hostility.

The long debate about the nosological status of puerperal
psychosis continues. The frequency of manic symptoms suggests a
close relationship with manic depressive disease, but two studies
have shown differences between puerperal and non-puerperal mania.

Kadrmas et al (1980) found that puerperal patients had more first rank symptoms of Schneider, and Brockington et al (1982) found that they had more confusion and disorganised communication. The claim that puerperal psychosis is a specific entity rests mainly on this element of confusion, which has often been noted; but it has never been substantiated by psychological or neurophysiological testing. The time is ripe for a thorough evaluation of the relationship between puerperal psychosis and manic depression, comparing them across a wide range of clinical and biological parameters. The number and duration of episodes, the ratio of manic and depressive episodes, electroencephalographic parameters such as evoked responses, the reaction to endocrine challenge tests, and the output of catecholamine and serotonin metabolites are all of interest. The relationship to 'cycloid' psychosis also requires elucidation. There is the possibility that puerperal psychosis can be divided into a majority who have manic depression, and a minority who have a specific puerperal disease with marked lability and confusion, very rapid recovery and a family history of episodes limited to the puerperium. This requires testing by a combined clinical and genetic study.

Very little is known about the treatment of puerperal psychosis, except from unsystematic clinical experience. These patients appear to respond unusually well to electroconvulsive therapy. The role of tricyclic antidepressants of various kinds, and of lithium requires investigation, preferably in collaborative treatment trials. Some patients develop excessively severe extrapyramidal side-effects to neuroleptic drugs; if this impression is confirmed, it could provide a clue to the biological basis of the disease. It is also interesting that several patients have been reported to relapse, suddenly and dramatically, at the first menstrual period This reinforces the widespread belief that hormonal status has something to do with its aetiology, though there are few empirical studies of hormones in this disease.

Puerperal mental illness is the ideal psychosis to study by 'high risk' techniques, because we know within 2 weeks when the disease is going to begin, and who is at risk since women who have already suffered an attack of puerperal psychosis or mainic depression have a 1/5 risk of puerperal relapse. Eventually we will be able to study the psychosis during its development; but such cohort studies are expensive, and there is a need for preliminary case control studies, to develop some testable biological hypotheses.

References

Brockington I F, Winokur G, Dean C (1982)
Puerperal Psychosis.
Chapter in: Motherhood & Mental Illness. Academic Press, London

Kadrmas A, Winokur G, Crowe R (1980)
Postpartum mania. British Journal of Psychiatry 135,551-554

POSTNATAL DEPRESSION: AETIOLOGY AND CONSEQUENCES

R. Kumar

Institute of Psychiatry
De Crespigny Park
London   SE5 8AF

INTRODUCTION

Puerperal psychosis is a rare, but consistent, complication of childbirth; it occurs in one or two in every thousand mothers, beginning in the first few weeks following delivery (Cranville-Grossman, 1971; Paffenbarger, 1982; Brockington et al., 1982). During the past fifteen years, the importance of non-psychotic psychiatric disturbance, such as postnatal depression, has become increasingly apparent. Although neurotic disorders are more insidious in their onset and less severe in their immediate impact, in overall terms they are probably more important than puerperal psychotic breakdowns; one reason being that they occur about a hundred times more frequently. Several investigators (see review by Kumar 1982) have confirmed Pitt's (1968) original finding of an incidence rate of around 10%. In England, therefore, the expectation is that about 50,000 recently delivered women will experience clinically significant depressive reactions each year (the annual birth rate being a little over half a million); many will become depressed for the first time in their lives, some will remain prone to depression for a long time (Pitt, 1968; Kumar and Robson, 1984) and all will have passed through a phase in their lives that entails major adaptations of role and behaviour and of psychological adjustment. Depression in the mother may also have an undesirable impact on the infant as well as on the rest of her family.

Many important questions are still not fully answered and some have barely been addressed. Who is most at risk? What are the likely precipitants of postnatal depression? What are the long-term consequences of postnatal depression? What can be done to prevent or treat such disorders?

One obvious pointer is a personal or a family history of psychiatric disorder (Cox, 1983a) and investigations of twins may shed some further light on the question of constitutional predispositions (Stein - personal communication). Reliable biological markers would be invaluable in this setting particularly if they could identify potential "cases" in advance, i.e. during pregnancy. The dexamethasone suppression test (Carroll, 1982) is not likely to be of much use in non-endogenous depressions either as a trait or as a state marker. Sandler and his colleagues (Bonham, Carter et al., 1980) have reported preliminary findings which suggest that disturbances in the conjugation and excretion of tyramine may prove to be of predictive value and these findings require confirmation and elaboration. Dalton (1980) has argued that deficiences in progesterone may be responsible for postnatal depression but there is no evidence to underpin this hypothesis other than anecdotal data about therapeutic responses. Nott et al. (1976) were unable to relate mood changes with variations in circulating sex hormone levels and, in a different but relevant clinical context, Brockington (see Brockington et al., 1982) was not able to influence the course of post-partum psychotic depressions with a progestogen. Other intriguing questions concern the possible links between hormonal influences on mood in the menstrual cycle (Clare, 1983) and postnatal depression, or links between the immediate postnatal changes in the blues and subsequent persisting and severe dysphoria (e.g. Kendell et al., 1981; Stein, 1982).

Studies of personality traits such as neuroticism in child-bearing women (Eysenck and Eysenck, 1975) are of doubtful validity either because of the ways in which subjects selected themselves (Meares et al. (1976), or because measurements were made at a time when the women were depressed (Pitt, 1968). In a recent survey (Kumar and Robson, 1984) which attempted to avoid some of these pitfalls, such measures were not found to be predictive of postnatal depression. In conclusion, the question of biological or constitutional predictors of postnatal depression remains wide open for further investigation.

Early environmental experience and relationships with parents

Early childhood experiences may critically influence the ways in which adults react and respond to events. Becoming a mother, especially for the first time, is a process that is never really complete and which involves complex and shifting identifications. The pregnant woman must at one and the same time begin to negotiate changes in the separateness of her own

identity vis a vis her parents as well as in her relationship with
the child she is carrying. The work of Frommer and O'Shea (1973)
and Brown and Harris (1978) provides some empirical support for the
insights that have been derived from individual cases about the
long-term sequelae of disturbed parent-child relationships.
Emotional reactions following childbirth may therefore be
especially sensitive indicators of disturbances in the mother's
own relationships with her parents. Cox et al. (1982) found that
childbearing women whose own mothers were dead were more frequently
emotionally distressed in the first week after delivery; they did
not, however, remain depressed. Kumar and Robson (1984) found
that postnatal depression was found more often in women who had
lost, or had had prolonged separations from their fathers in early
childhood, and also in women who described recent difficulties in
their relationship with their mothers. Such studies do therefore
indicate that enquiries about early childhood and parental
relationships can be of help in picking out women "at risk" for
postnatal depression. These inferences are based upon associations
and do not, of course, imply unitary relationships. Paykel et al.
(1980), for example, were not able to find any links between
postnatal depression and childhood separation from the subjects'
own mothers.

Concurrent predisposing factors

The lack of a supportive relationship with the spouse has
been given prominence as an aetiological agent for depression in
the model of Brown and Harris (1978) although it is sometimes
difficult to separate cause from effect in such research. For
example Cox et al. (1982) have shown that postnatal depression is
associated with a deteriorating relationship with the spouse.
Kumar and Robson (1984) were, however, able to implicate marital
disharmony as an aetiological factor in postnatal depression. The
extent of marital conflict was assessed in early pregnancy, that
is before the likely onset of postnatal depression.

Social adversity is commonly correlated with the occurrence
of depression, particularly in interaction with stressful events.
However, studies of postnatal depression have almost uniformly
shown that middle and upper class women are as prone to become
depressed as are working class mothers (see review by Kumar 1982).
Such observations suggest that it may be an oversimplification to
regard the birth of a child as an aetiological factor in postnatal depression simply as something adding to the "disappointment
and hopelessness of her position" (Brown and Harris, 1978).

Stressful life events and depression after childbirth

Paykel et al. (1980), Playfair and Gowers (1981) and Dean
and Kendell (1981) have all pointed to some association between

the occurrence of stressful events and postnatal depression, thus supporting the hypothesis put forward by Brown and Harris (1978). In the prospective survey by Kumar and Robson (1984) life events (undesirable and others) were recorded by interview in each trimester of pregnancy as well as three months after delivery. Two individual associations between events and depression were found: firstly between bereavement and depression in pregnancy, but not postnatally, and the second association was between preterm birth and postnatal depression. There was no support for the view that women who became depressed following delivery were likely to have experienced a greater number of stressful events in the preceeding months. Interactions with "vulnerability" factors such as marital conflict or working class status were tested by means of log-linear analyses and were also not found. This kind of prospective research model provides a more rigorous test for socially based theories of depression than do retrospective enquiries (see Henderson, 1981). More prospective studies are needed and with an emphasis on events that may have special relevance to childbearing women (see Barnett et al., 1983).

Postnatal depression - pregnancy and obstetric variables

Kumar and Robson (1984) found that conflict about the pregnancy, manifested by thoughts about obtaining a termination was significantly associated with subsequent postnatal depression. Neither Cox et al. (1982) nor Kumar and Robson (1984) were able to confirm earlier reports of an association between the presence of anxiety during pregnancy and the development of depression after childbirth (see Kumar 1982).

Obstetric complications have occasionally been implicated in severe postpartum mental illness (Paffenbarger, 1982; Kendell et al., 1981b) and while the contribution of such variables to post-natal depression may be critically important in individual cases there are no consistent general associations e.g. there are reports both for and against links with previous miscarriage (Blair et al., 1970; Playfair and Gowers, 1981) or with concurrent obstetric complications (Tod, 1984; Pitt, 1968; Paykel et al., 1980; Cox et al., 1982; Kumar and Robson, 1984). Obstetric practice may also exert unexpected influences on the ways mothers initially react emotionally to their babies (Robson and Kumar, 1980).

CONSEQUENCES OF POSTNATAL DEPRESSION

Effects on relationships

Cox et al. (1982) found that depressed mothers described a deteriorating relationship with their husbands and Kumar and Robson (1984) reported substantial levels of marital disharmony on more prolonged follow-up. These data must however be interpreted with caution because of the lack of controls. Both groups of investigators found that the sexual relationship was impaired to a greater extent where mothers were depressed. Kumar and Robson (1984) further reported that depressed mothers were more likely to describe feelings of detachment or dislike for their babies. There was, however, no increase in physical acts of aggression in this sample.

Long-term consequences

Pitt (1968) reported that in a proportion of women, depressions that began after childbirth persisted for at least a year. In the longitudinal survey by Kumar and Robson (1984), 50% of the "cases" at 3 months postnatally were still depressed by 6 months but none were rated as cases by the time the babies were a year old. It was clear, however, that the occurrence of depression either in pregnancy or after delivery, was the start for many women of prolonged emotional difficulties as evidenced by consultations with family doctors or specialists for such problems.

Postnatal depression and effects on the child

There have, so far, been two systematic investigations, following up the children of mothers who became depressed soon after delivery; these women and their children were compared with the mothers who remained well (see Cox et al., 1982; Kumar and Robson, 1984). Data from the children (as yet unpublished) have been described by Wrate et al. (1983) and by Caplan et al. (1983); both studies point to associations between maternal emotional disturbance after delivery and later psychological and/ or behavioural problems in the children. These are potentially very important findings.

CONCLUDING COMMENTS

There seems little doubt that postnatal depression is a serious health problem with important implications for the mother, her partner and possibly for the baby. Most investigations have emanated from the U.K. and apart from the pioneering work of Cox (1979; 1983b) in Ugandan women, there is very little in the way of systematic information about the incidence, manifestations and correlates of postnatal depression in cultures with different family and social structures. Any future work should aim to include data from fathers and also to combine psycho-social with biological enquiry. The time is also ripe to begin research into ways of preventing and treating postnatal depression.

REFERENCES

Barnett, C.E.W., Hanna, B. and Parker, G., 1983, Life event scales for obstetric groups, J. Psychosom. Res., 27:313-320.

Blair, R.A., Gilmore, J.S., Playfair, H.R., Tisdall, M.W. and O'Shea, C., 1970, Puerperal depression: a study of predictive factors, J. Roy. Coll. Gen. Pract., 19:22-25.

Bonham Carter, S.M., Reveley, M.A., Sandler, M. et al., 1980, Decreased urinary output of conjugated tyramine is associated with lifetime vulnerability to depressive illness.

Brockington, I.F., Winokur, G. and Dean, C., 1982, Puerperal psychosis, in: Motherhood and Mental Illness, I.F. Brockington and R. Kumar, eds., Academic Press, London. pp. 37-69.

Brown, G. and Harris, T., 1978, Social Origins of Depression, Tavistock, London.

Caplan, H., Cogill, S., Alexandra, H., Robson, K.M. and Kumar, R., 1983, Impact of maternal depression on the cognitive and emotional development of the young child. Abstracts of VII World Congress of Psychiatry - Vienna, p. 136.

Carroll, B.J., 1982, The dexamethasone suppression test for melancholia, Brit. J. Psychiat., 140:292-304.

Clare, A.W., 1983, Psychiatric and social aspects of premenstrual complaint. Psychol. Med. Monogr. Suppl. No. 4.

Cox, J.L., 1979, Psychiatric morbidity and pregnancy: a controlled study of 263 semi-rural Ugandan women, Br. J. Psychiat., 134:401-405.

Cox, J.L., 1983a, Postnatal depression, Hospital Update 9:1271-1275.

Cox, J.L., 1983b, Socio-cultural aspects of postnatal depression and postnatal 'blues'. Abstracts of VII World Congress of Psychiatry - Vienna, p. 136.

Cox, J.L., Connor, Y. and Kendell, R.E., 1982, Prospective study of the psychiatric disorders of childbirth. Brit. J. Psychiat., 140:111-117.

Dalton, K., 1980, Depression after Childbirth, Oxford University Press, Oxford.

Eysenck, H. and Eysenck, S.G.B., 1975, Manual of the eysenck Personality Questionnaire, Hodder and Stoughton, London.

Frommer, E.A. and O'Shea, G., 1973, Antenatal identification of women liable to have problems in managing their infants, Brit. J. Psychiat., 123:149-156.

Henderson, S., 1981, Social relationships, adversity and neurosis: an analysis of prospective observations, Brit. J. Psychiat., 138:391-398.

Granville-Grossman, K., 1971, Psychiatric aspects of pregnancy and the puerperium, in: Recent advances in clinical psychiatry, K. Granville-Grossman, ed., Churchill, London. pp. 266-310.

Kendell, R.E., McGuire, R.J., Connor, Y. and Cox, J.L., 1981, Mood changes in the first three weeks after childbirth. J. Affective Disorders 3:317-326.

Kendell, R.E., Rennie, D., Clarke, J.A. and Dean, C., 1981, The social and obstetric correlates of psychiatric admission in the puerperium., Psychol. Med., 11:341-350.

Kumar, R., 1982, Neurotic disorders in childbearing women, in: Motherhood and Mental Illness, I.F. Brockington and R. Kumar ed., Academic Press, London. pp. 71-118.

Kumar, R. and Robson, K.M., 1984, A prospective study of emotional disorders in childbearing women, Brit. J. Psychiat., (in press).

Nott, P., Franklin, M., Armitage, C. and Gelder, M.G., 1976, Hormonal changes and mood in the puerperium, Brit. J. Psychiat., 128:379-383.

Paffenbarger, R.S., 1982, Epidemiological aspects of mental illness associated with childbearing, in: Motherhood and Mental Illness, I.F. Brockington and R. Kumar, eds., Academic Press, London.

Paykel, E.S., Emms, E.M., Fletcher, J. and Rassaby, E.S., 1980, Life events and social support in puerperal depression, Brit. J. Psychiat., 136:339-346.

Pitt, B., 1968, Atypical depression following childbirth, Brit. J. Psychiat., 114:1325-1335.

Playfair, H.R. and Gowers, J.I., 1981, Depression following childbirth - a search for predictive signs, J. Roy. Coll. Gen. Practitioners 31:201-208.

Robson, K.M. and Kumar, R., 1980, Delayed onset of maternal affection after childbirth, Brit. J. Psychiat., 136:347-353.

Stein, G., 1982, The maternity blues, in: Motherhood and Mental Illness, I.F. Brockington and R. Kumar, eds., Academic Press, London. pp. 119-154.

Tod, E.D.M., 1964, Puerperal depression, a prospective epidemiological study, Lancet ii:1264-1266.

Wrate, R.M., Rooney, A., Thomas, P., Cox, J.L., 1983, Postnatal depression and later child behaviour. Abstracts of VII World Congress of Psychiatry - Vienna, p. 136.

POST-NATAL DEPRESSION AND SUBSEQUENT CHILD DEVELOPMENT:

A THREE YEAR FOLLOW-UP STUDY

R.M. Wrate, A.C. Rooney, P.F. Thomas and J.L. Cox

University Department of Psychiatry
(Royal Edinburgh Hospital), Morningside Park
Edinburgh   EH10 5HF

The study reported in this paper was established to explore the possibility that three year old children of mothers who suffered from post-natal depression following their birth may demonstrate increased rates of behavioural difficulty. Hitherto, the relationship between childhood disturbance & maternal depression is well established only for current depression (Weissman et al., 1972; Richman, Stevenson & Graham, 1982).

A prospective study in Sweden on sixty-nine women by Uddenberg & Englesson (1978), found an association between post-natal depression and the subsequent behaviour of the children four and a half years later. These authors did not, however, employ measures of proven reliability, nor were sufficient details available of the psychiatric diagnosis; the loss of 28% of cases in the follow-up period was a further disadvantage.

The follow-up study described in this paper is a continuation of the prospective study of 103 childbearing women in Edinburgh carried out by John Cox & his colleagues (Cox et al., 1982). In the original study many mothers suffered the "blues," but none developed a functional psychoses. On the other hand, 13% of mothers were found to have a depressive illness (fulfilling Spitzer, Endicott, & Robins' Research Diagnostic Criteria for Major or Minor Depressive Disorder) that lasted until the fifth month post partum. A second group of 16% were found to have depressive symptoms which lasted more than four weeks but were not present four months after delivery. Post-natal depression was not found to be associated with age, parity, or social class.

METHOD

Only twelve of the original 103 could not be interviewed again
three years later. Two refused, eight had moved abroad, and no
information at all was available about a further two. Almost all
interviews were conducted by A.R., who had not known any of the
women previously, nor which had previously suffered a post-natal
depression.

Behaviour disturbance of the child was assessed by questioning the mother using the well tested Behavioural Screening
Questionnaire of Richman & Graham - the BSQ - (1971), which
includes ratings of appetite & sleep disturbance, encopresis,
enuresis, mood, temper control, over-activity, dependency, non-
specific anxiety & specific phobias. The questionnaire does not
include direct observation of the child, nor is the phantasy life
of the child examined. Additional items were added to the interview
concerning general health of the child, the number of secure care-
givers, as well as opportunities to mix with local children and of
nursery school or playgroup attendance.

The mother's current mental state was then assessed using
Goldberg's semi-structured interview (1970). Following this, the
mothers' own account was obtained of whether she remembered any
depressive symptoms in the puerperium, and of the frequency and
duration of any other depressive episodes since (the severity of
any symptoms were rated using items from the SPI). Blindness was
only broken after these ratings were made, to determine the duration
of puerperal depression, as well as the use made of medical services
and to rate any family difficulties.

Obstetric & Paediatric case records were obtained for all but
two of the 91 mothers and their child, and a Post-natal Complications
Score (Littman & Parmelee, 1978) derived to assess the severity of
any health complications in the infant's first week of life. In
addition, the mothers also completed the Behavioural Checklist, BCL,
(Richman et al., 1982), as well as the Eysenck Personality Inventory.

RESULTS

All but three of the 30 women who had been depressed in the puerperium were successfully re-interviewed; two of the 13 women with
depressive illness could not be traced and one mother with depressive symptoms could not be interviewed. Those women whose depressive episodes had occurred since the puerperium are referred to as
having depressive episodes, whilst a further group consisted of
those women who had not been depressed at any time since delivery.
Three women were found on follow-up to have depressive symptoms, but
only one was considered clinically depressed; two women had personality disorders and one woman was recovering from a longstanding
hysterical paresis. Only the last had a disturbed child.

166

Table 1.   Mean BSQ Scores & Post-natal Depression

Sample:	Not Depressed	Later Depressive Episodes	Post-natal Depressive Illness	Post-natal Depressive Symptoms
	n = 48	n = 15	n = 11	n = 16
BSQ $\bar{x}$ Score =	4.6	4.3	4.6	7.3

$$F = 3.08, \text{d.f.} = 4, p = < 0.02$$

It should be noted that the blind code was not effective in a substantial number of those who had previously suffered a depressive illness, but was effective for all but one of the 16 who had suffered depressive symptoms in their puerperium.

Table 1 shows that the children's BSQ score was significantly higher only for those children of women who previously had post-natal depressive symptoms. For each subscale of the BSQ children of the depressive symptoms group had slightly higher mean scores, which was significant only for temper tantrums. It was clear also that the increase in BSQ total score was not caused by a few highly abnormal children.

Nevertheless, the overall behaviour disturbance in the total sample of children was not marked, and in only five (6%) was the BSQ total score above Richman's cut-off point for disturbance (the comparable figure for a much larger sample of less stable families in London was found by Richman & her colleagues to be 14.3%).

Similar differences to that found with the BSQ were evident for the BCL, although the differences did not reach statistical significance. Finally, as a low total symptom score would not betray a circumscribed but handicapping disorder, the BSQ interview protocols were also reviewed by R.W. using clinical criteria, but no significant difference was found between children whose mothers had been more severely depressed and those without any post-natal depression. Thus, our first hypothesis that women with more prolonged post-natal depressive illness were more likely to have behaviourally disturbed children at three years was not supported by our findings. The association found between less persistent forms of post-natal depression and later child behaviour disturbance on the other hand was quite unexpected.

Comparisons of women in the depressive illness & symptoms groups were, therefore, carried out (see Table 2). In addition to the differences demonstrated, mothers with depressive symptoms were also more likely to discontinue breast feeding. The women with a depressive illness on the other hand were much more preoccupied with their difficult marital relationship than worried about their child. These women who had had a post-natal depressive illness also had significantly higher neuroticism scores (mean score of 15.6), and had significantly higher SPI total scores at the three year follow-up (F = 5.65, d.f. = 4, p = < 0.001).

Table 2.   Differences Between Depressive "Illness" and
           Depressive "Symptoms" Mothers.

a)   Commoner in depressive symptoms group:

    Long childhood separation from mother $p < 0.01$
    Post-natal depressive preoccupation
    with new baby/maternal role $p < 0.01$

b)   Commoner in depressive illness group:

    Considered termination $p = 0.07$
    Marital relationship less often
    improved by pregnancy $p < 0.001$

  Marital relationship at 3 - 5 months post partum:

    Deteriorated $p < 0.001$
    Sexual dissatisfaction $p < 0.001$
    Sexual deterioration $p < 0.01$

  Maternal neuroticism $p < 0.05$

Examining the Secure Caregiving Scale, no significant differences were found between the two groups of post-natal depression; the total score was found to be significantly associated with current maternal mood (Spearman rank correlation, $r = 0.22$, $p < 0.02$), but not with maternal neuroticism nor with child behaviour at three years old.

The additive effect between puerperal depression and other variables is shown in Table 3. A first born child, post-natal complications, and maternal neuroticism all increased the mean BSQ total score in women who were also depressed, but this was only significant for post-natal depression and having a first child.

Table 3.   Post-natal Depression & Primiparity:
           Symptoms & Illness: n = 27
                                    BSQ

Ordinal Position	Mean	s.d.	n
Not depressed/Not a first child	4.16	2.66	31
Not depressed/First child	4.88	2.79	33
Depressed/Not a first child	5.09	3.33	11
Depressed/First child	6.88	2.50	16

$F = 3.42$, d.f. $= 3$, $p < 0.02$

The total score on the BSQ was not associated with maternal personality, as measured by the EPI, but as others have found (Richman, 1975), was significantly associated with current maternal mood, as measured by the SPI (Spearman rank correlation - $r = 0.23$, $p < 0.02$). Child behaviour was poorly predicted by an increased post-natal complications score & low birth weight.

DISCUSSION

Our findings were unexpected and did not confirm our original hypothesis. Instead an association was found between less prolonged post-natal depression and the subsequent behaviour of the child. In view of the additional differences found between these two groups of women, it seems likely that post-natal depression is not in fact a homogeneous clinical entity, and the failure of other studies to distinguish between different types of post-natal depressed women may prevent important associations emerging. Thus in Kumar & Robson's study (1980), where depressed women were examined as a homogeneous group, no association was found between depression and a mother's ambivalent attitude towards her baby.

Examination of the characteristics of the two groups of women with post-natal depression suggests that women in the present study with less prolonged post-natal depressive symptoms were much more anxiously preoccupied with their baby, which was more often their first, and much more frequently discontinued breast feeding. Although Winnicott (1965) & Kohut (1971), argue that maternal responsiveness in infancy is extremely important for healthy emotional development, if a depressed mood in the puerperium did have some general effect on mother-baby interaction it was clearly not enduring, except perhaps where in the depressive symptoms group the focus of the depressive preoccupation lay with the child itself and the mother's own maternal role identification. It is possible that such an episode may then disrupt the relationship a mother establishes with her infant, in much the same way that a period of separation in the infancy of monkeys may disrupt the mother-infant relationship (Hinde, 1977; Hinde & McGinnes, 1977). The alternative hypothesis of some general disturbance in the personality of these mothers contributing to their child's difficulties seems unlikely, as these women do not have neurotic personalities, nor was there evidence of a general disturbance in their other relationships. The significant increase in temper tantrums may indicate that some of the infants sense a need to control their previously depressed mother, still regarded as omnipotently withholding.

However, as these findings are derived from the study of a small sample and no direct observation of these mothers and their infants was carried out, until the work is replicated interpretation of the present findings must be made with considerable caution.

REFERENCES

Cox, J.L., Connor, Y., Kendell, R.E., (1982), Prospective Study of the Psychiatric Disorder of Childbirth, British Journal of Psychiatry, 140, 112 - 118.

·Goldberg, D.P., Cooper, B., Eastwood, M.R., Kedward, H.B., Shephard, M., (1970), A Standardised Psychiatric Interview for use in Community Surveys, British Journal of Preventive & Social Medicine, 24, 18 - 23.

·Hinde, R.A., (1977), Mother-Infant Separation and the Nature of Inter-Individual Relationships: Experiments with Rhesus Monkeys, Proceedings of the Royal Society, London, 196, 29 - 50.

·Hinde, R.A., & McGinnes, L., (1977), Some Factors Influencing the Effects of Temporary Mother-Infant Separation: Some Experiments with Rhesus Monkeys, Psychological Medicine, 7, 197 - 212.

Kohut, H., (1971), The Analysis of the Self, Monograph number 4, The Psychoanalytic Study of the Child, International University Press, New York.

·Kumar, R., & Robson, K., (1978), Neurotic Disturbances During Pregnancy and the Puerperium: Preliminary Report of a Prospective Study of 119 Primigravidae, in "Mental Illness in Pregnancy and the Puerperium," M. Sandler (Ed.) Oxford University Press, 40 - 51.

Littman, B., & Parmelee, A.H., (1978), Medical Correlates of Infant Development, Paediatrics, 61, 470 - 474.

·Richman, N., & Graham, P.J., (1971), A Behavioural Screening Questionnaire for use with Three Year Old Children: Preliminary Findings, Journal of Child Psychology & Psychiatry, 12, 5 - 33.

·Richman, N., Stevenson, J.E., Graham, P.J., (1975), Prevalence of Behavioural Problems in Three Year Old Children: An Epidemiological study in a London Borough, Journal of Child Psychiatry & Psychology, 17, 75 - 78.

·Richman, N., (1977), Behavioural Problems in Pre-School Children: Family & Social Factors, British Journal of Psychiatry, 131, 523 - 527.

·Richman, N., Stevenson, J., Graham, P.J., (1982), Pre-School to School, Academic Press, London.

Uddenberg, N., & Englesson, I., (1978), Prognosis of Post-Partum Mental Disturbance - A Prospective Study of Primiparous Women and their Four and a half Year Old Children, Acta Psychiatrica Scandinavia, 1958, 201 - 212.

·Weissman, M.M., Paykel, E.S., Klerman, G.L., (1972), The Depressed Woman as Mother, Social Psychiatry, 7, 98 - 108.

Winnicott, D.W., (1965), The Role of Maternal Care in "The Maturational Process & the Facilitating Environment," International Psychoanalytic Library, Hogarth Press, London.

ACKNOWLEDGEMENTS

This work was supported by a grant from the Scottish Section of the Mental Health Foundation.

MATERNAL MENTAL ILLNESS AND

MOTHER-CHILD BONDING DISORDERS

Frank Margison

Manchester Royal Infirmary
Gaskell House
Manchester 13, U.K.

Specialised psychiatric units for mothers with their babies have
been developed in several countries since the 1950's. One such unit
is a 9 bedded ward at the University Hospital of South Manchester
within the Department of Psychiatry. This unit serves the population
of the North West Region of England admitting mothers with severe
psychiatric illnesses with their babies. The unit has been in existence for about a decade and has been the site of a number of clinical
research studies.

This study describes the effects of severe psychiatric morbidity
on the developing mother-child relationship. The most dramatic
adverse effects are described by a summary of the findings about the
mother-child relationship as measured by affectionate behaviour,
practical competence and recordings of statements made by the mothers
about their babies.

Violent Behaviour Towards the Babies

There has rightly been concern to avoid violence or even infanticide in the setting of puerperal psychotic illnesses and severe
post-natal depressive neurosis. Psychoanalytic studies have
frequently assumed an aetiological relationship between post partum
psychiatric illness and hostility towards the baby. In this study we
will give an account of the violence occurring within a specialised
unit where very close observation of the mother and baby can take
place.

A descriptive account of each episode was recorded based on
extensive case notes and observational material on 245 consecutive

admissions between 1974 and 1979 (Margison 1981). In addition a number of episodes for each mother and an estimate of severity was made based on the likely <u>risk</u> to the child as follows:

TABLE 1 Risk Category for Violence to Baby

Nil	No attack occurred
Minimal injury likely	Trivial slapping, rough handling of baby with no evidence of injury
Moderate injury likely	Throwing baby onto bed violently, shaking or slapping baby violently. Attempting to smother baby when nurse present
Severe injury likely	Smothering baby away from nurses, throwing baby to floor or wall, assault leading to visible injury any use of a weapon or sexual assault, scalding, poisoning or burning.

The mothers were also diagnosed for the purposes of this and the following studies into 3 main mutually exclusive groups.

<u>Non Psychotic Depression</u>   i) Excluded if hallucinations or delusions present.
  ii) Fulfils Research Diagnostic Criteria for Major Depressive Disorder.

<u>Puerperal Psychosis</u>   i) Onset less than four weeks post partum.
  ii) Presence of delusions and/or hallucinations.
  iii) Excluding mothers with previous psychotic illness.

<u>Other</u>   Includes all other psychiatric illness.

TABLE 2 Risk of Violence in Most Serious Episode

<u>Risk Category</u>	<u>N</u>	%
Nil	224	(92)
Minimal	10	(4)
Moderate	8	(3)
Severe	3	(1)

The episodes of violence were infrequent. Of the mothers who were violent, 8 were violent on 2 occasions, 1 on 4 occasions and 1 on 6 occasions; a total of 37 episodes in 5 years of which nearly half were of minimal risk to the baby.

Analysing the degree of risk by the number of episodes, 8 of 11 single episodes were of minimal risk whereas only 2 of the 10 multiple episodes were of minimal risk. (p<0.05). Mothers with puerperal psychosis were significantly less likely to be violent than mothers with other diagnoses, (only 3 of 93 mothers with puerperal psychosis compared to 18 of 134 for other diagnoses, ($X^2 = 4.42$, d.f = 1, p<0.05).

This very low level of violence however needs to be seen in the context of the nursing care offered on the unit (Margison 1981).

TABLE 3 Nursing Care Required for Baby

Level of Care Required	N	%
Required no or minimal support	36	(15)
Considerable nursing help required	66	(27)
Extremely close supervision required	77	(31)
Extremely close supervision plus need to separate from baby	66	(27)

It can be seen that many of the mothers required very close observation for at least part of their stay on the unit. In view of this, more information is needed on the nature of the mother-baby relationship abnormalities.

The Mother-Baby Relationship

One effect of severe psychiatric disorder might be to reduce the mothers' practical competence during their illness. Mother with puerperal psychotic illnesses were significantly more likely than other diagnoses to require extensive nursing supervision for at least part of their stay. However, when duration of practical incompetence was examined, 80 of the 92 mothers with puerperal psychosis showed impairment lasting less than 8 weeks.

Although the analysis of data here was retrospective we had extensive records of the mothers' interactions with their babies. We thought it likely that recording of the mother-baby interactions would be selective but that any bias would be likely to favour recording of abnormalities rather than normal behaviours. (For this reason we have gathered prospective systematically recorded data on a further 80 mothers which will be reported elsewhere).

In measuring affectionate behaviour we were able to distinguish predominantly affectionate behaviour from behaviour showing hostility and/or rejection. In addition, we distinguished a form of abnormal contact characterised by neutrality or disengagement from the baby. We compared these categories for the two major diagnostic groups.

TABLE 4 Affectionate Behaviour to Child During

Most Severe Period of Illness Episode

	Predominantly Affectionate	Neutral or Disengaged	Hostility/ Rejection
Puerperal Psychosis	39	51	1
Depression (Non-Psychotic)	47	25	5

$$X^2 = 11.41, \text{ d.f.} = 2, \text{ p} < 0.01$$

It can be seen that hostility/rejection was uncommon particularly in the puerperal psychosis group, although this may be partly an artefact of looking at the typical behaviour in an illness episode rather than the most abnormal single sample of behaviour recorded.

These tentative findings are supported by an analysis of the overall type of statement of the child. For this measure all available recorded statements were categorised as positive, negative or uncertain/mixed. If more than 70% fell into the positive or negative category this was recorded as 'predominantly positive' or 'predominantly negative', the remaining mothers being classified as 'inconsistent'.

TABLE 5 Affectionate Statements About Child

	Predominantly Positive	Inconsistent	Predominantly Negative
Puerperal Psychosis	82	7	0
Depression	27	28	23

$$X^2 = 63.2, \text{ d.f.} = 2, \text{ p} < 0.001$$

Although this analysis of retrospective data must be considered tentative, there was a striking difference between the two main clinical groups, with puerperal psychosis mothers never stating <u>predominantly</u> negative feelings although negative statements were recorded.

A further analysis was carried out of the abnormal statements made according to content, preliminary findings of which were recorded elsewhere (Margison 1982). These results have been reanalysed for each category independently rather than by predominant category as previously.

TABLE 6 Abnormal Ideas Expressed

Content	Puerperal Psychosis (n = 82)	Depression (n = 73)
Delusional/ Idiosyncratic	50 (61%)	NA
Preoccupation with child's health	18 (22%)	13 (18%) NS
Feeling incompetent	25 (30%)	44 (60%) $p<0.001$
Lack of feelings	6 (7%)	14 (19%) $p<0.05$
Hostility/Rejection	13 (25%)	39 (53%) $p<0.001$

There were no differences for ideas about the child being ill and delusions only occurred in one group by definition. The delusional ideas were commonly that the baby had special powers or special meaning or was changing in some magical way. Three categories occurred more commonly in the depression group; i) feelings of incompetence ii) lack of feelings and iii) ideas of hostility and/or rejection.

From these preliminary data it is clear that a global concept of "abnormal bonding" during psychiatric illness is inadequate. There may be abnormalities in what is said about the baby or, rarely, in the form of violence or neglect towards the baby. There are also important behavioural abnormalities particularly a lack of normal affectionate behaviours (eg playing, cuddling) and/or other abnormal behaviours such as avoidance of the baby and lack of eye contact.

We have suggested that these areas should be described separately and then an estimate of the degree of bonding failure can be made in addition.

Preliminary Description of Bonding Failure

Bonding disorders may include:
1) Abnormal statements about the child (including hostility or re-jection.
2) Lack of affectionate behaviour (eg playing, cuddling)
3) Other abnormal behaviour (including avoidance and lack of eye contact.
4) Episodes of violence or neglect.

TABLE 7 Degree of Bonding Failure

Stage 1 No relationship problem noted

Stage 2 Isolated area of difficulty eg expressing abnormal ideas. No hostility, rejection, violence or neglect present.

Stage 3 Difficulty in several areas eg expressing abnormal ideas plus lack of affectionate behaviour. No hostility, rejection, violence or neglect.

Stage 4 Violence, neglect or hostility and rejection in presence of above stages.

Even during severe psychiatric illness, mothers were able to care for their babies with low levels of physical injury when adequate nursing support was provided. A number of relationship difficulties including transient disruption of emotional and practical competence during puerperal psychosis and more complex difficulties often involving negative feelings during depressive neurosis were present. Tentative results about the mother's ideation showed differences between the clinical groups studied.

Acknowledgements

The nursing staff of the Mother and Baby Psychiatric Unit, University Hospital of South Manchester have contributed greatly to the collection of data for these studies.

References

Margison F R, 1981, Assessing the use of a psychiatric unit for mothers with their babies: Risks to the babies. MSc; University of Manchester

Margison F R, 1982, The pathology of the Mother Child Relationship, in "Motherhood and Mental Illness", Brockington I F; Kumar R. Eds., Academic Press, London.

PSYCHIATRY AND MENTAL RETARDATION:

A HISTORICAL PERSPECTIVE

Mohsen Mirabi

Texas Research Institute of Mental Sciences
1300 Moursund Avenue
Houston, Texas 77030

Since the beginning of time there have undoubtly been
individuals whose abilities were greater or less than others.
Their apparency and level of disability however, would have been
(and to a great extent, still is) relative to the sociocultural
needs, expectations, values, and consciousness of their societies.
I would like to address the historical background of mental
retardation - the development of understanding, social care and
treatment of mentally retarded individuals - from ancient Greece
and Rome to the present.

The ancient Greek and Roman civilizations were characterized
by the practice of infanticide and eugenics. The importance of
intelligence, physical strength, and beauty were only secondary
to the four cardinal virtues advocated by the ancient greek
civilization: courage, temperance, justice and wisdom. Clearly,
there was no role for the deformed or disabled in Plato's
Republic, and in ancient Rome historians tell us that "defective"
and "unwanted" children were thrown into the Tiber by their
parents to relieve themselves of the burden of support (Rosen et
al, 1976). For those who survived, their lives would be subject
to the sociopolitical atmosphere of the times - highly influenced
by parentage, class, and existing culture. Those of wealthy
families probably received some sort of medical treatment; the
poor, however, were often sold into slavery, became beggars, or
worked endless hours in the mines (Scheerenberger, 1982).

The dawn of Christianity brought a new humanism for the
retarded. Many hospitals and orphanages were established during
this time. A large number of people were faced with the extreme
hardships of wars and plagues - less than half the population

survived to maturity - it is not surprising to learn that fear
and superstition abounded, as did healing through faith and mir-
acles and the promise of a rewarding afterlife.

The mentally retarded served as fools or jesters in medieval
times or were referred to as "les enfants du Bon Dieu"(children of
God), wandering about the streets of Europe, unharmed. They were
not, however, regarded by physicians as part of their medical
responsibility, and no attempts were made to educate them (Rosen
et al, 1976).

The Renaissance brought a flourish of exploration into the
arts and sciences. The growing interest in the human body and
anatomy led to the development of surgery; and medical care in
general improved. Divinity, witchcraft, spells, and amulets,
however, were still used to a great extent in the treatment of
disease. This superstition continued well into the Reformation;
both Luther and Calvin proclaimed the retarded as "filled with
Satan".

The 17th and 18th centuries are characterized by periods of
"reason" and "enlightment". There were significant changes in
philosophy; Galileo and Newton attempted to understand nature
through empirical observation. For Descartes, Pope, Hobbes, and
Locke, the "study of mankind is man". Another important 18th
century precedent of the mental retardation movement was the work
of Pinel. In 1792 he was appointed director of the Bicetre, the
institution for the insane in Paris. Widely known for striking
the chains from the insane, he was convinced that mentally disturbed individuals were diseased rather than sinful or immoral.

The 1800's witnessed great strides in medicine and education
and the generation of interest in the retarded. Medical concern
began with the physiologically oriented educational achievements
of Itard and Seguin.

The attempts of Itard in early 1800 to teach Victor, the
"wild boy of Aveyron", were well known to contemporary European
educators. Although Itard was unsuccessful his objective to
completely socialize Victor, his methods, based on sensory training and embodying much of what is now called behavior modification, did produce substantial improvement (Crissey, 1975).

Edward Seguin, a french physician and educator, is noted as
having a great influence in the field of mental retardation. He
was convinced that education was a universal right, that society
was obligated to improve the lot of all its members, and that the
mentally retarded were among those greatest in need (Crissey,
1975). Seguin worked under the supervision of Itard, who was by
then an old man, in the teaching of an idiot child. Not content

with Itard's sensory training approach, Seguin incorporated all the available educational and psychological methods into his own program which he eventually extended to a large number of children.

Beginning about 1866, "idiocy" ceased being regarded as a unitary and homogeneous condition. The British physician Down first described what he called the "Mongolian type of idiocy". Unfortunately though, he based the label upon physiognomic characteristics and an ethnic classification system. Another important contribution during this time was William Ireland's textbook "On Idiocy and Imbecility" published in 1877, which described twelve subclassifications of mental deficiency and ushered in an era of medical discovery of such conditions as Tuberculosis and Tay-Sach's Disease. The unitary concept of mental retardation was finally broken.

The impact of the theory of evolution had a significant effect on the view of mental illness which continued well into the early part of the twentieth century. From Malthus' Essay on Population, in 1803 which hypothesized an excess of population - some of which must be eliminated by war, starvation, or disease, to Darwin's concepts of survival of the fittest and natural selection - which conceived of human behavior and mental processes to have biological antecedents. Social Darwinism provided justification for the eugenics movement a half a century later and was Hitler's rationale for the extermination of 100,000 "incurables and mental defectives" in Germany (Rosen el al, 1976).

Darwin also influenced Francis Galton, his most illustrious student, who emphasized the importance of studying individual differences, setting the stage for the mental testing instruments of Cattell and Binet, and his studies of hereditary genius along family lines influenced Goddard's future investigation of the Kallikak family in 1910. This study utilized the much criticized pedigree method and attempted to demonstrate that mental deficiency was inherited as a Mendelian recessive trait. The Kallikak family, of which there was two branches: one illigitimate - began through Martin Kallikak's encounter with a feeble-minded barmaid. They produced several hundred retarded persons over six generations. In the other branch, Kallikak married a normal colonial maid and, though they produced a much smaller number of off-spring, the line was embellished by judges, teachers, and eminent persons all of normal intelligence or brighter. The differences between the two branches was striking. As a result, matters of health, nutrition, child care, community status, and early stimulation were interpreted as products of genetic differences, rather than the producers of the difference in life success (Crissey, 1975). This concept was an extremely persuasive and influential force during the early part of the 20th century (Rosen et al, 1976).

By the turn of the century, the mentally retarded began to be regarded as a menace. Laws forbidding the marriage of mentally retarded persons were enacted in several states. Laws were also passed permitting or mandating sterilization and permanent custodial care for the retarded. The presumed association between idiocy, pauperism, insanity, and crime gained popular acceptance, lasting well into the twentieth century.

Although the first half of the twentieth century was characterized by sterilization and segregation, there were some important advances that had significant impact on the future treatment and care of the mentally retarded. One major influence was the development of individual intelligence testing. In an attempt to devise an objective means for identifying and classifying children's intellectual ability, Binet and Simon developed the "measuring scale of intelligence" in 1905. This scale brought into existence a concrete and reliable method of helping educators place students in appropriate classes and adapting instruction to fit the child's individual needs and abilities.

It is instructive to consider Binet's original concepts of the relationship between retardation and intelligence quotients - he said "an individual is normal when he can conduct himself without having the need of the tutelage of others, when he earns sufficient income for his needs. Retardation is an idea related to a host of circumstances that must be kept in mind in judging each particular case"[*]. Binet considered his scale as only one of a number of indicators of developmental status or rate. It provided a means for studying individual learning processes and encouraged the view that mental retardation is a heterogeneous condition (Crissey, 1975).

Unfortunately, when this measuring scale began being studied by others, Binet's philosophy was lost. Studies done with the use of this tool concluded that retardation was hereditary and irreversible and furthermore, that most criminals, vagrants, alcoholics, and prostitutes were mentallly retarded. It was unfortunate that the Binet-Simon scale was used by some to verify the prophesies of hereditability and irreversibility, but the concepts were consistent with the social values of the time and were agreeably accepted.

The history of the care and study of the mentally retarded is expansive; from the days of Itard and Seguin, we have seen incredible advances in special education; we have witnessed the

---

[*] Wolf, T.H., *Alfred* *Binet*, Chicago. University of Chicago Press, 1973, p.194

realization of Pinel's dream through deinstitutionalization; developed standard diagnostic and classification systems that are in use throughout the world; and have improved treatment for the mentally retarded through multidisciplinary intervention; clearly we have come a long way. It is in the spirit of our predecessors, whose insight and ingenuity have collectively paved the road for our work today, that we move toward the future and come closer and closer to our goal of improving the quality of life of the mentally retarded.

REFERENCES

Crissey, M. Mental Retardation Past, Present, and Future. American Psychologist, August: 800-808, 1975.

Kanner, Leo. A History of the Care and Study of Mental Retardation. Charles Thomas, Publisher, 1964.

Rosen, M., Clark, G., Kintz, M., (eds). The History of Mental Retardation, Vol. 1, Baltimore: University Park Press, 1976.

Scheerenberger, R.C. A History of Mental Retardation. Paul H. Brookes Publishing Co., 1983.

Wolf, T.H. Alfred Binet. Chicago: University of Chicago Press, 1973.

PSYCHIATRIC SYNDROMES AFFECTING RETARDED PERSONS IN RESIDENTIAL

CARE

Michael Mulcahy

Medico-Social Research Board
73 Lower Baggot Street
Dublin 2, Ireland

Despite the encouraging trend towards community care in many
countries residential centres of varying size for the retarded
are likely to persist for some time in the future.   It is worth
reporting therefore an experience with those termed severely
emotionally disturbed in a residential setting.   The period
covered by these observations extends from 1972-83.   Initially
it was difficult to assign a psychiatric diagnosis in individual
cases.   Many had been admitted because of behavioural problems.
Others had acquired these from institutional deprivation.   As
beneficial changes were introduced in the hospital the amount of
disturbance decreased and it became possible to identify the
existence of true mental illness in individuals.   True in this
context refers to illness whose origin is presumably more genetic
than environmental, or if environmental has occurred at such an
early stage of development and with such severity, that later
environmental manipulation, could not alone effect an improvement.

    Stewart's Hospital was the first residential centre for the
mentally retarded in Ireland and was founded in 1868.   In common
with other institutions of its type it has a varied history and
with the continuing pressure for residential accommodation, it
gradually became overcrowded.   The patient population in 1972
was accommodated either in the main building or in a later
pavilion style addition dating from 1950 referred to as the New
Unit.   Altogether the hospital was arranged in 11 wards or units
averaging about 33 patients each.   At that time a proportion of
the patients were considered on clinical examination to be severely
emotionally disturbed.   The term was used to describe persons who
were consistently upset in their behaviour either with themselves,

their peers or the staff, who regularly required tranquillising medication and who demanded a large amount of the time of the medical and nursing staff. A feature of the hospital in 1972 was that day activity programmes were unavailable for the majority of residents. In effect, the handicapped spent most of their day in the ward situation, with only a minority attending school, in occupational therapy or working in the gardens. All, however, benefited from walks in the extensive grounds and had other recreational outings.

During the next decade systematic improvements were carried out in the residential environment. Staff numbers doubled, numbers in each ward decreased and activity programmes are now available for the majority of residents. The final stages of the upgrading programme envisage that all residents will be living in small chalet like buildings or in community based homes. An occupational cum recreational programme will be available to all on a structured basis. The new pool, gymnasium and activity centre are already operational and fifty residents have moved to the new chalet residences accommodating ten each.

The effect of these better conditions on the frequency of disturbance and its magnitude is evident. There are fewer broken windows, unexplained accidents and simply less noise. The number of residents deemed severely emotionally disturbed however remains much the same. The main difference is that they are now better managed and more accessible to accurate clinical diagnosis.

Of course in the eleven year interval the population has changed in several respects. Some have died and a smaller number have been admitted. Everybody there in 1972, staff included, is now eleven years older. The main finding is that the numbers considered to be severely emotionally disturbed are unchanged and

Table 1. Stewart's Hospital

Residents	No.	Emotionally Disturbed	No.	Emotionally Disturbed
		1972		1983
Under 16 years	133	37 (28%)	40	5 (12%)
Over 16 years	223	40 (18%)	292	65 (22%)
Total	356	77 (21%)	332	70 (21%)

Table 2.   Stewart's Hospital 1983. Clinical Psychiatric
           Syndromes

Code		
296	Affective Psychoses	14 (20%)
299	Psychoses Specific to Childhood	12 (17%)
314	Hyperkinetic Syndrome	7 (10%)
300	Neurotic Disorders	4 (6%)
295	Schizophrenic Psychoses	3 (4%)
312	Conduct Disorders	3 (4%)
293	Transient Organic Psychotic Conditions	2 (3%)
294	Other Organic Psychotic Conditions	2 (3%)
311	Atypical Depression	1 (1%)
	Unclassified	22 (31%)
		70(100%)

represent 21% of the total population (Table 1).

A firm clinical diagnosis could be made in 49 or (70%).
The greatest single category is that of affective disorder.
The prevalence reported here of 4.2% of the total compares with
a prevalence of 2.8% reported by Wright (1982) from a much larger
hospital population.   The difficulty in assigning relative
importance to environmental as opposed to endogenous factors is
best illustrated in the case of the affective psychoses.   Wright
drew attention to the importance of "vegetative criteria" in the
diagnosis of this condition in the severely retarded.   These
criteris include sleep problems, diurnal variations in mood or
behaviour and changes in appetite and weight.   It is in just
such areas, however, that the retarded person may be effected
entirely on account of extraneous causes.   For example weight
loss in an overcrowded, poorly supervised ward can be due to
somebody not getting enough to eat! (Table 2).

The largest group is subsumed under unclassified because no
ICD category is entirely satisfactory.   The main characteristic
of this group is disordered, aggressive behaviour, coupled with
severe to profound mental handicap.   Only 27% were epileptic.
Terms such as personality disorder and conduct disorder are not
particularly suited because the patients so described bear no
comparison with persons of average intelligence who are categorised
with these labels.   Corbett (1979) found in the Camberwell Survey
that a similar group whom he designated behaviour disorder, was
the largest diagnostic category, 25% of a total population of 402.
The disordered behaviour in this group resembles the "primitive"
behaviour described by Menolascine (1983).   All our cases are
severely or profoundly retarded and are mainly a management problem

Table 3. Stewart's Hospital

1972	Order of Priorities	1983
1	Optimal Physical Environment	4
2	Adequate Recreational and Occupational Outlets	2
3	Adequate Staffing	5
4	Continuity of Staff	1
5	Psychiatric Treatment	3

because of aggressivity. I suspect that environmental factors are of paramount importance in these patients in the sense that their underlying organic pathology renders them more easily susceptible to acting out under stress. Most of the behaviourally disordered, unclassified group at Stewart's still reside in unsatisfactory conditions and the diagnostic problem will not be resolved till the full improvement plan is implemented.

The only other comment one could make in the diagnostic breakdown is the low frequency of schizophrenia. However, it is notoriously difficult to make the diagnosis in persons who have not acquired language.

All of the group described are receiving psychotropic medication. A further 29 are on medication but are not considered seriously disturbed. Altogether 30% of the hospital population receive psychotropic medication, other than anti-convulsants. Night sedation is rarely if ever employed.

I suspect from the observations here reported that even despite an optimal living situation, whether in the home, in small community residences, or in larger residential centres a proportion of the mentally retarded will continue to manifest serious psychiatric disorders. This proportion may be smaller however than was first thought. Its true prevalence must await more whole population studies along the lines reported by Reid (1980) and others

Meanwhile it appears that certain environmental factors are more important than others in the prevention and management of psychiatric illness in the hospitalized retarded. Our experience has led to a change in the order of priorities as viewed by the management (Table 3). Continuity of staff now appears more important than total staff numbers. The contribution of skilled psychiatric care has become accentuated. The introduction of depot neuroleptics alone has contributed a great deal to the general environment by controlling the disruptive behaviour of individual patients. Whatever the different priority accorded in different situations there will be a continuing need for the deployment of psychiatric expertise.

SUMMARY

A hospital population of emotionally disturbed mentally retarded persons were observed over an eleven year period. During that time their environment was gradually improved. The frequency and amount of disturbance has diminished, yet the numbers involved remained the same. Clinical diagnosis becomes easier as the living situation of the retarded is ameliorated.

ACKNOWLEDGEMENTS

I wish to express my thanks to Dr. Eithne Davern, Consultant Psychiatrist, Stewart's Hospital and to my secretary Miss Maureen O'Dwyer of the Medico-Social Research Board.

REFERENCES

Corbett, J.A., 1979. Psychiatric Morbidity and Mental Retardation in Psychiatric Illness and Mental Handicap. Royal College of Psychiatrists, London, 11-25.
Menolascino, F.J., 1983. Mental Health & Mental Retardation - Bridging the Gap. University Park Press, Baltimore, U.S.A.
Reid, A.H., 1980. Psychiatric Disorders in Mentally Handicapped Children: A Clinical and Follow-up Study. J. Ment. Defic. Res., 24, 287.
Wright, E.C., 1982. The Presentation of Mental Illness in Mentally Retarded Adults. Brit. J. Psychiat., 141, 496-502.

AUTISM AND DISTURBANCE OF SOCIAL CONTACT IN MENTALLY RETARDED

CHILDREN

Anton Došen
Observation Centre for children with developmental
disorders " de Hondsberg"
5062 JT OISTERWIJK; The Netherlands

INTRODUCTION

Diagnosticians are aware of the fact that disturbances of
social contact occur in children with specific sensory disorders,
in infantile autism, in infantile psychosis and in mental
deficiency.
Since with retarded children the disturbance of social contact
comes frequently to the fore (Wing and Gould, 1979) and puts a
specific stamp on the child's behaviour as a whole, with these
children it is often very difficult to distinguish between
infantile autism and contact disorder due to other reasons.
Certain authors (Corbett, 1977; Haracopos and Kelstrup, 1978;
Wing and Gould, 1979) signalize higher frequency of autism and
psychosis in retarded children. These authors attribute this
finding to the frequent organic cerebral abnormalities in
retarded children. An organic abnormality, giving rise to a
mental handicap, according to these authors, affect specific
cerebral areas leading to symptoms of autism and psychosis.
It is our experience, gained in working with mentally handicapped children, that the contact disturbances in these children
often mislead the diagnosticiand to the diagnosis of autism and
psychosis, while the reason for this discord can lie in an
inappropriate interaction between the child and its environment
and in inadequate stimulation of the child to the social contact.

OUR POPULATION AND THE METHOD

Among 184 retarded children admitted in our observation
clinic, we diagnosed a serious disorder of the social contact
in 13 children.

The mean age of these children was 5 years and 9 months (range 3 - 12 years). 11 of them had an I.Q. between 20 and 50 and 2 of them between 50 and 70.

Most of them were incapable to speak, and a few had a very limited number of words which they sometimes used.

These children could not tolerate bodily contact with other persons. Some of them could be kept on the lap or in the arms for a few minutes but longer-lasting contact rendered them excitable, aggressive or auto-aggressive. Others did not markedly repel bodily contact. They passively allowed themselves to be handled by a nurse, but it was obvious that they did not feel any pleasure in this contact. Eye contact with these children was not possible. They had little interest in material. Some of them played with a particular object in a stereotyped manner. The others played with their body parts or made stereotyped movements. They would react with fear or even with panic and fits of anger towards all changes in their environment. Their mood would change without demonstrable cause.

The parents of six children noted this "strange behaviour" from the birth of the child. Further 7 began to be found strange during their 2nd or 3rd year.

Upon medical examination all children had neurological and/or EEG abnormalities.

On the basis of DSM III criteria the diagnosis of infantile autism could be made in all these children. We diagnosed these children in the first instance as "disturbed in the primary contact".

All children were given a psychotherapeutic treatment. This treatment was administered in a "therapeutic milieu" of a ward where the children lived day and night. Within this therapeutic milieu they received an intensive individual treatment, which was conducted by a nursing staff intensively counselled by qualified therapeutists (Došen, 1983).

Theoretically the treatment was based on a psychodynamic model and inspired by studies of the development of the attachment between the mother and the newborn child (Spitz, 1945; Bowlby, 1969; Ainsworth, 1962).

We saw the disturbance of primary contact in these children as a stagnation in the first phase of their social and psychological development. The child cannot organize and integrate the stimuli which it receives from its environment through its senses.

It has no realization of its bodily limits and no concept of the objective world.

In our therapeutical concept we try to organize the environment of the child and to dose the stimuli in such a manner that the child can accept and integrate them in its own cognitive system. In this way the child is stimulated to the emotional and social development.

The therapy starts with the organization of the environment in the spatial and temporal sense. It means that the changes of the environments or in the environments must be avoided.
The living room must not be too exitable for the child. The activation of the child occurs within a stable daily rythm which is determined by its mental capability. The child had to grow familiar with its space. In such organized environment the child receives an offer of the bodily contact always with the same nurse, within a well-planned day program and with a constant daily frequency.
Initially the treatment is aimed at estabishing contact with the child through its tactile senses and its kinesthesie. The guiding principle here is that of gradual development of the receptivity to external stimuli. The proximal senses such as tactility and kinesthesia would be sooner capable of adequately receiving and integrating of external stimuli than distal senses such as hearing and sight (Spitz, 1945; Freedman, 1979).
The nurse tries to establish a pleasurable bodily contact with the child and avoids communication through hearing or sight (speech or play with material) as much as possible. Not earlier than that the child has accepted the bodily contact, the treatment goes to the next phase in which the nurse stimulates the communication via material and speech. This treatment we call "contact therapy".
The therapy lasted approximately 6 months.

THE RESULTS

Nine children showed a distinct improvement of their social contact. They clearly liked being handled by the nurses, they grew less anxious and less labile in mood and their eye contact was better. Their fits of anger, their aggressive or auto-aggressive tendencies diminished considerably or disappeared entirely. Some showed improvement of their verbal communication and were able to cope better in the group. They showed more interest in play with material and their stereotyped activities decreased.
The social contact in these children was comparable with their mental age.
Examined comparatively according to DSM criteria for childhood autism, these children could no longer be classified as autisitic on the basis of their behacioural symptoms. Four children in this group showed slight improvement in the course of the treatment. Although their refusal of primary contact diminished, they continued to exhibit the symptoms on the basis of which, according to DSM criteria, the diagnosis of childhood autism still could be applied.

DISCUSSION

Our experiences in the therapy accentuate the role of the environment factors in the development of a mentally deficient child.

A baby with CNS anomalies is often too quiet and apathetic. The stimulation threshold in these children may be very high. Such children inadequately initiate the bond with the mother.

A similar situation may develop when a child impairs the attachment bond by its restlessness and hyperactivity. Occasionally, such children are hypersensitive to certain sensory stimuli, (acoustic, visual, tactile) rendering them irritatble and easily frustrated. Organic cerebral lesions and prematurity of neonates may necessitate a longer hospital stay and pronlonged separation from the mother. A number of authors have observed that such a separation immediately after birth may severely impair the development of the attachment bond.

Owing to deficiency of their cerebral functioning and/of problems during the first few months of life, these children are unable to cope adequately with and work from the contact with the mother and are unable to establish contact with the mother.

In severe cases, deprivation and isolation may grow so bad that the child begins to lead an autistic existence.

We donot quite agree with some authors (Wing and Gould, 1979; Haracopos and Kelstrup, 1978) if they state that organic pathology of CNS in these children is the reason of their impair-ments of social contact. In our opinion the organic pathology is but one factor in the development of this disorder. The other factor which may be juust as important is an adequate stimulation of social development form the surroundings of the child. Unfavourable environmental circumstances in this case may be comparable with the effect of social deprivation of the child. The children who showed good results to the contact therapy could be compared with children called by Menolascino (1970) "children with developmental arrest".

The children who did not respond to the therapy could suffer in our opinion, apart from difficulties mentioned above, from the other more specific neurobiological or genetic underlying pathology, which may cause a specific abnormality such as infantile autism, schizophrenia or atypical psychosis. Owing to the mixture of symptoms the differential diagnosis may be very difficult and is, in our opinion, often possible only after clinical therapeutic exploration. Diagnostic differentiation is still very important because of an adequate treatment and the prognosis of further development of the child. Our therapeutical experiences with children with disturbances in social contact could be useful in the prevention of psychiatric disorders in retarded children. Special attention should be given to the timely detection and early guiding and counselling of mothers of these children.

Qualified workers could teach the mothers how to establish primary contact with their handicapped children.

CONCLUSION

Moderately and severely retarded young children often are not adequately stimulated during the development of their attachment, resulting in an arrest of emotional and social development. Such condition of a child is often misdagnosed as infantile autism or psychosis. Timely detection and diagnosing of the developmental arrest can make a basis for an adequate treatment and guiding of the mothers in their attachment behaviour towards these children.

SUMMARY

Lack of social contact is often a symptom of young, moderately and severely retarded children. When this lack of social contact is linked with a lack of language development, these retarded children are often classified as autistic.

Thirteen children, who upon admission to our clinic were diagnosed as 'infantile autistic' according to the DSM III criterion, received "contact therapy". This therapeutic approach is aimed at establishing primary body and eye contact between the therapist and the child. Following approximately six months of therapy, nine of the children showed an improvement in social contact and the symptoms of autism decreased or disappeared.

On the basis of this experience, the author suggests that monderately and severely retarded young children are often not adequately stimulated during the development of their attachment to the care provider, resulting in stagnation of social and emotional development.
The author advocates a better differential diagnosis of disturbed social contact and autism in these children.

REFERENCES

AINSWORTH, M.D. (1962): The effects of maternal deprivation:
        Public Health papers - Geneva: World Health Organization.
BOWLBY, J (1969): Attachment and Loss; Vol I Attachment; Basic
        Books New York.
CORBETT, J.A.(1977): Mental Retardation, psychiatric   aspects;
        in: M. Rutter, L.Hersov: Child Psychiatry - Modern
        Approaches, p.829-858, Blackwell Sc.Publ.
DOSEN, A.(1983): Experiences with individual relationship therapy
        within a therapeutic milieu for children with severe
        emotional disorders; Proceedings IASSMD congress, Toronto;
        Univ. Park Press, Baltimore, vol. II.
FREEDMAN, D.A. (1979): The sensory deprivation; Bulletin of
        Menninger Clinic 43,29-68
HARACOPOS, D. KELSTRUP, A (1978): Psychotic behaviour in children
        under the institutions for the mentally retarded in Denmark
        J. Aut. Ch. Schizo. 1, 1-12
MENOLASCINO, F.J. (1970): Infantile autism, descriptive and
        diagnostic relationship to mental retardation, in:
        Menolascino:Psychiatric approach to mental retardation,
        New York.
SPITZ, R.A. (1945): Hospitalism; Psycho-analytic study of the
        child; New York, International Univ. Press.
WING, L. GOULD, D. (1979): Severe impairments of social inter-
        action and associated abnormalities in children:
        epidemiology and classification: J. Aut. Dev. Dis. 9,
        11-29.

Schizophrenia in the Mentally Retarded

Frank J. Menolascino

University of Nebraska Medical Center
602 South 45 Street
Omaha, Nebraska

The historical relationship between the symptoms of mental retardation and mental illness will initially be reviewed. The interrelationships between the symptoms will then be illustrated by
presenting one of our recent studies in a community-based sample
of retarded citizens. Specific focus on the clinical diagnosis
of schizophrenia in the retarded, and its differential response
to treatment modalities, are reviewed through the author's recent
study on the efficacy of psychopharmacological agents. Lastly, the
current and future challenges which this "dual diagnosis" presents
will be underscored.

Psychiatric Aspects of Mental Retardation

Historically, the relationship between schizophrenia and mental
retardation has been described since the very beginning of psychiatry.
Indeed, the descriptive clinical picture of Victor, the "Wild Boy
of Aveyron" who was described by the French Psychiatrist Jean-Marc
Itard[1] in that mid-nineteenth century, would today be considered
that of an adult psychotic. Despite this clinical picture of both
psychosis and severe mental retardation, Itard was able to effect
very beneficial developmental and behavioral results with the "Wild
Boy" and thus initiated five decades of hope for the retarded. In
1896, Kraeplin[2] delineated the relationship of psychosis and mental
retardation as one wherein demential praecox (i.e.,schizophrenia)
was typically engrafted upon previously existing indices of mental
retardation. In 1911, Bleuler[3] proposed the term "Propf-schizophren-
ia" to describe this same relationship. Despite these early excellent descriptions of schizophrenia in the mentally retarded, it has
not been widely discussed in the psychiatric literature until the
last two decades.

Prior to the Sixties the frequently noted behavioral and personality aspects of retarded citizens were commonly attributed to their basic developmental delays; the behavioral signs or symptoms noted were viewed as expressions of central nervous system abnormalities. However, the Kennedy legislation of 1963 and its resultant University Affiliate Programs in mental retardation initiated in the United States a national network of multi-disciplinary teams to study more closely the overall cognitive-behavioral functioning of retarded citizens. Their goal was also to take a fresh look at mental retardation and at the ways in which retarded patients function in institutions, families and workplaces. It soon became apparent, through increasing contributions to the psychiatric literature, that there were a large number of mentally retarded citizens who had concurrent mental illness--which has been termed the "dual diagnosis" in the field of mental retardation[4]. For example, studies have noted consistently that 25-30% of the mentally retarded persons have been deinstitutionalized and as public advocacy for the retarded has become stronger and more effective. Because of the deinstitutionalization movement, we now have many retarded individuals living in the community who once were, or would have been, locked away. These findings are born out today as the deinstitutionalization of the retarded brings more of these individuals to the attention of psychiatrists in the community. In addition, strong parental advocacy voices demand mental health services for their retarded sons and daughters.

The Nature of Mental Illness in the Retarded

The nature and frequency of mental illness in the retarded has been illuminated in several large clinical studies, including one we recently completed involving patients served by a community-based program for the retarded in Nebraska. During a three year period, we found that 114 (14.3%) of the 798 retarded individuals in this program had identifiable evidence of mental illness. Table 1, which employ the DSM III nomenclature system, shows the type of frequency of mental disorder we encountered by patient age in this study.

As noted in Table 1, schizophrenia is a common mental illness in the retarded, and was noted in all age groups but the youngest. Schizophrenia is noted at all levels of retardation and this diagnostic point has prompted much debate in the literature, and the recurring clinical questions is: How can one make the diagnosis of schizophrenia in very low functioning and essentially non-verbal individuals‾ This professional concern must closely focus on the etiological, developmental and phenomenological dimensions of the majormental illness in the retarded. We have summarized our clinical experiences on this topic in Figure 1.

In the psychopharmacological study to be described herein, we noted four individuals who displayed both severe mental retardation and schizophrenia. The presence of bizarre behavior, persistent withdrawal, echolalia, and blunted affect in adults who had clearly regressed from an earlier higher level of functioning was striking. These four individuals illustrate the superimposition of schizophrenia upon etiologically clear instances of mental retardation (i.e., one had Down's syndrome, one had fetal rubella, and two had major cranial malformations causing mental retardation.) According to their personal-clinical histories, all four of these individuals developed schizophrenia between the ages of 18 and 22 years.

Table 1   Types of mental illness in a community-based sample of 114 mentally retarded individuals by age

Chronological Age (Years)

Diagnosis	6-10	11-20	21-30	31-40	41-50	51+
Schizophrenia (N=24)		7	14	2	1	1
Personality Disorder (N=31)		5	14	7	4	1
Generalized Anxiety Disorder (N=1)			1			
Adjustment Disorders (N=24)	5	11	4	3	1	
Organic Brain Syndrome (N=34) With Transient Behavioral Reaction	2	15	3			
With Transient Psychotic Reaction		9	1	3		

Similarily, it has been our clinical experience that the markedly primitive behaviors noted in severely retarded adults (e.g., severe retardation with associated poor language development) can be readily separated from schizophrenia superimposed upon primary mental retardation. For example, we noted instances of paranoid schizophrenia in two non-verbal adult patients who drew on paper their "attackers", complete with non-verbal gestures. One such individual would label his separate fingers as the "source" of his common delusions which he would portray symbolically in crude drawings. Paranoid and catatonic features were the most frequently noted hallmarks of the acute chronic schizophrenia, the altered affective responses, bizarre rituals, and persistent use of interpersonal distancing devices are clearly schizophrenic behaviors.

197

I. Etiological and Developmental Dimension	
Developmental Arrest: Primary or Congenital	**Acquired: Non-psychotic--psychotic**
The individual never had a functional ego. There is no distinct concept of the self; instead, there is an amorphous and formless personality (essentially a minimal personality structure). The reasons why these patients never developed a functionally complex ego early in life: may be due to a primary integrative problem (e.g., cerebral dysfunction, mental retardation, specific mid-brain deficits; or possible secondary integrative problems (e.g., secondary to a negative intake process such psychotoxic mothering, deprivation syndromes, combined sensory-general environmental input difficulties, etc.).	(1) Regressive dynamic; primary (childhood schizophrenia). (2) Secondary (Propf-schizophrenia: Organic congenital cerebral insult/dysfunction (e.g., infantile spasms syndrome and its residuals; traumatic or post-infection etiologies, etc.). (3) Toxic psychoses (e.g., phenylketonuria). A toxic metabolic disorder can literally disintegrate the personality' relationship to reality.

II. Phenomenological Aspects		
A	B	C
Organic Brain Syndrome with Behavioral Reaction	**Organic Brain Syndrome with Psychotic Reaction**	**Schizophrenia**
1. Distinct (and early indices of retardation ("untutored").	1. History of MR/major developmental delays	1. Long history since early in life with withdrawn and regressive behaviors (less than 6 months): primary mental retardation disinterested in tutoring.
2. Benign autism: limited ability to respond to interpersonal stimulation.	2. Isolated and lonely; long standing personality posture of rigidity.	2. Autism (motoric and interpersonal distancing: not of recent onset).
3. No island of intact personality functioning at chronological age level.	3. Some scattered islands of intact personality functioning (not disorganized).	3. Disorganized personality-chronically so!
4. Minimal stress anxiety-initially turned inward toward self (abuse), then negativism and diffuse motoric overactivity.	4. With minimal stress: Repetitive behaviors; if stress mounts; out of contact (psychotic) behaviors, poor language development.	4. Ritualistic behaviors: initially utilized to avoid interacting with others as demands for appropriate behaviors mount: he becomes more bizarre, affectively unavailable, and secondary signs of schizophrenia become more prominent.

Figure 1   Clasification of psychotic reactions in the mentally
retarded: etiological, developmental, and phenomenomo-
logical factors

The majority of these dual diagnosis individuals whom we have
examined were in need of inpatient psychiatric care. Our treatment
program consists of a balanced approach (including psychoactive
medications) by a multi-disciplinary team. We have continued to explore the psychoactive agents which may have potential clinical
advantages in providing earlier or increased treatment efficacy. In
the past, the author has been involved in psychoactive drug research
studies on thioridazine (Mellaril) and haloperidol (Haldol) for this
dual diagnosis group. Yet these two of my "standby favorites" still
do not produce the degree of treatment-outcome results I would like
to obtain; thus my ongoing search for more effective major psychoactive agents, Navane (thiothixene) began to impress us in our daily
clinical work; we decided to do a formal research study to see

whether our impressions of its superior clinical efficacy were valid.

Clinical Study: Thiothixene vs. Thioridazine in Retarded and Non-Retarded Schizophrenic Patients

Our recent study was designed to provide a clearer picture of the efficacy of specific psychoactive drugs with the mentally retarded-schizophrenic patients. We decided to conduct a rater-blind comparison of Navane (thiothixene) and Mellaril (thioridazine) in a sample of retarded and non-retarded schizophrenic individuals. Specifically, the present study was designed: 1) to see if there was a differential response to thiothixene and thioridazine in retarded schizophrenics; 2) to determine which drug might offer enhanced short-term treatment response 3) to determine whether the type and/or number of side effects of these two psychoactive agents was the same in the mentally retarded schizophrenic as in the non-retarded schizophrenic patients; and 4) to provide a clinical trial of the overall efficacy of these two psychoactive agents in these populations.

To reach these goals, this rater blind study compared the effects of these two medications on randomly assigned retarded and non-retarded schizophrenics in an inpatient psychiatric hospital setting. Medication was given to patients by psychiatrists who knew which medication the patient was on, in order to maximize the simularity of this trial to real clinical situations. However, the raters of the medication effects did not know the identity of the two drug groups, and the patients were unaware of the nature of their medications. In brief, the research methodology employed was the following: Sixty one male and female inpatients with a diagnosis of schizophrenia (according to DSMIII criteria) of any subtype participated. Thirty-three received thiothixene and 28 received thioridazine. The study participants, classified on the basis of I.Q. (using the Wechsler Adult Intelligence Scale) and social adaptive assessment, were divided in two groups. Those with the WAIS score below 70 were classified as retarded, those who scored within the normal range were so designated. The subjects were then randomly assigned to the two study medications. Patient evaluations were made at weeks 1,2,3,4,8 and 12 by observers who were blind to the medication assignment and dosage(s). Each subject was evaluated by the same observer throughout the study. At the conclusion of treatment, a five point Therapeutic Effect Index was completed for each subject in the study.

Study Findings

Our study demonstrated that treatment with either thiothixene or thioridazine produces significant improvement of schizophrenia in both groups as reflected in standard psychiatric rating scales. Clinically, the patients in both groups showed improved social adjustment, improved attentivensss, less inappropriate behavior, and increased approachability. Interestingly, to achieve optimum therapeutic effects, non-retarded patients required higher doses of both study medications than did their retarded counterparts.(see Figure 2).

Our study's most striking finding was the difference in time required to achieve maximum therapeutic effect between the two drugs under investigation. We found a significantly p. < .05) more rapid onset of therapeutic effect in retarded-schizrenic patients treated with thioridazine. The mean treatment time needed to produce the optimal therapeutic effect in thiothixene-treated retarded-schizophrenic individuals was 12 days, while 28.8 days were required to produce similar effects in the retarded-schizophrenic thioridazine group.

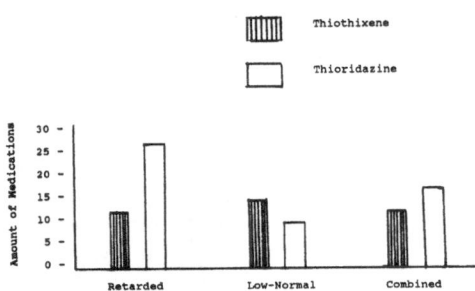

Figure 2 Dosages required for optimal therapeutic response

Across the board, both drugs produced the same number of predictable side effects. However, in the thiothixene group, extrapyramidal symptoms were common and usually responsive to symptomatic therapy while drowsiness are observed much more frequently in the thioridazine group.

Discussion

I have reviewed some of the special diagnostic treatment challenges presented by retarded individuals who are also schizophrenic. It is underscored that schizophrenia in retarded individuals is a distinct, treatable entity, just as it is in non-retarded individuals. This is not an academic point, since, in the future, we can expect increasing numbers of retarded persons to be living among us in the mainstreams of our communities rather than in the large public institutions to which they were once co-signed as "helpless and hopeless". I believe this increasing trend is going to stimulate an enhanced interest in studying the psychiatric aspects of mental retardation. Future research efforts need to be directed at refining diagnostic criteria to better predict which mentally retarded patients with allied schizophrenia are most likely to benefit from balanced treatment approaches which include the judicious utilization of the major psychoactive agents.

In summary, it is my prediction that we will see increasing clinical attention to the psychiatric aspects of mental retardation--both in the general mentally retarded population and those with the dual diagnosis of both mental retardation and schizophrenia. Concurrent with this widening attention will be an increased focus on the utilization of specific psychoactive agents, such as thiothixene, which hold great promise for promptly quelling the major psychiatric disorders which so often complicate the retarded citizens adjustment to the interpersonal world of everyday life. It is my hope that the foregoing study will add to our professional understanding of one of these major mental illnesses--schizophrenia-which so often complicates the lives of retarded persons who are trying to "make it" in our world.

REFERENCES

1. Itard, J. The wild boy of Aveyron (Translated by G.& M. Humphrey). New York: Appleton-Century-Crofts, 1962.
2. May J., May, J. and Menolascino, F. Mental Illness in the Mentally Retarded. In: F. Menolascino and J. Stark (Eds.) Mental Illness and Mental Retardation. New York: Plenum Press, 1983.
3. Menolascino, F.: The research challenge of delineating psychiatric syndromes in mental retardation. In Psychiatric Approaches to Mental Retardation. New York: Basic Books, 1964.
4. Menolascino, F.& McCann, B.: Mental Health and Mental Retardation: Bridging the Gap. Baltimore. University Park Press, 1983.
5. Menolascino, F. Psychiatric Aspects of Mental Retardation. New York: Basic Books, Inc. 1970.
6. Szymanski, L. & Tanguay, P.: Emotional Disorders of Mentally Retarded Persons. Baltimore: University Park Press, 1983.
7. Eaton, L. & Menolascino, F.: Psychiatric disorders in the mentally retarded: Types, problems and challenges. American Journal of Psychiatry, 139:10, October, 1982.

PSYCHIATRIC CONSULTATION TO A RESIDENTIAL

FACILITY FOR THE MENTALLY RETARDED

Stephen L. Ruedrich

Nebraska Psychiatric Institute
University of Nebraska College of Medicine
602 South 45th Street
Omaha, Nebraska 68106

The last thirty years has witnessed an explosion of interest in psychiatric consultation. Most authors have focused on scientific description of the consultation, others have chosen to examine its "art." Caplan separated consultations according to their primary focus, and the extent to which the consultant is interested in educating the consultee.[1] Solomon noted that the psychiatric consultant represents both himself <u>and</u> the entire field of psychiatry, and thus must be sensitive to both its contributions and its limitations.[2] Nowhere is this more true than in the area of mental retardation. However, until recently the need for psychiatric consultation for retarded persons has been generally unrecognized or under-valued. Groups such as the GAP (Group for the Advancement of Psychiatry) have noted that psychiatric trainees have more personal than professional knowledge of mental retardation, and that consultants who care for such "devalued persons" may have status problems.[3,4] This is tragic in view of the evidence that the mentally retarded suffer a variety of psychiatric disorders, and benefit from treatment of these conditions.[5,6] For these reasons, interest has surfaced regarding the treatment of psychiatric disorders in the retarded, with the focus on diagnosis, prevention, and treatment. Few have addressed the <u>role</u> of the psychiatrist, fewer the consultation itself. This paper <u>will</u> examine the role of the psychiatric consultant in a residential facility for the mentally retarded.

Although there has been a recognized need for consultation services for the retarded, little has been written in the area. Menolascino described successful consultation utilizing contact, crisis intervention and staff training.[7] Crisis intervention within an institution, involving behavior modification, was outlined by Pierce.[8] Beitenman noted the need for psychiatric servies in the institution, where admission was often selectively based on the presence of psychiatric disorders, and the <u>lack</u> of such services. He emphasized the importance of involving the daily care-givers in all consultation activities, and advocated a case seminar format as most effective for staff education.[9] More recently, the GAP has highlighted psychiatric consultation for the retarded, and identified the residential facility as an area that can benefit.[10] Interactions between the psychiatrist and the institution are many and often over-lapping. In general, however, the consultant may function as: 1) a confidant/therapist for the patient or staff; 2) a synthesizer and mediator for the interdisciplinary treatment team; 3) an expert/teacher; 4) a supportive motivating force for both the primary care-giving staff and professional staff; and 5) an advocate/ally for the retarded individual and institutional personnel.

CONFIDANT/THERAPIST

The primary purpose of the psychiatric consultant may be that of providing direct medical consultation. Sandt and Leifer have argued that the "sender" of the consultation request is <u>the</u> crucial factor in the consultation process, charging that the psychiatrist becomes the agent of the sender, who is invariably a staff member.[11] Additionally, mentally retarded persons are rarely able to seek con-sultation on their own. Hence, the psychiatrist must be aware that he is essentially working for the consultee, and is seen as such by both patients and staff. This often makes it difficult to gain more than token rapport with patients. Occasionally the care-giving staff are even reluctant to allow the consultant to see the individual alone, for reasons of concern for safety or fear of disclosure of past inter-actions. Additionally, the consultant may not attempt to examine the patient in confidence based on his fears, misconceptions, or feelings of inadequacy. Together these rarely allow for the one-to-one inter-action that characterizes psychiatric consultation. The patient may be viewed as superfluous, deaf, uncomprehending, or absent. Thus, modeling by the consultant that addresses the patient as an individ-ual with unique qualities and needs is mandatory. Time and attention directed at forming a therapeutic bond with the retarded individual can be utilized to promote communication and trust, and lead to on-going relationships in psychotherapy. A dividend is that such activ-ity serves as modeling and facilitates confidant-type contacts by the staff. This makes more credible recommendations for staff-led indi-vidual and/or group psychotherapy; the consultant can then assume a supervisory role. In all, this produces a more favorable climate for recognition of mentally retarded persons as individuals, who can benefit from traditional psychotherapeutic approaches.

MEDIATOR

A second major assignment is that of mediator. The psychiatric consultant must be sensitive to predominantly hidden agendas in the consultation request, and attempt to tease out issues of authority diffusion, communication blocks, and group dynamics that are a hallmark of institutional treatment. Caplan has characterized this "consultee-centered administrative consultation" as one of the more difficult tasks for most consultants.[12] Within the institution there are multiple complex relationships among the players, providing the consultant with numerous opportunities to act as synthesizer or mediator. Generally conflicts occur in four areas, whose characteristic problems result in requests for help when impasses develop.

The first concerns disagreements between members of multidisciplinary treatment teams, involving issues which seemingly fall between disciplinary cracks. When a patient's problem does not fit nicely into one disciplinary area, or overlaps several, questions of authority, competence, and decision-making procedures occur. Thus the psychiatrist may be presented questions whose covert content is one of therapeutic turf. The consultant, unaware of these submerged issues, may fail to address them and effect no resolution, or choose sides and become enmeshed in the conflict. There are no simple guidelines; most authors advocate an approach that balances the consultant's personal ethics with the goal of improvement of the mental health climate. The best interests of the mentally retarded individual must be tantamount; the consultant cannot allow conditions to exist which compromise optimum medical treatment. A subset of this conflict can erupt between professional and nonprofessional caregivers. Psychiatric consultation is sometimes sought when a retarded person is not responding to treatment. The overt message to the consultant is "why isn't it working?"; however, the covert request is to make the nonprofessional staff work harder. Conversely, the direct care-givers often view the professional staff as insensitive, "too scientific," or not willing to get their hands dirty. This bidirectional denigration can be viewed as projection based on frustration by both sides. The consultant's failure to anticipate such conditions will lessen his effectiveness, and may lead to changes in treatment, when what is needed is promotion of realistic expectations. Similarly, conflicts may form between staff and institutional administration. The psychiatric consultant can pursue either direct mediation, moderating face to face discussion of programatic needs, provide direct program consultation, or function indirectly by supporting staff at all levels. Rarely is direct interpretation necessary or helpful; rather, gentle nudging of both sides proves most beneficial.

Finally, the consultant may have to deal with disagreements or open warfare between the institutional staff and the family or guardian of the mentally retarded individual. Often these struggles surround issues of control and responsibility, with guilt, subsequent scapegoating, and real concern for the welfare of the family member on both sides. Investigation often reveals a family who has not worked through the separation, guilt, and grief accompanying the institutionalization of their relative, who then resists mutual cooperation in treatment. The psychiatric consultant can provide opportunities for ventilation, support, and model an atmosphere of optimal sensitivity to such needs. This is especially true at the point of institutionalization itself, where psychiatric consultation can facilitate ongoing cooperation rather than a series of confrontations. Thus, the mediator role is inescapable for the psychiatric consultant who should identify and embrace this consultation activity.

EXPERT/TEACHER

Third, the psychiatrist will be expected to assume the traditional role of expert and teacher. This occurs at several levels, including personal instruction and group presentation. As previously stated, the pressing need for psychiatric services in institutions has been outlined, but not yet met. The consultant himself must often identify exactly what range, method, and volume of psychiatric treatment is needed. Primary in his initial contacts then, should be education regarding the presence, types, frequencies and treatments of psychiatric disorders in the retarded, with the clear message that abnormal behavior should not be ascribed solely to the retardation itself without examination for concurrent psychiatric disorders. This needs to occur at several levels, but primarily with those persons most likely and most able to facilitate consultation - generally the physician or psychologist within the treatment team. Of particular importance, however, is fostering similar acceptance and sophistication in the primary care-givers. Numerous authors have addressed the stereotyping, irrational expectations, and fantasies that surround psychiatric consultation in general; the same is true in work with the retarded.[13] Hence, psychiatrists must have repeated and meaningful contact with the frontline staff, avoid jargon, promote teamwork, and expect testing of his expertise and effectiveness.

Of particular interest in terms of teaching is assessment of the retarded patient. Often disorders are overlooked because of unique problems associated with lack of language development in the patient, or lack of knowledge on the part of the staff. Teaching basic interviewing skills, and special techniques or equipment applicable to retarded persons (for example, signing or language boards), fosters closer interaction and increased sensitivity to the presence of symptoms. Instruction and demonstration of assessment in the areas of suicide, psychosis and sexuality can lead to routine questioning about these topics and improve diagnosis.

Finally, consultants often have a covert role (as defined by institutional administration) as "experts" in social and legal activities of the patients, and legal and medical actions of the staff. Consultants should address formally whether they will be called upon for expert testimony; in this way they can assess expectations of institutional administrators and limit or modify the scope of their consultative activity accordingly.

SUPPORTER/MOTIVATOR

A fourth role available for the consultant is that of supporter and motivator for the institutional staff. This function is often neglected and under-utilized as a method for increasing staff esteem and as a result, optimal patient care. Ignoring this activity may be a reflection of the consultant's doubts or therapeutic pessimism with the retarded. Employment and employees in institutional settings may be as "devalued" as the retarded persons they serve, and psychiatrists are not immune. Activity and energy in this area may be exceptionally fruitful, if the ultimate goal is to provide the most benefit to the most patients.

Specifically, the consultant should avail himself of opportunities to support, praise, and value the treatment staff. They are continuously faced with difficult or unresponsive patients, interdisciplinary conflicts, administrative bureaucracies, cost constraints, and uninterested or hostile family members. Requests for psychiatric services may represent frustration with any or all of the above, along with a general sense of discouragement. Psychiatrists sensitive to these issues can provide needed empathy, sense of self worth, and motivation. Recognition of past efforts, present energies, and future plans disrupt the therapeutic inertia that often characterizes institutions. Overt cheerleading is not recommended; it is as important to help staff form realistic expectations as it is to strive for maximum efforts. However, commentary which provides realism can also encourage continued efforts and increase individual self esteem and staff cohesion. Active support and encouragement to engage in research, or share expertise through publication, may provide the energy necessary for renewed interventions, and can take place in the context of patient-centered consultation.

Finally, formal group psychotherapy for staff can be helpful for brief periods (often crisis situations) in which discovery of common frustrations, disappointments, and goals can increase cohesion and improve care. In all, the psychiatrist should pursue opportunities to function as supporter and motivator for the staff, which may be among his most important consultative efforts.

ADVOCATE/ALLY

The final assignment for the clinician consulting to the mentally retarded individual is less traditional, for it reverses basic psychiatric precepts having to do with maintenance of therapeutic distance and patient autonomy. This is the important role of advocate and ally, in which the psychiatrist steps outside his usual role in promoting the social, legal, medical and economic welfare of the person.

Within the institution the consultant can lobby on behalf of individuals or groups in promoting common objectives of optimal treatment, increased autonomy and community-based programs. Most institutions are already committed to these goals; in others, the consultant can serve as a source of sufficient energy, authority, and conscience to begin the process.

The role of the consultant as advocate need not end at the institutional wall. The same characteristics that enable the psychiatrist to be effective inside the institution can make him or her successful on the outside. In fact, a position as an unaffiliated consultant may make more credible any efforts in this direction. Often the institution for the retarded citizen is isolated from psychiatric and medical organizations; liaison to these groups can rally powerful forces for change. Communities which are reluctant to support community-based programs can benefit from education, reassurance and direction about these sensitive issues.[14] Again, the specific ability, credibility, and independence of the consultant can be helpful. Formal contact and coordination with parent and other advocacy groups, such as NARC (National Association of Retarded Citizens), can also help and should be investigated.[15]

SUMMARY

The need for psychiatric services, particularly consultation, within residential facilities serving the retarded has been recently recognized, but remains under-utilized, under-valued, or absent. Consultation is likely to improve patient care in institutions, and can provide for the treatment of psychiatric disorders occurring in residential patients. The psychiatrist will find himself filling at various times and in varying combinations, the roles of confidant/ therapist, mediator, expert/teacher, motivator, and advocate/ally. Failing to consider one or more of these can seriously limit the potential effectiveness of the consultation process; addressing and embracing them can serve to open and expand the role and with it, increase the benefit to the patient.

REFERENCES

1. G. Caplan, "The Theory and Practice of Mental Health Consultation," Basic Books, New York (1970).
2. P. Solomon, An Overview, Summary, and Conclusion, in: "The Psychiatric Consultation," W. M. Mendel, ed., Grune & Stratton, New York (1968).
3. Group for the Advancement of Psychiatry, "Psychiatric Consultation in Mental Retardation," GAP #104, New York (1979).
4. N. R. Bernstein, ed., "Diminished People," Little Brown, New York (1979).
5. L. R. Eaton and F. J. Menolascino, Psychiatric Disorders in the Mentally Retarded: Types, Problems and Challenges, Am. J. Psycl 139:1297-1303 (1982).

6. M. S. Adams, Psychiatric Consultation to a Mental Retardation Program, J. National Med. Assoc. 68:213-216 (1982).

7. F. J. Menolascino, Psychiatric Long Distance Consultation for the Mentally Retarded, Ment. Retard.9:23-25 (1971).

8. P. S. Pierce, Crisis Intervention in a State Institution for the Mentally Retarded, Hosp. and Community Psychiat. 28:9-13 (1977).

9. E. T. Beitenman, The Psychiatric Consultant in a Residential Facility for the Mentally Retarded, in: "Psychiatric Approaches to Mental Retardation," F. J. Menolascino, ed., Basic Books, New York (1970).

10. Group for the Advancement of Psychiatry, "Psychiatric Consultation in Mental Retardation, " GAP #104, New York (1979)

11. J. Sandt and R. Leifer, The Psychiatric Consultation, Comprehen. Psychiat.5:409-418 (1964).

12. G. Caplan, "The Theory and Practice of Mental Health Consultation," Basic Books, New York (1970) pp 19-34.

13. Ibid, pp 48-79

14. F. J. Menolascino, "Challenges in Mental Retardation," Human Sciences Press, New York (1970) pp 310-316.

15. Ibid, pp 62-103

SPECIALISED NEEDS OF THE RETARDED:

EPIDEMIOLOGICAL SURVEYS

T.L. Pilkington

Consultant Psychiatrist
Whixley Hospital
York, England

There have been many surveys carried out on the mentally retarded in the U.K. Some classic ones were by:

Tredgold, in 1908, for a British Royal Commission, which
indicated the prevalence as 4.8: 1,000 population.

Lewis, in 1929, for a Government Department in England and
Wales, showing the prevalence as 8.7:1,000 population.

Penrose, in 1938 (The Colchester Survey of 1,280 in-patients
for the Medical Research Council)

McKeown and Leek, in 1967, of 1,652 in-patients (British Medical
Journal, 1967, 3 573-76)

There have been many similar surveys in other countries and attempts have been made to carry out cross-cultural surveys (the W.H.O. Technical Report No.392 in 1968 reported general rates of 1-3% of the population as being mentally retarded). Different criteria are used and the results often rely on questionnaires filled up by other people. How reliable are they?

The Wessex criteria of dependency, Fig.(1), are widely used, for example, by the National Development Team, an Inspectorate for England set up by the Government in 1975. In consequence, many hospital populations have been surveyed in accord with these scales; fig. (2) shows a typical profile. The excessive number of Down's syndrome patients, especially in hospital "A", will be noted.

GROUP I

Criteria Competent in all areas of self-help, ambulant, continent, no behaviour problems, not disruptive in any way.

GROUP II

Criteria Continent, ambulant, almost completely self-sufficient with mild problems of behaviour which could be corrected with a short period of treatment and self-help training. A number could be considered for self-care training-units.

GROUP III

Criteria Continent with lapses at night. Some are mildly over-active with occasional mild behaviour problems. All are said to be easily managed and would benefit frcm specific training. If discharged to a hostel, staff ratios would need to be higher than for those in Groups I and II.

GROUP IV

Criteria Severe double incontinence, multiple physical handicaps, severe epilepsy, extreme hyperkinetic behaviour, aggression to self and others.

Fig. 1. Based on the Wessex Dependency Scale

	BEDS	WESSEX				DOWN'S SYND.
		I	II	III	IV	
HOSPITAL A	291	32	42	70	147	55
HOSPITAL B	156	55	17	50	34	11
HOSPITAL C	28	3	19	13	3	6
HOSTEL D	21	15	1	5	0	0
HOSTEL E	18	6	3	6	3	5
TOTALS	514	109	72	144	182	77

Fig. 2.

This survey was carried out in 1981. Fig. (3) compares the (nursing returns on the Downs' patients with similar returns on the same patients two years earlier; there is a considerable discrepancy. The return from hospital "X", a neighbouring hospital, is shown for comparison. Fig.(4) shows, for interest, the age span of the hospitalised/

hospitalised Down's syndrome patients. It is suggested that surveys such as these, relying on subjective judgements, are liable to wide variations which limit their reliability.

Combined Hospitals	NOS.	W E S S E X I II III	IV
Survey 1979	77	59	18
Survey 1981	77	70	7
Hospital X (270 beds)	16	16	0

Fig. 3. Down's Syndrome

What of the special, and particularly psychiatric needs of the retarded? Fig. (5) shows the number of in-patients considered by the nursing staff to have additional mental illness. It is significant that considerably more are on psychotropic drugs. Fig.(6) shows the predominance of severe behaviour disorders, of which about a half had a mental illness component, in referrals to the consultant psychiatrist from both hospital and community. Estimates of the prevalence of mental illness in the retarded vary widely, as the comparisons in Fig.(7) show. It would seem reasonable, however to assume a prevalance of at least 20% in the institutional population, possibly increasing as the attention of the general psychiatric services move away from long-stay hospital populations. It is important, therefore, to look at the availability of specialist staff.

AGE	12-21	22-31	32-41	42-51	52-61	62-71
NUMBERS	6	22	18	11	8	1

Fig. 4. Down's Syndrome (Hospitals A + B)

	BEDS	MENTALLY ILL	PSYCHO-TROPIC DRUGS
HOSPITAL A	291	12	108
HOSPITAL B	156	7	41
HOSPITAL C	28	3	13
HOSTEL D	21	6	1
HOSTEL E	18	2	6
TOTALS	514	30	169

Fig. 5.

	SEVERE BEHAVIOUR DISORDERS	ADDITIONAL MENTAL ILLNESS
O.P. Clinics (4) (pop. 600,000)	84%	48%
I.P.S (Hospitals and hostels - 600 places)	96%	36%

Fig. 6. Consultant Referals 1980-82

8%	Primrose	1971	Institutions
14%	National Development Team	1980	"
15%	Tibbets	1979	"
33%	Penrose	1938	"
37%	McKeown and Leck	1967	"
40%	Sykes	1977	"
58%	Williams	1971	"
(46%	Corbett	1979	Population Study)

Fig. 7. Mental Illness in the Mentally Retarded

The Bulletin of the Royal College of Psychiatrists (U.K.) in February, 1982, reported an excess of consultants (mental handicap) aged 50-60, and a rise in those from overseas to nearly 40%. The number of unfilled posts rose by 400% between 1970 and 1980 and 25% of all the training posts are presently unfilled. Fig. (8) shows the number of vacant consultant posts, 41 out of 150 in England and Wales, six months ago. Half of these are occupied by locums, generally without appropriate qualifications, and half are not even being advertised.

Specialty	NO.	(Whole Time Equiv.)	Occupied by Locums	NO.	(Whole-Time Equiv.)	Occupied by Locums
Mental Handicap	41	(40)	13.4*	25	(24.5)	6.1*

*Total Locums = 19.5

Fig. 8. Vacant Consultant Posts in England and Wales, September, 1982 (Dept. Health and Security)

(9) is part of a survey recently distributed by the Royal College of Psychiatrists. Thirteen out of the eighteen Regions have less than one consultant per 200,000 population (the recommended minimum), some being grossly in excess of this. Fig.(10) shows the position in England about two months ago, wherein it is seen that the situation is in fact worsening; the regional variations are not readily explained, although there is some North-South bias.

	Consultant Establishment	Population	Population Per Consultant
S.W. Thames R.H.A.	19	2,905,000	152,947
South Western R.H.A.	18	3,025,000	168,278
East Anglia, R.H.A.	11	1,863,000	169,364
Mersey R.H.A.	8	2,458,000	307,250
Oxford R.H.A.	7	2,340,000	334,286
N.W. Thames R.H.A.	10	3,460,000	346,000
Wessex R.H.A.	6	2,740,000	457,334
Yorkshire R.H.A.	7	3,577,000	511,000
North West R.H.A.	7	4,339,000	619,852

Fig. 9. Dept. Health and Social Security, April 1982 (Selected)

REGION	ESTAB	VACANT	OCC BY LOCUM	UNOCC
S.W. THAMES	19	5	2	3
SOUTH WESTERN	18	3	1	2
EAST ANGLIA	11	3	1	2
WEST MIDLANDS	17	6	2	4
MERSEY	8	2	2	0
OXFORD	7	2	1	1
N.W. THAMES	10	0	0	0
TRENT	13	7	3	4
N.E. THAMES	10	4	1	3
NORTHERN	8	3	3	0
S.E. THAMES	9	1	1	0
WESSEX	6	3	2	1
YORKSHIRE	7	5	3	2
NORTH WEST	7	5	1	4
TOTALS	150	49	23	26

Fig. 10. Survey, March, 1983

It is clear that there is some psychiatric retreat in progress. What of training for the future? In "The Future of the Consultant in Psychiatry" (a draft paper from the College of Psychiatrists) the possibility of joint appointments is considered. The questions are asked: "Is the general psychiatrist a viable and useful entity for the future or should most 'generalists' have a special interest? Should the bulk of mental handicap practice be in the hands of 'pure' specialists or of special general interest psychiatrists?" Joint appointments have been practised in many areas (notably in Dundee in Scotland) with some success for some time and it is suggested that they/

they might be encouraged in "Mental Handicap Services - The Future", a recent definitive document from the College of Psychiatrists. Both College documents, incidentally, while acknowledging the value of the multidisciplinary approach, take the view that the ultimate responsibility rests with the consultant.

It does not seem that in the "pure" specialism of mental retardation, specialist training and qualification in psychiatry are required; in one area of England, for example, with a population of $1\frac{1}{2}$ million (North Yorkshire and Humberside) there has been only one substantive consulting psychiatrist with appropriate qualifications, for the past five years. What, then, of the nursing staff?. The new Training Syllabus for the Register of Subnormality Nurses (1982) runs to 70 pages and over 10,000 words, of which the following 0.17% represent the total reference to psychiatric skills; "recognise the signs and symptoms of psychiatric disorders and, with others, enable effective management of the conditions". It is of interest that the parallel syllabus for mental illness nurses (not usually employed for the mentally retarded) only runs to 29 pages, and includes the incidence, causation, training and education of the mentally retarded, and the psychiatry of mental disorder in relation thereto.

There may be a pointer to the future in the curriculum for community nurses (Joint Board of Clinical Nursing Studies, 1982), which prompts the nurse to "identify the psychiatric problems of the patient ....establish therapeutic management programmes ...apply individual and group therapeutic skills......and explain research". As a supporting text-book (Carr, Butterworth and Hodges, 1980) gives headings such as "The Community Nurse as Consultant ....as Clinician... as Therapist", it may be that some off-shore islands of Europe are also subscribing to the notion of "bare-foot doctors", which one may argue, is no bad thing.

It appears that there is a growing gap between the services for the mentally retarded and services of significant psychiatric orientation, which may be leading to the increasing neglect of potential patients in the "grey areas" between. It is significant that a large independent (private) psychiatric hospital in the U.K. (St. Andrews, Northampton) has developed a flourishing behaviour modification unit for the mentally retarded, and MENCAP (the parents organisation) has expressed its concern over the comparative lack of psychiatric facilities for the retarded in the National Health Service to other independent hospitals.

Perhaps the new challenges of the 1980's and onwards may be met by a re-orientation of specialist initiative in the mental handicap field from within general psychiatry, but we should note the comment of the late Professor Penrose; "Some of my general psychiatry colleagues appear to believe that I deal with conditions that are highly contageous!"

PROBLEM CONCERNING THE RELATIONSHIP BETWEEN PARENTS

AND THEIR HANDICAPPED CHILDREN

Andreas Rett

Ludwig Boltzmann-Institut for the
Handicapped Children
Riedelgasse 5, A-1130 Vienna

The societal position of mentally handicapped children
has no doubt improved over the past years. Mainly because of
rapidly progressing causal research that unearthed a variety
of factors related to brain-damages. The causes for many syndromes
known for decades or even centuries were pulled out of the
mystical darf of bygone ages and stripped off their magical
surplus-meaning.

In that way an important complex clouding the parent-child
relationship, namely that of guilt could be cleared out. It
was the question of guilt, its locatiotion and attribution
which presented a problem of existential import for the familiy.

It is known that the most important and decisive event
in the life of the handicapped child and its family is the
first interpretation of a disfunction by a physician. Attitudes
of the parents toward their child are heavily dependent upon
the way they are being informed about possibilities and limitations
for their child and hence for themselves. Nihilism and utopianism
are extremes to be rejected in prinicple. The truth most likely
lies somewhere in the middle. Information for the parents does
not merely entail explanation and diagnosis, but means thorough
information about the physical and mental consequences of the
handicap for the development of the child, his behavior and
social existence.

Clearly, this information has to be conveyed in a form
both understandable and lucid. Further, information does not
end there with the first diagnosis, but in fact has to be added
to, supplemented and enlarged which is a consequence of the

dynamics of development of the handicapped child from infant
via juvenile to adult. Also dynamic is the position of the
parents toward the handicapped child and its problems. Often
we find vast differences between the attitude of mother and
father toward their child. The larger this differences become,
the greater the problems will be, the more uncertain the
educational strategies employed, the more insecure the handicapped
person himself and the more discrepant and changing in his
daily behavior. The sound and the content of the mother's
utterances become worn out, heard by the child much more often
than the father's voice, which leads with the more intensive
physical contact of the mother to an inefficiacy of her educational
measures. The burden on the parents becomes greater. An example
is the fact that about 62 percent of the handicapped children
known to us sleep in the marital bed. The consequences for
the marital community are on the long run serious if not
disastrous. Here we are not only thinking about the sexual
life of the parents but also about their social and human companionship and their needs. As an additional problem we recognise
the aging of the handicapped and of his parents. Observations
of more than 5000 families with handicapped children over a
period of 10 years let us sharply discern how educational and
social activities are slackening, how social isolation is growing
and how the restriction of family life is beginning and increasing.
The relationship of the mentally retarded to his human invirons
is best mapped by a model envisaged as a triangle and published
first in 1960.

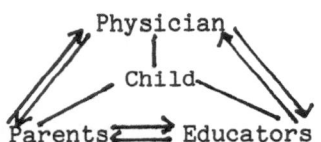

The child is in the center of the triangle and in optimal
circs under the influence of the significant others in his
surrounds: the parents, the educators and the physician. Only
if an equilibrium prevails between the functional areas of
these cornerstones, can the mentally handicapped stay in the
center of attention and care. The balance, however, is quickly
destroyed if one of the three agents alters his relationship
to the child by diminution, enhancement or by moving towards
another direction.

The isosceles triangel becomes a vastly deformed geometrical
shape and the position of the mentally retarded loses its anchoring
and security.

The basic contition for a full and optimal functioning
of the triangle is reciprocal trust among the three agents:
the knowing that the other is always seeking the right and

pursuing the essential course of action. The respective activities have to be properly geared and finely tuned to each other. Questions the parents ask themselves might be e.g., did the physician come up with the correct diagnosis, did he prescribe an optimal therapy, does he care enough for my child? Do teachers, educators, therapists emply all the methods that promis success?

Vice versa the questions become - do the parents follow the advice given by physician and teacher and apply it in practice? Do they understand and do they want to understand what is being said about their child? Today it is clear that the triangle is subject to the influence of a multitude of unknown factors, not only acting presently but extended in time over the years throughout the process of growing-up of the child. A change of physician or teacher often brings about complete reorientation of the force-field of the triangle. We know enough about exhaustion processes between teacher, parents, educators and the child, about fascinating initial successes and their ebbing-out as a function of time and the wear and tear in human relationship. Attrition, of course, is also evident in parent-child relationships and it is the task of the physisican and of the educator to detect it and compensate for it by application of new mehtods. The mentally handicapped grown up and grown old gradually but inevitably reduces his sphere of interests. First the language contacts are being reduced and concomitantly the social contacts.

Sooner or later the question arises whether the handicapped can still be cared for in the fold of his family. The question is often prompted by sickness of the parents, by the loss of one parent or when the behavior of the handicapped becomes unbearable for the family. We know that many aging parents entertain the wish to die after their mentally handicapped offspring. This is understandable knowing that the care for the aged is not everywhere optimally provided for and the parents naturally worry where their child will keep on living.

This surely is a question of utmost importance and we shall have to answer it if we are to live up to our social ideal to better the life of the mentally handicapped. Despite of all modern educational systems, special schools, occupational therapy and financial security for the families affected the mentally handicapped remains a permanent problem for his parents, a sore that never heals.

Gottfried Benn, the reknown German poet aptly wrote:
"Durch jede Stunde, durch jedes Wort
blutet die Wunde der Menschheit fort."

MENTAL HEALTH TREATMENT MODALITIES

FOR THE MENTALLY RETARDED

Jane L. Holtzclaw Bottlinger

Clinical Director of Children and Adolescent Services
University of Nebraska College of Medicine
Omaha, Nebraska 68106

Contemporary literature is replete with information concerned
with the rehabilitation of the mentally retarded and an infinite
fund of knowledge exists regarding the treatment of mental illness
per se. However, little attention has been focused upon the problems and challenges inherent in the treatment of the individual who
possesses the dual diagnosis of mental illness plus mental retardation. The mentally retarded account for roughly three percent of
the population. Available statistics suggest that at least thirty
percent of these individuals suffer from some form of mental illness
compared to an estimated sixteen to twenty percent of the general
population.

Factors which may predispose the mentally retarded to experience
emotional disturbances are important to consider for it is these elements which impart a unique dimension to their treatment needs. So-
ciologically the mentally retarded are more likely to be exposed to
those environmental stressors which are known to precipitate interpsychic turmoil--lower socioeconomic status, rejection by family,
lack of an effective peer group, and paucity of social supports. The
mentally retarded generally exhibit deficiencies in communication
skills with the result that they may experience difficulty in commu-
nicating their needs, feelings, or inner drives in an effective exter-
nalizing mode. The result may often be an excessive internalization
or an inappropriate choice of external expressions. From a psychodynamic point of view the retarded individual is compromised in his
ability to define, integrate, and discharge drives and impulses.
Though basic primitive drives which he experiences are no different
in content or quantity his inability to effectively respond may in
part be due to a diminished repertoire of defensive mechanisms. His
responses are most likely based upon developmentally primitive modes

which are discharged on a concrete operational level. Hence, available defensive mechanisms may not be sufficient to adequately respond to more complex drives. In addition, the retarded individual has fewer outlets for social expression or age appropriate models of interpersonal adaptation. Expressive abilities, (often manifest by delayed language comprehension and expressivity) are often impaired as are abilities to integrate or modulate cognitive, sensory, and motor phenomena--resulting in a personality wherein experiences may be perceived and felt, but can not be adequately externalized and appropriately handled. This may result in an increase in confusion, frustration, and interpsychic discomfort at different developmental epochs. Finally, the ability to sublimate or discharge drives appears to be a function of intelligence which in turn, may directly relate adversely to the expected behaviors in our technologically advanced civilization.

There are a number of additional factors which place the retarded at greater risk for the development of emotional disturbances. These individuals frequently suffer from a multitude of physical or neurological problems resulting not only in a variety of handicaps and illnesses but also in the involvement of a large number of professionals. Parental concern may result in overprotectiveness or rejection and family or peer group expectations may be inappropriate. Feelings of humiliation from failed expectations, fears and anxieties from life's complexities, and a constant push to vocationally and socially achieve all result in additional sources of potentially stressful areas for the retarded individual.

In treating the mentally ill mentally retarded individual one must look not only at the nature of the mental illness per se but also at the limitations which the individual's level of intellectual functioning imposes. Most important however, one must assist the individual in developing appropriate mechanisms by which he may attempt to overcome those variables which initially put him at greatest risk. Enablers of such an end include the following goals:

1. Remediation of identifiable and specifically treatable mental illness (psychosis, endogenous depression, etc.).
2. Stabilization of, and concrete conscious awareness of, physical problems and limitations.
3. Ability to consciously identify feelings and impulses in conjunction with the development of appropriate and socially acceptable means of expression of feelings and emotions.
4. Development of effective peer interactional skills.
5. Comprehension on the part of family mem-

bers as to appropriate expectations.
6. Facilitation of use of community supports.

As a result of the multiplicity of components precipitating and perpetuating mental illness in this group of patients the most effective treatment will be a multidimensional program. A balanced treatment approach will incorporate three principle aspects--medical, psychological, and social-family dimensions followed by extensive follow-up considerations.

The medical treatment of the patient will include treatment of any medical conditions which are present, many of which may not have previously been identified but may in fact be significant factors in the patient's presentation (i.e. treatment of occult hypothyroidism, management, judicious use of psychotropic medication, physical therapy for motoric dysfunction, etc.). In many cases the use of psychotropic medication may be indicated but careful consideration should be given to the assessment of indications before instigation. Medications are most likely to be useful in the treatment of uncontrolled aggression, of behaviors resulting from drastically diminished impulse control, and of excessive anxiety, affective disturbances, or psychotic behavior. The tendency to simply medicate undesirable behaviors should be avoided. Careful consideration must be given to identification and specification of problematic behaviors, intensity, and frequency of behaviors, the presence of absence of identifiable antecedents, the degree to which the behaviors are disruptive and/or disabling, and the degree to which modification of subsequent reinforcers have been effective.

The treatment of the individual with psychotropic medication can be conceptualized as falling into three phases. In Phase I (Induction Phase) medication is introduced and titrated to an effective level--that is, dosage will be adjusted so that target symptoms are alleviated. As a result the individual becomes more available behaviorally and emotionally to participate in the learning process. During Phase II, medication dosage may remain stable or may be decreased as the individual's response to therapeutic interventions facilitates a stabilization of responses. During this phase, the Primary Treatment Phase, there is continued competition between desirable and undesirable behaviors with positive behaviors and emotional responses becoming more predominant as therapy progresses. In Phase III (Maintenance Phase) desirable behaviors replace undesirable behaviors. Medication needs will likely decrease during this phase so that dosage may be titrated downward to the lowest effective maintenance dosage.

Psychological needs of the patient will best be addressed through a variety of modalities including behavioral modification, psychotherapy, family therapy, and development of communication skills. Behavioral modification programs may take a variety of approaches and must be designed to specifically meet the needs of the individual. Important considerations include the use of a highly structured environment where expectations are clearly and concretely defined and where consequences and contingencies can be consistently enforced. Positive reinforcers administered in close proximity to the evaluation of desired behaviors will generally be more productive than negative enforcers. Any program once instigated should be given an adequate trial time as behaviors may initially worsen or the Initiation Phase may be prolonged. Close supervision by interested and empathetic staff is an important element enabling the individual to develop the degree of internal motivation requisite to the success of any program. Psychotherapy should focus on a concrete, goal directed, reality based supportive approach to the individual's problems and interpsychic conflicts. Therapy may take place on an individual basis or in a group format and may be quite instrumental in allowing the individual to develop internal as well as external controls. The development of communication skills is an additional component essential to the psychological development of the individual. For many the need to communicate far outweighs the ability to do so verbally. Hence the development of alternate modes can be vitally important. A variety of alternatives exist depending upon the needs and abilities of the patient and include signs/gestures, communication boards, or the use of drawings.

Family therapy is an important aspect of treatment as it provides a vehicle by which family members may come to better understand the nature of the individual's difficulties, his specific needs (as well as abilities), and ways in which they may most appropriately and effectively meet those needs. In addition family members may be experiencing guilt, confusion, or anger which may compromise their relationship with the patient but which can be alleviated through therapy or information sharing.

Finally, one must focus on the social and educational dimension of the patient's treatment. The notion that the mentally retarded individual is incapable of learning promotes a grave disservice. However, impaired intellectual functioning, diminished self concept, and an enhanced potential for psychological disorganization when stressed may be significant obstacles to acceptable vocational performance. Education should focus upon the attainment of those skills which will allow the individual to function maximally within the community as well as upon those learned behavioral responses which will help him function more appropriately under stress. Survival skills and appropriate vocational training will enable the individual to function more effectively within the community and will serve to increase his sense of self esteem. In many cases residential alternatives may need to be considered. The mentally ill mentally retarded individual will generally function most effectively in a structured, predictable, supervised environment. Independent living may not be viable and residing at home may place excessive stress upon the family unit. Alternatives such as intermittent respite care or group home living may provide environments which most appropriately meet the individual's needs. Hospitalization may be necessary when the degree of emotional disturbance or behavioral impairment is severe enough to mitigate against less restrictive options. Social skills training as well as active involvement in recreational pursuits will enhance the individual's ability to relate effectively to peers and authority figures. Community resources should be tapped in regards to available support systems for patient or family, vocational opportunities, recreational resources, and residential options.

Vitally important to the successful treatment of the mentally ill mentally retarded individual is the provision of ongoing follow-up. The individual as he responds to treatment will require continued support, encouragement, and reinforcement in order to maintain and adapt behaviors and responses learned in one environment to a variety of situations and experiences. Without such support the individual would be at risk to find himself facing an experience with which he would be unable to cope and which might subsequently precipitate a return to pretreatment behavioral and emotional responses.

In summary, the treatment of the mentally ill - mentally retarded individual, though complex and multidimensional in nature, is always a major challenge for the psychiatrist. To be effective, therapy must focus not only on the patient's emotional needs but also on his concurrent medical, social, family, educational, and vocational needs. Treatment and management goals include the development of learned behavioral responses as a means of diminishing neurotic conflict, the realization of realistic goals and expectations on the part of the patient and family, and the mobilization of community support systems to further facilitate the individual's emotional development.

REFERENCES

Group for the Advancement of Psychiatry, 1979.
    Psychiatric Consultation in Mental Retardation.
    Mental Health Center, Washington D.C.
Lipman, R.S. 1970. The use of psychopharmacological agents in
    residential facilities for the retarded. In: F.J. Menolascino,
    (ed.), Psychiatric Approaches to Mental Retardation. pp. 387-398.
    Basic Books, New York.
Lott, G. 1970. Psychotherapy of the mentally retarded. In F.J.
    Menolascino, (ed.), Psychiatric Approaches to Mental Retardation.
    Basic Books, New York.
Menolascino, F.J. 1977. Challenges in Mental Retardation: Progres-
    sive Ideology and Services. Human Sciences Press, New York.
Mental Health and Mental Retardation: Bridging the Gap, Edited by
    F.J. Menolascino and B.M. McCann. Baltimore: University Park
    Press, 1983.
Perry, M.A., and Cerreto, M.C. 1977. Structured learning training

of social skills for the retarded. Ment. Retard. 15:31–34.

Rivinus, T.M. 1980. Psychopharmacology and the mentally retarded
    patient. In: L.S. Szymanski and P.E. Tanquay (eds.), Emotional
    Disorders of Mentally Retarded Persons. University Park Press,
    Baltimore.

Roos, P. The Handling and Mishandling of Parents of Mentally Retarded
    Persons. In (above). 83–115.

Scanlon, P.L. 1978. Social Work with mentally retarded client.
    Social Casework, 59:161–166.

Serrano, A. 1979. A Child-centered family interview. In: J. Noshpitz
    (ed.), Basic Handbook of Child Psychiatry, Vol. I. Basic Books,
    New York.

Szymanski, L., and Tanquay, F. (eds.), 1980. Emotional Disorders
    of Mentally Retarded Persons. University Park Press, Baltimore.

AN ADAPTIVE HANDICAP: BORDERLINE PERSONALITY DISORDER IN THE MENTALLY IMPAIRED

Richard L. Rubin

University of Miami School of Medicine
Suite 202, 7741 S.W. 62 Avenue
Miami, Florida 33143

This paper continues from previous work on applying individual psychotherapy to people underserved because of mental retardation handicap (Rubin, 1983). There I broadly reviewed modern definitions of mental disorder, current issues in developmental disabilities, and applications of counseling and psychotherapy with the retarded. Specific approaches for choosing methods, selecting patients, and pursuing treatment techniques were examined. A systems approach to collaboration with family and the primary handicap program was emphasized as necessary for effective individual treatment. I will present here a more specific view of psychodynamic factors that contribute to borderline personality disorder and produce need for psychotherapy treatment. The general term mental handicap is used to encompass both intellectual impairment and organic dysfunction, and to include severe learning disabilities (previously called borderline retardation) as well as DSM-III mental retardation.

A Modern Approach to Psychodynamic Issues

The term psychodynamic is based in the traditional concept that normal and pathological human behavior can result from interacting and opposing forces. Both innate and environmental factors affect development of personality structure; the resulting structure becomes the agency for continuing management of these forces (American Psychoanalytic Assoc., 1968). The study and application of psychodynamics in the mentally handicapped have suffered from clinicians' emphasis on the cognitive deficits and organicity. However, the modern concept of adaptive functioning provides a basis for integrating cognitive and organic problems with personality development and psychotherapy. Adaptive functioning is defined by the American Association on Mental Deficiency as "the effectiveness of an

227

individual in coping with the natural and social demands of the environment." An adaptive assessment has become increasingly important in evaluation and therapy with the mentally handicapped. Skills and deficits are described relative to age norms from a diverse handicapped population. Going beyond IQ, it is now a necessary criterion for retardation diagnosis in DSM-III. An adaptive approach draws added value from its direct application to modern normalization goals that handicapped people develop the skills necessary for successful home and community life (Knapp and Salend, 1983). This view of adaptive functioning is consistent with psychodynamic concepts. The American Psychoanalytic Association (1968) defined adaptation similarly, as "the capacity to cope reasonably, yet advantageously, by intrapsychic changes or by modifications in the environment through activity." To love and work seems similar to coping with natural and social demands.

Recent research does not support the exclusive role of organic factors for determining development and psychopathology in the mentally handicapped. Michael Rutter's (1981) studies are showing that organic injury and deficit contribute much less than believed to specific psychiatric disorders and syndromes. Adverse perinatal events also seem less influential. The stability of mother - child interaction can be more powerful in early childhood disorders when organic trauma has occurred (Hertzig, 1983). Similarily, it is becoming more difficult to consider mental handicaps as static. Cognitive reorganization with improved concept formation and symbol use has been observed in severely learning disabled children (Smith and Phillips, 1981). Both internal developmental events and environment variables such as the quality of family care and education are critical factors.

While organic characteristics appear less controlling, psychodynamic forces may now be more important as handicapped children are growing up in different circumstances from the past. The degree and quality of their developmental opportunities are markedly improved. The last three decades' progress with individual rights, the deinstitutionalization movement, the expansion of community school and living programs, and the changing goals of families toward home parenting have created an environment of greater human interaction and complexity for mentally impaired children. Psychodynamic thinking was influential in promoting these changes. The work of Spitz and Bowlby exposed the personality damage from institutional deprivation and parenting loss. Modern family living produces potential for greater personality growth, but may also increase the incidence of certain dynamic psychological disorders. Study and documentation of these psychodynamic changes are not available in the literature.

Borderline Personality Syndrome

Opportunity for study of such psychodynamic effects is presented by the interaction of mental handicap problems with ego development. Modern concepts of the borderline personality and self psychology provide an example of such interaction.

The association of borderline personality disorder and organic impairment has received recent attention. In a descriptive diagnostic study using DSM-III criteria, Andrulonis et al (1980) distinguished three sub-groups among 91 hospitalized borderline children, adolescents, and adults: non-organic, major organic (brain trauma, encephalitis, epilepsy), and minimal organic (ADD, LD). The combined organics made 39% of the total sample. Minimal organics tended to show severe adaptive problems earliest, at about age 8. The major organics had onset of severe psychiatric problems at around age 13 and the non-organics at age 15. Childhood adaptive problems were important in bringing the organic patients to psychiatric attention.

In their effort to clarify criteria for borderline personality syndromes in children, Bemporad et al (1982) described extreme fluctuations of adaptive functioning interfering with all life areas, pervasive and severe anxiety, distortions in thought content and process, markedly disturbed relationships, and poor impulse control. Some degree of cognitive or neurologic abnormality was found in two-thirds of their 24 cases. Interpersonal and environmental factors were also prominant, particularly family history of abuse, neglect, bizarre parent behavior, or inconsistent care. Bemporad inferred a multifactor borderline etiology including organicity deprivation of early socialization, and chronic exposure to an inconsistent or chaotic environment.

Data on the relationship between borderline personality and mental retardation is difficult to find. Eaton and Menolascino's (1982) comprehensive study of psychopathology in a community population found similar types of disorder as in the non-retarded. Although previously regarded as rare, neurotic and personality disorders appeared common, particularly in the higher intelligence levels. In the borderline and mild retardation ranges, 44% of the psychiatric diagnoses were neurotic or personality disorders, while only 17% among the moderate and 8% among the severely retarded. Although the borderline personality syndrome was not specifically identified because DSM-III format was used, the four cases of emotionally unstable personality suggest a borderline diagnosis. These figures present several psychodynamic implications. First, the higher functioning retarded may have the intrapsychic capacity to develop the defensive operations and ego patterns of both health and disorder. Secondly, as similar to the general population, such neurotic and personality disorders may include psychodynamic factors, in addition to cognitive deficiency and organic dysfunction. Third, comparison of the mildly retarded to borderline personality syndrome patients with other forms of organic and cognitive disorder appears justified.

Psychodynamic Etiologic Factors

This mentally handicapped group - including the mild MR, organic LD, MBD, ADD, and other impaired - is at high risk for the major psychodynamic causes of borderline personality as described by modern American self psychology. The first is ego abnormality in self and object relations. The infant with organic disorder often has a disturbance in neurophysiologic state, either irritable or apathetic (Chethik, 1979). These characteristics disrupt and diminish the child's experience of comforting by parent care. As a result, the self begins with more intense impressions of dysphoria and uncertainty. In the toddler, these neurophysiologic dysfunctions become more specific as deficits in perception, attention, and memory. Paulina Kernberg (1982) has described their effects on ego development as impairment of the internal mental representations of self and others. Whatever the objective quality of parent care, the organic dysfunctions can cause distortions, disturbance, or deficiencies in the child's subjective experience of self and other. Otto Kernberg (1975) places the developmental failure in borderlines at the transition from primary narcissism to involvement with people in the outside world of reality. Personality arrest and pathological defenses pull the child to maintain an inner world of immature self-gratification to ameliorate the early painful experiences. Concurrently, the perception and memory deficits of the mental handicap can foster the developmental fixation. The child will have problems discriminating gratifying situations in the real world, adding to the sense of deprivation and frustration.

The mental handicap also predisposes to borderline ego abnormalities by interfering with active efforts of the child for influencing the environment. The irritable or apathetic infant has decreased deliberate and effective efforts at self-gratification from the object world, such as reaching and smiling. Normally, in addition to intraphysic changes such as defense development, the ego fulfills the task of adaptation by modifications in the environment through activity, not just passive adjustment (American Psychoanalytic, 1968). The success of such actions contributes to stable and satisfying introjects of the self and object world. The combined interaction of these handicap and psychodynamic development forces can result in the borderline personality syndrome with fragile ego structure, distorted sense of self, pathological relationships with others, and primitive defensive operations, such as projection, devaluation, splitting, omnipotence, and denial (P. Kernberg, 1982). Measured in adaptive terms, the resulting deficits in age appropriate functioning can be substantial.

The second psychodynamic cause of the borderline personality syndrome is exposure to impaired parenting at critical phases of ego development. The literature on this has been extensive. Mahler (1975) concluded that borderline formation results from failed resolution of the rapprochement sub-phase of separation-individuation occurring between 16 and 24 months. Usually the abnormal care is attributed to the mother's pre-existing pathology. However, an organically impaired child may distort a good enough mother's efforts. Medical illnesses, feeding disorders, sleep disturbance, irritable resistance to soothing, and apathetic unresponsiveness to smiles and play can provoke parent feelings of anger and loss with harmful effects on relating with the child. Because these children often otherwise appear fine and are not identified early as dysfunctional, parents can respond with anxiety and guilt, leading to depressive and obsessive compulsive reactions. If the child is more visibly handicapped or medically involved, other dynamics will operate, such as shock to value expectations and stresses of extensive reality demands. Parent reactions of affective neglect, angry abuse, and infantilization are possible and common under these circumstances. Even without parent psychopathology or harmful emotional reactions, most good enough mothers are severely challenged by the mentally handicapped child's variable, resistant, and disguised needs. These abnormal interactions between the handicapped child and mother can interfere with resolution of the autonomy and independence issues central to the rapprochment phase. Resulting helplessness and dependence cause adaptive deficits. In addition, these can be misinterpreted as due only to the mental handicap. Consequently, a lower level of expectation will be set for the child, with continuation of the fixation in personality development.

Clinical Cases

The form of psychiatric presentation for borderline personality problems in the mentally handicapped requires study. My current experience suggests that among children raised at home, demand in adolescence for greater autonomy and independence can exacerbate borderline problems. The following illustration cases were both raised in stable, upper middle class urban families.

A 16 year old girl was referred for increasing anger at parents, agitated episodes, jealousy of siblings, and nocturnal fears. Having attended a residential school since age 15 because her parents sought improved independence skills, these problems were most intense on vacations home. She had a persistent belief that her parents would never allow her to return home. She resisted school and community program efforts towards adaptive improvement, often denying her handicap. Attempts to childishly please her parents in an overdependent, merging fashion alternated with defiant, omnipotent threats to sign out of school at age 18. She often expressed devaluation of herself and others, including family, peers, and adults at school. Labile emotion problems, separation fears, and unstable relationships had been present episodically lifelong. Her mental handicap had unknown etiology; "MBD and probably mild retardation" were diagnosed at age 3. IQ at age 15 was 53. A Rorschach showed some thought disorder signs and much subjective turmoil, but not full psychosis. The AAMD Adaptive Behavior Scale revealed an average of 58th percentile skills on part one and 78th percentile severity of behavior problems on part two, suggesting the psychiatric disorder was decreasing her level of functioning.

A 21 year old young woman was brought by her parents for increasing emotional outbursts characterized by anger at herself as well as others, intense but vague fears of harm, hitting herself, and psychotic thinking with a duration of episodes up to 30 minutes. These were always precipitated by criticisms or performance expectations from others, occurring with family, peers, and other adults. Crucial current developmental stresses were imposed by her graduation from high school special education program and parents' increasing anxiety over her lack of independent abilities "up to her potential." For ten years at least, her level of anxiety had been high with low frustration tolerance, impulsivity, fears of failure and rejection, and shifting levels of adaptive functioning in both home and community activities. At present, she attempted to minimize her handicap and ambivalently considered fantasies such as that Burt Reynolds might help her learn to be an actress. A psychotic diagnosis was not evident on this or previous evaluations. Her mental handicap resulted from encephalitis at age 4 months with several days' coma and severe developmental sequelae. Partial motor seizures were active until age 6; she was off anticonvulsants by age 8, and EEG's have subsequently been normal. Efforts to habilitate her motor and language functions were intensive over several years with significant disruption of relationships with parents. Weschler IQ at age 19 was 78. At age 21, her AAMD Adaptive Scale part one (skills) averaged 68th percentile, below expectations from her IQ and the quality of her education and training program. On part two (behavior problems), she averaged at the 76th percentile, with four scales over the 90th percentile of severity, clearly in the psychopathological range.

Conclusion

This paper has explored the role of certain psychodynamic factors in personality development of the mentally handicapped. This is warranted by new psychiatric knowledge of mental disorder, changing circumstances of family and community living opportunities, and new approaches in ego psychology. The next step is study of psychotherapy approaches to these psychodynamic factors and borderline processes. Goals of cure for the ego structure problems seem unrealistic. Masterson (1981) found organic impairment a poor prognostic factor in his intensive psychoanalytic program with borderline adolescents. More appropriately, work might focus on the three psychodynamic etiologic factors that operate after the organically vulnerable infant has begun to internalize distorted perceptions of others. These are 1) early childhood-mother interaction disturbances, 2) stresses at later developmental stages, and 3) family and environmental obstacles to personality growth and corrective development. The handicap and its adaptive consequences will continue present and limit complete change in ego deficits. At best, the handicap can be "objectified" and managed by more realistic and adaptive psychological process (P. Kernberg, 1982).

REFERENCES

American Association on Mental Deficienty (1975), <u>Adaptive Behavior Scale Manual</u>, Washington, D.C.

American Psychoanalytic Association (1968), <u>Glossary of Psychoanalytic Terms and Concepts</u>, New York.

Andrulonis, Paul et al. (1980), Organic Brian Dysfunction and the Borderline Syndrome. Psychiatr. Clin. No. Am., 4:1.

Bemporad, Jules et al (1982), Borderline Syndromes in Childhood: Criteria for Diagnosis, Am. Jnl. Psychiatry, 139:5.

Chethik, Morton (1979), The Borderline Child, in J. Nosphitz ed., <u>Basic Handbook on Child Psychiatry</u>, Vol. II, Basic Books, New York.

Eaton, Louise and Frank Menolascino (1982), Psychiatric Disorder in the Mentally Retarded: Types, Problems, and Challenges, Am. Jnl. Psychiatry, 139:10.

Kernberg, Otto (1975), <u>Borderline Conditions and Pathological Narcissism</u>, Jason Aronson, New York.

Knapp, Samuel and Spencer Salend (1983), Adapting the Adaptive Behavior Scale, Mental Retardation, 21:2.

Mahler, Margaret, F. Paine, A. Bergman (1975), <u>The Psychological Birth of the Human Infant</u>, Basic Books, New York.

Masterson, James (1981), Review of Borderline Adolescent Treatment, Central States Conference, Am. Soc. Adolescent Psychiatry, Galveston.

Rubin, Richard (1983), Bridging the Gap thru Individual Counseling and Psychotherapy, in F. Menolascino and B. McCann eds., <u>Mental Health and Mental Retardation: Bridging the Gap</u>, Univ. Park Press, Baltimore.

Rutter, Michael (1981). Psychologic Sequelae of Brain Damage in Children, Am. Jnl. Psychiatry, 138:12.

Smith, Beryl and C.J. Phillips (1981), Age-Related Progress Among Children with Severe Learning Disabilities, Devel. Med. Child Neurol., 23: 465-76

COMMUNITY BASED PROGRAMS FOR THE MENTALLY RETARDED

Akihiko Takahashi

Aichi Prefectural Colony
Kasugai, Aichi 480-03
Japan

TYPES OF COMMUNITY CARE

Two examples of the community plan in Japan are presented showing differences in their program development and quality of services. Actually, there are many different types of practice in the community plan, but if one takes typical examples among them, there seems to be two kinds of program. The first is a pre-designed system of service program provided with detection, diagnosis and treatment services. Those services are integrated consistently into a system. The second is a group of multiphasic and multidisciplinary services each of which was developed as a counter-measure for particular need in the community. Services of this type are administered by existing resources in the community, and are co-related with each other.

Typical example of the first type is seen in Zushi city in Kanagawa Prefecture. In 1973, a public children's medical center in Yokohama city, which is located about 30 kilometers apart from Zushi, started an experimental study in order to establish a model system for effective detection of congenital anomalies and for improving maternal and child health care program. They selected Zushi as an experimental field of study. The system was planned and developed by Dr. I. Matsui and his co-workers and was called as "the Zushi Model".

The aim of this model was "to collect all information concerning health and diseases of pregnant mothers, neonates and children under school age, to find any high-risk group among them, to follow up mothers and children at high-risk, and to provide proper care for handicaps."

This experimental project is a typical example of "Pre-designed system". Previously, there were many different services function-

ing independently in Zushi city. Under this project, those existing services were re-examined and integrated into single service
system which has the aim as mentioned above. (Fig. 1.)
     Presumed reasons for the success in this system-developing
project are;
(1) to have children's medical center backing up the system as being the secondary or tertail care center,
(2) to have relatively limited size of the city in terms of population and area,
(3) to have active and enthusiastic work of Public Health Nurses
since many year in advance, and
(4) to have citizen of higher cultural and intellectual standard.
     Matsui and Kato, active members of the project, proposed an
evaluation scale to examine the level of systematization of maternal
and child health care program in the community as shown in Fig. 2.
According to this scale, total surveillance of pregnancy, and detection and follow-up of all pregnancy at high-risk composes Unit I,
total surveillance of live-birht infant, and dectection and follow-
up of all infants at high-risk composes Unit II-A, and supportive
service programs compose Unit III. When those three Units will be
established and linked in line, a system will have been completed.
The Zushi Model, being provided with Unit I, II and III, can be
taken as a good example of the complete system.
     An example of the second type of service program can be seen
in the Community Plan of Higashimurayama city in Tokyo Metropolis.
(Fig. 1) There are neither general hospital nor university in the
city. A national neuropsychiatric hospital and a public children's
hospital located in an adjacent city are serving as tertial treatment center for this area.
     The first movement for the care of retarded children in the
city was initiated in 1962 when several mothers wanted to have
special class in public school for their retarded children. This
demand was well taken by local Board of Education, and officers
in charge cooperated with local professional people to open first
special class for retarded children in a public school.
     This was the first experience of citizen movements which has
been settled as the basic pattern of movement for community care
program after that. The patter is that parents ask for particular
service for their child, then professionals make it into realizable
needs and plan countermeasures to be developed, and city administrators develop new service under the cooperation of parents and
professionals.
     Several services have been improved and started since then
such as maternal and child care program, diagnostic and treatment
clinic for preschool children in general, counseling service for
mothers at the same clinic, nursery care for handicapped preschool
children, technical advice to nursieries accepting handicapped
children, day-care center for preschool children, special education
programs, workshop for yound retarded adults and group home for
retarded adults. Those services are mainly carried on by local

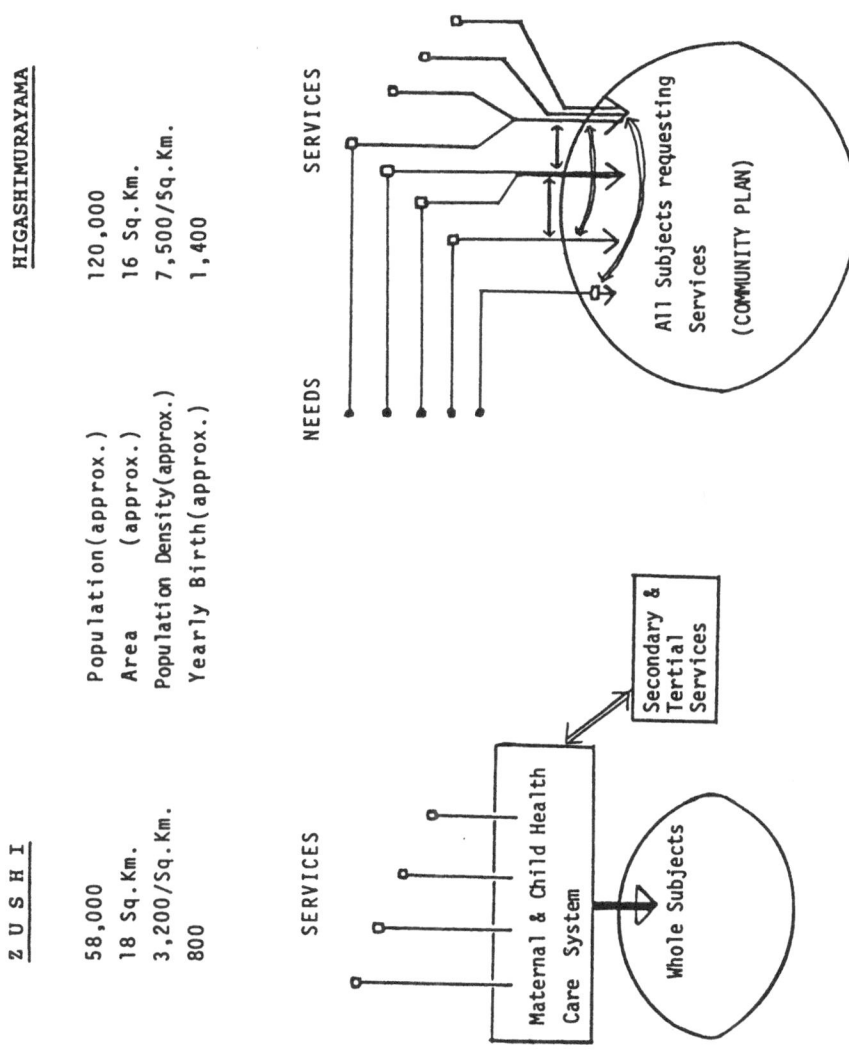

HIGASHIMURAYAMA

Population(approx.)	120,000	
Area (approx.)	16 Sq.Km.	
Population Density(approx.)	7,500/Sq.Km.	
Yearly Birth(approx.)	1,400	

Z U S H I

58,000		
18 Sq.Km.		
3,200/Sq.Km.		
800		

SERVICES

NEEDS SERVICES

All Subjects requesting Services
(COMMUNITY PLAN)

Secondary & Tertial Services

Maternal & Child Health Care System

Whole Subjects

Fig. 1 Programs in Zushi and Higashimurayama

237

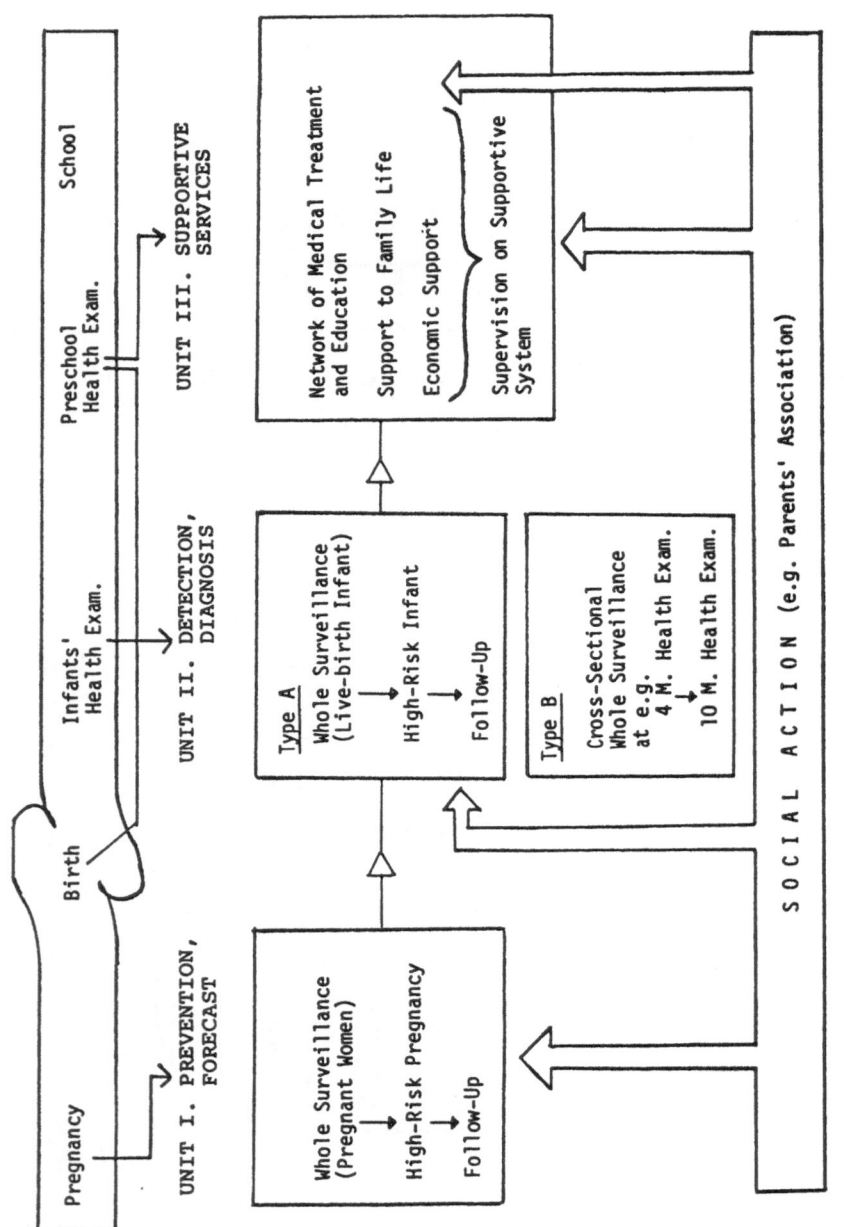

Fig. 2   Evaluation scale of health care program

(I.Matsui & H.Kato, 1982)

manpower. Services are loosely connected with each other, and not integrated yet. In short, service system in Higashimurayama is multiphasic and multidisciplinary and this system contains functions of the Unit III of Matsui's scale. Presently, what is going on concerning early detection of handicapping conditions in the city is that majority of cases with handicap are first mentioned their abnormality by either family or medical clinics, and infant's health examination is playing relatively small part. Then, the next goal of the Higashimurayama Plan will be to reach the level of the Unit II-B regarding case finding function.

DISCUSSION

It is widely supported by specialists involved in the community care program in Japan that whole surveillance of pregnancy and live-birth and the follow-up service of high-risk group must be the best way for early detection and intervention instead of focussing on picking up cases with the mark of handicap among general population. Zushi Model has realized this principle in the field. This system is fundamentally health-oriented in its nature since it was originated from health care program. It seems to have some connection with a difficulty within the system mentioned below.

Although the Zushi Model is superior compared with any other types of program, there are some deficits with it as follows;
(1) Risk-factors taken in this system are basically of medical, health oriented in nature. Degree of caseness of high-risk case in this system, therefore, may not always coincide with degree of worry on the side of parents. Parents usually worry about daily problems which may not be so serious from medical point of view. This kind of discrepancy in the judgment on seriousness of porblem between professional examiner and parents may cause disharmonious relationship between the two. This gap should be taken to be very important and way to bridge it must be studied.
(2) Primarily, this system has been planned by a group of professional people and is operated as a part of municipal administration. This fact easily leads to such a situation that citizen under the system sees it as being given by someone else, that is, municipal authority, and they remain as merely a passive recipient of service of the system. Under such circumstances, parents hardly can participate themselves actively in the operation of the system. Moreover, general public who are screened out by screening of the system shows less interests in this business. Thus, the system may be in danger of being isolated from generic service network and of being apart from citizen consumer.

Contrary, in the Higashimurayama Plan, parents of retarded child are actively involved in the program. Parents' association digs up needs of retarded people and their family, and professionals and administrators work together to develop services to meet the needs. In the program, parents also play an important role of giving support and adviceto other family with handicapped children. In doing this, parents are no longer a passive recipient of services but are a service provider for other client and take part in citizen advocacy services. This makes parents of retarded child possible to go on the main stream of the community. However, Higashimurayama Plan has several deficits in it as follows;

(1) As for the level of systematization and specialization, this plan is still at the stage of early development. It lacks the Unit I program in the evaluation scale of Matsui, and has primitive form of the Unit II-B.

(2) Program corresponding the Unit III has multiphasic activities, but those services are not well integrated yet. Therefore, quality of services are relatively low.

(3) There are some difficulties in the process of formation of needs through direct demands and requirements from parents of retarded children, and in setting priority among different needs. The program needs to have coordinating function such as liaison person proposed by Coda, or expeditor or case manager of Scheerenberger, or key-person of Takahashi.

CONCLUSION

Through my observation of several community programs, it is found that the level of systematization of efficiency of program seems to be in reverse correlationship with the range and extent of participation of people in the area regardless of being handicapped or non-handicapped; that is, to what extent the program is community-based.

Final aim of our study is to establish system with high quality of service which is carried on not only by limited number of professional people but also by the community itself, that is, people in the community. It must be a real "community-based" service program.

240

MENTAL HEALTH SERVICES TO COMMUNITY-BASED RETARDED CITIZENS

W. H. Lo and T. Lo

Mental Health Service
Hong Kong

Before World War II mental health services to the mentally retarded were virtually non-existent in Hong Kong and the task of caring for them remained the sole responsibility and burden of family members, (1). The latter tended to conceal their problems to avoid stigma and shame and confined the retarded at home segregating them from the rest of society.

In 1960 special education emerged as a separate service within the Education Department the expansion of which has been outlined by Rowe, (2). In 1964 a school for the mentally handicapped together with a speech and hearing centre was first established, followed later by a programme of screening and provision of special classes for slow-learners in ordinary schools. The Social Welfare Department opened the first rehabilitation centre in 1962 and another in 1963 and later day-centres, boarding centres, sheltered workshops and social clubs. In addition a job placement unit for the disabled was set up.

Until very recently rehabilitation services for the mentally retarded were provided in a tripartite system with the Medical and Health Department catering for the severely retarded, the Social Welfare Department for the moderately retarded and the Education Department for the mildly retarded. However, this system was not so well integrated at working levels and in 1977 a Rehabilitation Development Co-ordinating Committee was formed to integrate inter-departmental multidisciplinary activities. Since 1979 education and training of all grades of the retarded have been centralised under the Education Department. This is in line with the U.K. system where no child is regarded as 'ineducable' or 'unsuitable for education in school since 1971, (3).

Prevalence of Mental Retardation and the Central Registry for the Disabled

The 1976 By-Census found that the mentally retarded constitute 1.66% of the population. The figure can be broken down into broad age groups as appear in Table I. However, this is thought to be an underestimate and for planning purposes the prevalence rate taken is shown in Table II. The Central Registry for the Disabled was established in 1981. It will help arrive at a more reliable figure in due course. This is important not only for planning resources and providing data for further research but also to enable a better co-ordination of rehabilitation services and avoid their duplication to clients.

Table I.   Age Group Distribution of Mentally Handicapped in Hong Kong - By-Census 1976

0 - 9	20.9%
10 - 19	52.2%
20 - 29	20.4%
30 - 39	3.4%
40 - 49	2.2%
50 - 59	0.6%
60 and over	0.3%

Table II.   Prevalence Rates of Mental Retardation Adopted for Planning Purposes

Mental Retardates	Age Bracket	Prevalance Rate (per 10,000)	Estimated Population
Severely Handicapped	0-39 40 and over	10.00) 0.40)	3,000
Moderately Handicapped	All ages	40.00	19,000
Mildly Handicapped	All ages	150.00	71,000
All Grades	All ages	200.40	93,000

Prevention and Early Detection of Mental Retardation

Genetic counselling service - This was established in 1981. Apart from providing genetic counselling to families at risk it has a cytogenetic laboratory as a back-up service, maintains a local chromosome register and stores relevant information.

Prenatal diagnostic service - This was also established in 1981. It provides special monitoring for infants with special risks of developing disabling conditions to ensure that congenital or acquired defects are detected and remedial action taken early e.g. hypothyroidism and G6PD deficiency.

242

It must be pointed out that these services are rudimentary at present. More emphasis is placed on improving skills for diagnostic procedures, training doctors and technicians and collecting as much information as possible on the incidence of various genetic diseases and abnormalities in Hong Kong.

Comprehensive observation scheme - This was introduced in 1978. It provides routine observation for all infants from birth to age 5, especially for those considered to be at greater risk. The main objective is to ensure that all congenital or acquired defects are discovered, and remedial action taken as early as possible so that the chances of restoring full function can be maximised. The observation is done by specially trained nurses at all family health centres.

Multi-disciplinary assessment clinic - The first child assessment clinic was opened in 1977. It carries out comprehensive tests on at risk children from birth to age 12. The multidisciplinary team consists of paediatricians, clinical psychologists and social workers. Referrals are made to child psychiatrists when required.

However, as children grow older reassessment in social, educational and vocational aspects become important. For retardates who are attending either special schools or resource/special classes in ordinary schools they go through periodic assessments built into their educational programmes. For retarded adolescents and adults attending day centres, boarding centres, vocational training centres and sheltered workshops, they are regularly reassessed with regard to their mental state, social and vocational capacities and suitability for employment as well as any special need for treatment of associated physical or mental illness.

Special Care, Education and Training

Pre-school care - Places are available for mildly handicapped children in ordinary pre-school centres promoting their integration with ordinary children in a normal setting. Other places are in special centres for more severely handicapped children providing general child care and special training and day-time relief for working mothers.

Autistic children's unit - There are 3 children's units for day care and treatment of retarded children with autistic features. The units are situated in mental health centres and are served by a team of speciality trained staff.

Group testing programmes - These are now done in Primary I Primary III school children. Of the lowest rated 10% of P. I and 10% of P. 3 pupils 6% and 30% respectively are found to be handicapped. They are referred to the psychological services for schools.

Psychological services for schools – The main functions of such services are to provide diagnostic and remedial measures for retarded children as well as those with behaviour and emotional problems and to give advice and guidance to both parents and teachers.

Special Education Section – Educational psychologists of the Special Education Section, apart from giving psychological assessments to children referred from various sources are also required to provide psychological services to children attending special schools and special classes as follows, (4).

(a) reassessment such as diagnostic educational assessment of children who are not functioning at their expected level or those having specific weakness which affects their learning;

(b) review of the educational programme of the individual child in accordance with individual developmental needs to ensure that educational programmes are properly tailored to suit different cognitive development patterns;

(c) treatment of children with behaviour problems involving the formulation and administration of treatment programmes for emotionally disturbed children who continue to exhibit adjustment and behaviour difficulties even in a small group situation; and

(d) advice to teachers on treatment plans and educational progress.

General and technical education – It is the Government's policy to provide all handicapped children with 9 years of free education and some will receive a longer period of such education. The mildly handicapped are encouraged to attend ordinary schools where resource/special classes are provided for them. The more severely retarded who cannot benefit in the ordinary education system are placed in special schools for the retarded. Vocational training will be provided beyond normal school learning age, to help them to achieve their potential.

Psychiatric Treatment and Rehabilitation

There are 4 mental health centres and 3 psychiatric units which offer a wide range of psychiatric treatment and rehabilitation services including counselling and medical social service, occupational therapy, industrial therapy and recreation. They are easily accessible to the community-based retarded citizens in various districts. Any associated mental illness or behaviour problems can be dealt with there.

Work Activities Centres

It is presumed in this paper that community-based services exclude institutional care. Therefore, hospital care for the severely retarded has not been mentioned. However, some moderately retarded school learners who may not benefit from vocational training or open or sheltered employment are provided with day care in work activities centres. The aim is to make them more independent in their daily life and to improve their basic skills. The programme contains daily living skills, social training including recreational and group activities and training in work habits and manual dexterity with simple work tasks. Some of the severely retarded may, if capable, attend such centre as well.

Social and Recreational Activities

Retarded persons have the same need for social life and recreation as normal persons. Indeed, their needs for organized activities are greater as they require extra stimulation to achieve their full potentials and they are less capable of arranging such activities themselves. By having such activities they are in a better position to enter meaningful group relationship.

Transport

The majority of severely retarded and some moderately retarded have serious mobility problems and transport facilities are provided for them to attend day programme of one kind or another.

Other Services

Apart from the Government departments a number of voluntary agencies are providing various services for the retarded and their families including counselling, home help, home nursing, day care centres, residential accommodation, transport, sports and recreations. The Association for Mentally Handicapped Children and Young Persons is among the most active agencies in this respect.

The Labour Department undertakes to place the disabled in open employment and to those who are severely handicapped a disability allowance is given.

The Parents Association for the Mentally Handicapped provides opportunities for parents to maintain frequent constant and mutual support to exchange ideas and discuss problems.

Even now facilities and services for the retarded are far from adequate to meet the demand but efforts by all concerned will significantly reduce the shortfalls in the coming decade.

A flow chart of screening assessment, treatment, training and placements is shown in Table III.

Table III. Flow Chart of Screening, Assessment, Treatment, Training and Placement

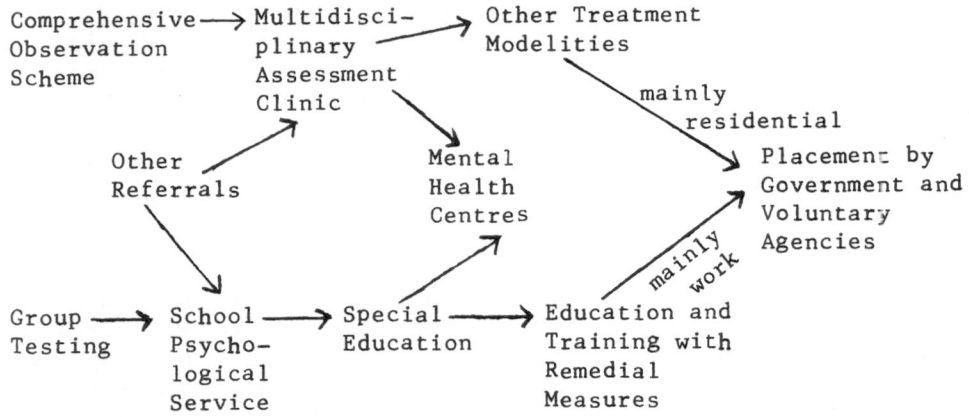

Summary

Integrated planning and orderly development for the mentally retarded were formulated for the first time in a Ten-year Rehabilitation Programme Plan for the Disabled in 1976. This is reviewed annually by the policy makers. As a result of co-ordinated efforts by all concerned significant achievements have emerged in the recent few years though facilities and services for the retarded are far from being adequate to cope with the demand. Nevertheless, essential areas covering their needs have been laid down and substantial expansion is expected in the coming decade.

REFERENCES

1. Lo, W. H., and Kwok, I., 1981, "History of Psychiatry in Hong Kong," Journal of the Hong Kong Psychiatric Association, vol. I, p. 14-17.
2. Rowe, E., 1971, "Special Education in Hong Kong" in Aspects of Mental Health in Hong Kong (ed. W. H. Lo). Published by the Mental Health Association of Hong Kong.
3. Mittler, P., 1975, "Education of the Mentally Handicapped" in Contemporary Psychiatry (ed. T. Silperstone and B. Barraclough) Headley Brothers Ltd.
4. Social Services Branch - "Identification and Assessment Services" in 1981 Review of Rehabilitation Programme.

ISSUES AND DAY TREATMENT
FOR THE DUAL DIAGNOSED:
MENTAL ILLNESS/MENTAL RETARDATION

Robert J. Fletcher

Beacon House
110 Prince Street
Kingston, N.Y. 12401

INTRODUCTION

The mentally retarded represent a high risk population for developing a wide range of mental and personality
disturbances as demonstrated by Eaton and Menolascino
(1982). Even in light of this vulnerability, the mental
health needs of the mentally retarded have historically
received inadequate professional attention as indicated by
Cushna "et al."(1980). Persons who have the co-existence
of mental retardation and mental illness may constitute
one of the most underserved populations in the United
States as indicated by Reiss "et al." (1982).

There are two fundamental reasons why this population
has been without the necessary mental health services.
One can be categorized under the rubric of the negative
professional disposition toward providing psychiatric
treatment to mentally retarded persons. Many professionals in the mental health field are vulnerable to what
Phillips (1967) labeled misconceptions as they relate to
psycho-pathology found in the mentally retarded. Potter
(1965) has indicated that there is a lack of interest in
the mental health field with respect to providing treatment services for the mentally retarded. Menolascino and
Bernstein (1970) have suggested that there is a poor
attitude on the part of mental health professionals working with this population. Additionally Syzmanski (1977)
has pointed out that the mental health professional
community is ignorant as a result of deficiency in formal
training in mental retardation.

The second major obstacle is related to a bureaucratic systems problem found in the United States. This impediment is that neither the mental health nor the developmental disability systems want to take responsibility for persons who have a co-existence of mental illness and mental retardation as shown by Rowitz (1980). Each care delivery system regards such services as the responsibility of the other. The dual diagnosed population frequently "fall through the cracks", as they have been largely unidentified, untreated and therefore underserved.

In response to the mental health service need for this population, Beacon House, a community based program under the auspices of Ulster County Mental Health Services, developed an innovative day treatment model which utilizes highly structured groups within an interdisciplinary treatment approach. This model treatment program is an adjunct to a larger existing day treatment facility for the mentally ill. This model uses a humanistic approach to treatment in which individual worth, development, and potential are the cornerstones of our philosophy. The program consists primarily of a group work method augmented by both individual therapy and medication treatment. The following will provide a description of this day treatment model for the dual diagnosed population.

TREATMENT GROUPS

Group Psychotherapy

This problem solving vehicle is effective in addressing a wide range of clinical issues such as object loss, interpersonal relationships, impulse control, and functional limitations. The group fosters social interaction, problem solving skills and has an effect on decreasing feelings of isolation, rejection and defeat. The group therapists need to take an active role in establishing structure, providing direction and facilitating group process.

Movement Therapy

A primary goal of movement therapy is for the expansion of a movement vocabulary to increase the ability to express attitudes, feelings and ideas. Body movements can be a cogent means by which to interpret behavior. Some of the treatment techniques utilized are psychodrama, gestalt and dance therapy.

Cooking Group

This experiential group consists of three phases, each with its own therapeutic functions. The initial phase, a process focusing on decision making, provides the group with planning responsibilities. The cooking phase fosters a sense of contribution and accomplishment. The third phase, that of consumption, provides positive reinforcement for a cooperatice effort.

Horticulture Therapy

This group provides an effective means of gaining emotional enrichment as members learn to cooperate, share, and relate to one another in a meaningful way toward common objectives. Members can gain a sense of success, as plants are non-threatening and respond in a demonstrative way to care and attention.

Arts and Crafts Group

The arts and crafts group is a task oriented approach through which members engage themselves in meaningful activity by making individual craft projects. The notion of follow-through, from concept development, through task completion, has great therapeutic value. Also, the internal satisfaction of creating for oneself, and the external reward for a completed project fosters ego development.

Music Therapy

Music therapy can be an effective technique to illicit emotional responses from individuals who have difficulty in expressing themselves verbally. Also, being part of a music group promotes feelings of belonging and contribution. In addition, music instills focus, organization, and structure in a manner which is experienced as pleasurable.

Photography Group

The photography group has demonstrated to be clinically valuable as it is enjoyable. The members derive a great deal of satisfaction from this group and use it creatively as a vehicle for expression. The photographic images of the members are useful tools of treatment as the group uses this material in identifying and processing group psycho-dynamics.

Recreational Therapy

Recreational therapy provides a forum for fun, relaxation and socialization. Through utilization of community resources there is an opportunity for year round recreation. Recreational activity is therapeutic, enjoyable and provides a normalizing experience.

Life Skills Group

This group is designed to provide supportive, therapeutic and instructional approaches to learning practical skills for daily living. The utilization of community resources such as the library, post office, and laundramat are useful means for acquiring practical skills and knowledge. Additionally, there are topical discussions and seminars in areas such as human sexuality and current events awareness.

Community Meeting

The community meeting is a brief early morning session which serves two functions. First it allows an opportunity for members to express immediate problems or issues of concern. Secondly, the community meeting is a decision making forum for planning trips and special events. This decision making process enhances feelings of autonomy and self-control.

PROGRAM EFFECTIVENESS

In order to test the effectiveness of the program, a research study was undertaken as demonstrated by Fletcher (in print). All the subjects in the program were evaluated by six different counselors as they appeared shortly after admission, and again after an average of fourteen months in the program. The evaluation consisted of rating each of the subjects on a scale from 1(poor) to 7(high) in six different categories: A) self-esteem, B)socialization, C)problem solving, D)impulse-control, E)ability to be at a group at the scheduled time or place, and F)degree of the member's involvement in the program.

An analysis of the study demonstrated that each of the six tests showed that the counselors as a group rated the subjects with mean scores which were significantly higher in every category after an average of 14 months of treatment. The results of this study have demonstrated the effectiveness of this day treatment model for these dual diagnosed individuals.

INTERDISCIPLINARY TEAM APPROACH

As an interdisciplinary approach in a team work effort each staff member provides a particular area of expertise and collaborates closely with other staff. In addition to the group method of treatment, each member is assigned a counselor who functions as the member's primary therapist and provides individual therapy and case management services.

The psychiatrist works closely with staff in a team work approach and provides direct services to members through which consultation, adjunctive therapy and medication treatment is provided. The psychiatrist's role as that of all other staff members is like a cog in a wheel, each piece dependent on the other to function effectively and synergistically.

SUMMARY

It is important to note that the emphasis is primarily on the process rather than the content of each group transaction. One's active involvement in the process is indeed, the treatment. The objective of the groups are to effect individual change in psycho-social functioning through personal involvement and commitment. Actual concrete skills that are learned as a result of involvement in a particular group are a secondary benefit.

The members have formed a cohesive group with corresponding group identity. Also, the sense of belonging to a peer group counteracts the pervasive feelings of isolation and inadequacy which are characteristic of these individuals. There is a tremendous amount of support and encouragement demonstrated by one member to another as modeled from staff to member. The quality of interactions demonstrated by staff towards members as depicted by warmth, concern and creative utilization of personal energy, have tremendous positive effects on members.

This model of providing day treatment services for the dual diagnosed population is both resourceful and creative. It enables members to develop therapeutic relationships, and work toward prescribed treatment goals in a non-threatening but structured enviornment. The interdisciplinary team approach utilizing both verbal and non-verbal therapeutic techniques have demonstrated their effectiveness.

REFERENCES

Cushna,B. Szymanski,L. & Tanguay,P., 1980,
    Professional roles and unmet manpower needs ,
    in:"Emotional Disorders of Mentally Retarded
    Persons",L.S. Szymanski & P.E. Tanguay,eds.,
    University Park Press, Baltimore.
"Diagnostic Statistical Manual III",1980, Am.
    Psychiatric Assoc. 3rd printing, Washington.
Eaton, L. & Menolascino,F., 1982 Psychiatric
    disorders in the mentally retarded: Types,
    problems and challenges, Am. Jour. of Psych.,
    139: 1297-1303.
Fletcher, R. in print, A Model service for the
    mentally ill/ mentally retarded population ,
    in:"Mental Illness In The Mentally Retarded",
    F. Menolascino and J. Stark eds., Plenum
    Press, New York
Menolascino,F. & Bernstein, N., 1970, Psychia-
    tric assessment of the mentally retarded
    child ,in:"Diminished People-Problems and
    Care of the Mentally Retarded",Norman
    Bernstein ed., Little Brown, Boston.
Phillips, I. 1969, Psychopathology and mental
    retardation, Am. Jour. of Psych., 124:29-35.
Potter, H., 1965, Mental retardation : The
    cinderella of psychiatry, Psych. Quart,
    39: 537-549.
Reiss,S., Levitan, G.,& McNally, R., 1982,
    Emotionally disturbed mentally retarded
    people: An underserved population, Am.
    Psychologist, 37: 361-367
Rowitz,L., 1980, Mental health services for
    the mentally retarded individual ,in: "A
    Community Mental Health Sourcebook for
    Professional Action",W. Silverman, ed.,
    Praeger, New York.
Szymanski, L., 1977, Psychiatric diagnostic
    evaluation of mentally retarded individuals,
    Jour. of the Am. Acad. of Child Psych., 16:
    67-68.

EPIDEMIOLOGY OF DEMENTIA

A. Michael Davies

Brookdale Institute of Gerontology and
School of Public Health
Jerusalem, Israel

Epidemiological studies of senile dementia are of considerable potential importance in the testing of etiological hypothesis,
evaluation of therapy and in the estimation of future service
needs. The need for such studies is made more urgent by the explosion of the elderly population and by the aging of the elderly
themselves.

Epidemiological Approaches to Senile Dementia

Population based surveys of moderate and severe senile dementia, of all causes, have been limited to a handful of developed
countries and report considerable variations in prevalence, from
3.8% to 14% of the elderly. Most of the differences can be explained by methods of case finding and criteria of diagnosis and
by the size and age distribution of the population studied.   For
series where the methods and criteria are similar, the differences
narrow, and the prevalence in the population aged 65 and over
ranges between 5 and 7.1% with a mean around 6.3% (1). Comparable
studies which permit computation of age-sex specific prevalence
rates, are limited to data from surveys in 5 countries, conducted
between 1956 and 1975 in a total population sample of 4,500. The
numbers of surveyed subjects age 80 and over, and particularly
over 85, are very small, with poor reliability of computed rates
for the oldest groups.

There is, however, firm support for a number of generaliza-
tions (Table 1). Prevalence of all forms of dementia increases
with age from 65 upwards (although the curve may flatten out after
80 or 85), and there are relatively fewer cases in women under 75
compared to men but more after the age of 80. Thus, the total

Table 1. Percentage prevalence of organic brain syndrome by sex in pooled data.

Age	males	females	both sexes
65-	3.9	0.5	2.1
70-	4.1	2.7	3.3
75-	8.0	7.9	8.0
80-	13.2	20.9	17.7
All ages	6.2	6.3	6.3

Pooled rates computed by Kay and Bergman (1) based on surveys of 2267 subjects reported by Nielson (2), Kay et al (3) and Kaneko (4).

Table 2. Computed annual incidence of age psychosis in Lundby for the two periods 1947-57 and 1957-72. Both sexes, medium and severe cases; rate per 1,000.

	1947-57		1957-72	
Age	cases	rate	cases	rate
50-59	1	0.3	1	0.2
60-69	11	5.0	13	2.9
70-79	29	18.8	36	14.8
80-89	23	58.0	31	33.0
90-99	1	44.8	5	39.3

Data from Hagnell et al (14)

combined prevalence is similar in the two sexes.

The excess in males under 75 may be partly explained by more arteriosclerotic (multi-infarct) dementia which accounted for 88% of the cases, compared to 43% for women, in a pooled data from 4 surveys (1). The proportions of cases of dementia with an arteriosclerotic etiology were similar (41% and 43%) in the two sexes at age over 75, but the samples were small. Of interest is the difference between the ratios in Kaneko's (Japanese) series (4) where 71% of the total of 38 cases at all ages were arteriosclerotic compared to 42% of the 175 cases collected from Denmark (2), England (5) and Sweden (6). The high frequency of hypertension in Japan suggests paths for future investigation and possible control programs. Populations with a high mortality from ischemic heart disease might show fewer survivors with a susceptibility to multiinfarct dementia, and thus a higher proportion of cases of the Alzheimer type.

An important factor affecting observed prevalence of senile dementia is the age structure of the older population: a higher proportion of old-old in a population would lead to a disproportionate increase in cases. Thus, the general application of a single prevalence figure (e.g. 6.3%) for those over 65, is not appropriate. The fastest growing sector of the elderly population in developed countries is the age group of 80 and over which will double in size between 1960 and 2000, and even faster in several European countries (7). Application of· the mean prevalence rate of 6.3% shows an anticipated increase in total cases by over a third within the next few decades and even more in individual countries where the proportion of the elderly is already higher. When the age make-up of the elderly population is taken into account and calculations are based on age-specific rates, the anticipated increase in total moderate and severe cases reaches 150%. Thus, those who will provide care for the elderly must take into account the consequences of the demographic transformation. These estimations assume a constant expectation of life after diagnosis and a steady age specific incidence rate. However, Gruenberg and Hagnell (8) have reported the increasing survival of even severe cases of dementia, leading to a greatly increased prevalence for the same incidence rates.

On the other hand, Fries (9) has presented a convincing case for progress towards a finite life span for all with compression of morbidity; so that more and more people should live a healthy life until death after little or no disability, at around the age of 85. The fall in cardiovascular and some cancer mortality in many countries supporters the hypothesis (10,11), as do the studies of Svanborg in Goteburg (12). For the near future, however, the fall in mortality will most probably yeild an increase in morbidity as sick people are kept alive (13). The future impact on senile dementia prevalence can only be guessed at. The fall in hypertension should decrease the cases of multi-infarct dementia, but the fall in premature death from other causes could increase the population of elderly susceptibles to Alzheimer disease.

It is assumed in this reasoning that age specific incidence rates for senile dementia will remain as at present and that case fatality will remain steady or improve. The first assumption is challenged by the work of Hagnell and his colleagues in their 25 year longitudinal follow-up of a complete population (14). They computed the annual age specific incidence for the 10 year period, 1947-1957, and for the 15 year period 1957-1972. Table 2 summarizes the incidence of "age psychosis" equivalent to Roth's (15) "organic brain syndrome", in the two periods. Because of the difficulty of standardizing the diagnosis of "mild" senile dementia, only the data for moderate and severe impairment are given here: severe cases constituted 75.7% and 81.4% respectively of the combined totals in the two periods and showed the same age-sex trends. The incidence,, like prevalence, increased with age although new cases in the highest age group were very few. However, the incidence in the second period was lower than that in the first period, at all ages. The cumulative life time risk in the second period was also lower, for both men and women.

There is clearly an urgent need for more such baseline studies of the incidence and prevalence of dementia in different population groups, using standardized screening tests of proven validity (1, 16). For purposes of planning services, it may be sufficient to have gross estimated rates based on screening tests of reasonable sensitivity and specifity, and one of the important questions is accurate assessment of the deficiencies of "quick and dirty" survey methods. But if epidemiological surveys are to be but the first step in case identification for further studies, such as the relationship of histo-compatibility antigens to sub-groups of Alzheimer's disease (17), then as Walford observes, "a relatively small proportion of incorrectly diagnosed cases among the patient population will greatly diminish the chances of finding significant differences" (18).

The development of diagnostic tests with clear discrimination between cases of different etiology is, thus, particularly crucial, and standard criteria must be established for different levels of severity if we are ever to unravel the natural history of the different components of the dementia syndrome (1, 16, 19).

The most pressing need is for the conduct of studies of incidence and prevalence of the different forms of dementia in different populations by standard methods. Does the incidence continue to increase in the 80 and 90 year olds? Is there a difference between populations, such as those of Sweden, with low premature mortality from other causes and those where the expectation of life at 45 is shorter? Advantage could be taken of difference in beliefs, family and community organization, socio-economic levels, nutrition, health services and patterns of infectious and chronic diseases in different populations to test hypotheses such as those listed below and to formulate new ones.

1. The Slow Virus Hypothesis. Should there be such a virus, by analogy with Kuru and Jacob Creutzfeld disease (20, 21), infection early in life might protect and infection late in life cause neurological damage by analogy with multiple sclerosis (22). There should thus be fewer cases of Alzheimer's disease in populations with poor sanitation, but there may be pockets of high incidence (cf. 23) and differences in different groups of migrants coming from countries of low prevalence to those of high prevalence and vice versa.

2. Genetic Associations. Whether the association of certain HLA types with Alzheimer's disease (18) holds true for non-American populations should be tested: a first clue would be the establishment of different frequencies of the disease in populations with different HLA distributions. Another approach lies in the similarity between the neuronal changes in Down's Syndrome and Alzheimer's disease (24) and in maternal age at birth in the two conditions (25). One might expect, therefore, a clustering of Down's and Alzheimer's cases in the same families or communities, and surveys of the latter should be undertaken in areas with high and low rates of Down's Syndrome (cf. 26, 27).

3. Social Support Systems. Contributory, rather than strictly causal, support of family, social group and familiar environment is crucial in the maintenance of mental health (28, 29) and withdrawal precipitates admission to hospital (29,30). The hospitalized population represents only a fifth to a third of the cases of SD (3,31), and these may have different personal and socio-economic characteristics from those who stay in the community. If the support system prevents the onset of dementia as has been claimed (though not proved, cf. 24), then there will be a lower incidence in those with spouse and family support. If such

support merely alters the manifestations of dementia and only delays the inevitable breakdown, then there will be the same incidence and a milder clinical picture. But if the family support serves only to delay the recognition of the disease by the health authorities, then the incidence will be the same but the cases more severe at detection. Measurement of the effect of social support systems is a priority for epidemiological studies.

In conclusion, therefore, epidemiological studies are fundamental to our understanding of senile dementia, both for the planning and design of long-term care and for the testing of hypotheses of etiology which could guide clinical care and laboratory studies. The standardization of diagnostic and survey tools is an essential prerequisite for cross cultural studies.

References

1. Kay, D.W.K. and Bergmann, K.
   Epidemiology of mental disorders among the aged in the community. in: Birren, J.E. and Sloane, R.B. (Eds)
   Handbook of Mental Health and Aging, Prentice Hall, 1980, pp.34-56.

2. Nielsen, J.
   Geronto-psychiatric period prevalence investigation in a geographically delimited population.
   Acta Psychiat. Scand. 38: 307-330 (1962).

3. Kay, D.W.K., Bergmann, K., Foster, E.M., McKechnie, A.A. and Roth, M.
   Mental illness and hospital usage in the elderly: a random sample follow-up.
   Comprehensive Psychiatry, 11:26-35 (1970).

4. Kaneko, Z.
   Care in Japan. in: Howells, J.C. (Ed)
   Modern perspectives in the psychiatry of old age.
   New York, Brunner-Mazel, pp. 519-530.

5. Kay, D.W.K., Beamish, P. and Roth, M.
   Old age mental disorders in Newcastle-upon-Tyne,
   I. A study of prevalence.
   Brit. J. Psychiat. 110:146-158 (1964).

6. Akessan, H.O.
A population study of senile and arteriosclerotic psychoses.
Human Heredity, 10: 546-566 (1969).

7. Siegel, J.S.
Demographic aspects of the health of the elderly to the year
2000 and beyond..
World Health Statistics Quarterly 36 (1) (1983).

8. Gruenberg, E.M. and Hagnell, O.:
The rising prevalence of chronic brain syndrome in the elderly.
in: Levi, S. (Ed.) Society, stress and disease: aging and
old age.
London, Oxford University Press, 1981.

9. Fries, J.F.
Aging, natural death and the compression of morbidity.
New Eng. J. Med. 303: 130-135 (1980).

10. Havlik, R.J. and Feinlieb, M. (Eds).
Proc. Conf. Decline in Coronary Heart Disease Mortality.
Washington, USDHEW, National Institute of Health
publication no. 79-1610, May 1979.

11. Ostfield, A.M.
A review of stroke epidemiology.
Am. J. Epid. 2: 136-152, (1980).

12. Svanborg, A., Bergstrom, G. and Mellstrom, D.
Epidemiological studies on social and medical conditions
of the elderly.
Copenhagen, WHO Regional Office for Europe.
(EURO Reports and Studies 62) 1982.

13. Gruenberg, E.M.
The failure of success.
Milbank Mem. Fund Q. 55:3-24 (1977).

14. Hagnell, O., Lanke, J., Rossman, B. and Ojesjo, L.
Does the incidence of age psychosis decrease?
Neuropsychiatry, 7:201-211 (1981).

15. Roth, M.
The natural history of mental disorder in old age.
J. Ment. Sci. 101:281-301 (1955).

16. Schoenberg, E.S.
Methodological approaches to the epidemiological study of
dementia in: Mortimer, J.A. and Schuman, L.M. (Eds).
The epidemiology of dementia
London, Oxford University Press, 1981, pp. 117-131.

17. Cohen, D., Eisdorfer, C. and Walford, R.L.
Histo-compatibility antigens (HLD) and patterns of
cognitive loss in dementia of the Alzheimer type.
Neurology of Aging, 2: 277-280, 1982.

18. Walford, R.L.
Immunological studies of Down's syndrome and Alzheimer's
disease.
Ann. New York Acad. Sci.396: 95-106 (1982)

19. Small, G.W. and Jarvik, L.F.
The dementia syndrome.
Lancet ii: 1443-1446 (1982).

20. Gajdusek, D.C.
Unconventional viruses and the origin and disappearance
of Kuru.
Science,197: 943-960 (1977).

21. Torack, R.M.
Adult dementia: history, biopsy, pathology.
Neurosurgery, 4: 434-442 (1979).

22. Leibowitz, U., Kahana, E. and Alter, M.
Multiple sclerosis in immigrant and native populations
in Israel.
Lancet, ii: 1323   (1969).

23. Dean, G., Grinaldi, G., Kelly, R.and Karhausen, L.
Multiple sclerosis in southern Europe.
I. Prevalence in Sicily in 1975.
J. Epid. Comm. Med., 33: 107-110 (1979).

24. Roth, M.
Aging of the brain and dementia: an overview.
in: Amoducci, L., Davison, A.N.and Antuono, P. (Eds).
Aging of the Brain and Dementia, New York, Raven Press
1980, pp. 17-21.

25. Eisdorfer, C., Cohen, D. and Buckley, C.E.
Behavioral serum immunoglobin relationship in the cogni-
tively impaired elderly. in:Katzum, R. and Terry, R.D. (Eds).
Alzheimer's disease, senile dementia and related disorders.
New York Raven Press, 1979.

26. Lilienfeld, A.M.
    Epidemiology of Mongolism
    Baltimore, Johns Hopkins Press, 1969.

27. Harlap, S., Davies, A.M., Haber, M., Rossman, H.,
    Prywes, R. and Samueloff, N.
    Congenital malformations in the Jerusalem perinatal study.
    Isr. J. Med. Sci. 7:1520-1528 (1971).

28. Brody, E.M.
    Environmental factors in dependency.
    in: Exton-Smith, A.N. and Evans, J.G. (Eds). Care of the
    elderly: meeting the challange of dependency.
    London, Academic Press, 1977, p. 81.

29. Butler, R.N. and Lewis, M.I.
    Aging and Mental Health, St. Louis, Mosby, 2nd ed., 1977.

30. Isaacs, B., Livingstone, M. and Neville, Y.
    Survival of the unfittest: a study of geriatric patients
    in Glasgow.
    London, Routledge, 1972.

31. Kramer, M.
    Application of Mental Health Statistics.
    Geneva, World Health Organization, 1969.

RISK FACTORS IN LATE LIFE DEMENTIA

Donna Cohen, Gary Kennedy, Sandra Nehlsen-Cannarella,
Mehendra Kumar and Carl Eisdorfer
Montefiore Medical Center
111 East 210 Street
Bronx, New York 10467

The dementias of later life, of which Alzheimer's disease is
the most common, have emerged as one of our most serious public
health problems. Throughout the world we are witnessing an
increase in the prevalence of the dementias of late life (Kramer,
1980) not only because people are living longer, but because the
population over age 75, who are at the highest risk for
Alzheimer's disease, are the fastest growing segment of the
population. The rapid relative growth of the aged population at
risk for Alzheimer's disease and related disorders forecasts a
significant burden on society unless ways are discovered to treat
and prevent them.

In an attempt to understand the cause or causes of
Alzheimer's disease, the identification of risk factors or
antecedent conditions must become an area of active research
(Cohen and Eisdorfer, 1983). Can we identify the risk factors
which cause an individual to develop or to be vulnerable to
Alzheimer's disease? Is there evidence that environmental factors
are important and that prevention may be possible? Does
Alzheimer's disease strike people at random as they age or can we
identify susceptible individuals before they manifest obvious
clinical symptoms? To what extent are we dealing with a single
disease entity as contrasted with a disease of multiple origins
albeit similar presentation.

The risk factors for primary neuronal degeneration of the
Alzheimer type are not well understood. However, we do know that
the risk of manifesting the disorder increases as a function of

263

advancing age past 60. Since chronological age is such an important predictor variable, age must be taken into account in the search for other risk factors. Death is a second important confounding variable in risk factor research. Death introduces an ascertainment bias resulting from the early mortality of gene carriers who might otherwise display the dementia in later life.

This paper will review the evidence for the best documented risk factor, family history, and several other hypothesized risk factors: Parental age, HLA associations, and altered immunoregulation.

At present, family history appears to be the best documented risk factor for Alzheimer's disease. The probability of manifesting the familial form of Alzheimer's dementia may be analyzed in two ways: (1) the probability of carrying the gene, and (2) the probability of the gene showing penetrance (Sinex and Merrill, 1982). If we assume an autosomal dominant mode of inheritance, as most investigators have reported, the probability of a first-degree relative carrying the gene is 0.50. The probability of the gene showing penetrance is a function of age, other risk factors as well as accurate diagnosis of the disease.

Although many investigators have examined the possibility that Alzheimer's disease has a genetic basis, to date, there have only been two large scale studies, one in Sweden by Larsson et al. (1963) and one in Minnesota by Heston et al. (1981). Heston and his colleagues (1981) confirmed the work of Larsson and associates (1963) who estimated that about 12 percent of the population may carry the "Alzheimer gene." In the early onset form of the disease (pre-age 65) half of the children of an affected parent or half of the siblings should manifest the disease. With later onset of the disease, this probability should decrease unless nongenetic factors are important.

What are the empirical genetic risks for parents, siblings, and second degree relatives of an affected person compared to the general population? Table 1 presents the age-specific risks as reported by Heston (1983). The cumulative risks show an increase of 4-5 percent among parents and relatives with each age interval. This increase is a feature of the relatives as well as the controls; the difference is in the age at which cases occur. Siblings and parents at all ages are at greater risk than second degree relatives, who, in turn, are at greater risk than the general population. The risk to parents is consistently higher than siblings. Finally, only 1/3 of all families had a secondary

Table 1. Empirical Risk for Alzheimer's Dementia Among Relatives
of Probands (Heston, 1983)

Cumulative Risk as Percentage for

Age Interval	Siblings	Parents	Second Degree Relatives	Population
50 – 54	–	0.1 + 0.7	–	–
55 – 59	0.4 + 0.3	–	–	–
60 – 64	0.9 + 0.5	2.7 + 1.2	1.1 + 0.7	–
65 – 69	3.8 + 1.0	6.3 + 1.9	2.2 + 1.0	0.4
70 – 74	7.7 + 1.5	11.8 + 2.6	2.9 + 1.2	1.2
75 – 79	11.5 + 2.0	13.6 + 2.8	4.1 + 1.7	2.5
80 – 84	15.1 + 2.6	17.7 + 3.6	7.0 + 3.3	3.7
85 – 89	19.5 + 3.5	22.7 + 4.8	–	6.4

case of Alzheimer's disease, suggesting that sporatic Alzheimer's
is more common than the familial form.

The risk to siblings varies as a function of whether the
proband has early or late onset and whether a parent is affected
or unaffected with Alzheimer's disease. The risk to relatives of
probands with onset after age 70 is similar to the risks for the
general population. The risk is increased for relatives of
probands who had earlier onset and who had an affected parent.
For relatives of probands with both early onset and an affected
parent, the risk approaches the 50 percent as predicted by the
autosomal dominant hypothesis.

The limited data available suggest that sporatic dementias
are more common than the familial form, and, here, we have no
conclusive evidence for any risk factors. Only advancing age
appears to have predictive value (Sluss, 1980). The risk for
Alzheimer's disease appears to increase, at least through age 80,
at which point the risk decreases.

Although there are a number of research strategies and
statistical models for estimating the risk of disease in persons
with different characteristics and past experiences, almost no
research has been done (Cohen and Eisdorfer, 1983). The limited
data we have are derived from hypotheses about the nature of the
disease and its association with other illnesses or conditions.

Whereas a prospective study of an older population with hypertension, arrythmias, and other stroke-associated risk factors has merit in the identification of risk factors for multi-infarct dementias, our paucity of knowledge about Alzheimer's disease makes a prospective study an expensive low yield investigation. A case-control study would be valuable to attempt a comparison of the frequency of occurrence of suspected risk factors.

The genetic association and similarities between Alzheimer's disease and Down's syndrome have generated a number of questions about their relationship. These two diseases may share aspects of the same pathogenesis, e.g., immune alterations, such that older maternal age might be observed in Alzheimer's disease as seen in Down's syndrome. Our laboratory first suggested that there might be a subset of children who develop dementia of the Alzheimer type in later life who are at increased risk as a result of being born to older mothers (Cohen, Eisdorfer, and Leverenz, 1980). Figure 1 shows the age distribution of mothers at childbirth by 5-year age groupings for several populations: Eighty clinically diagnosed cases studied in our laboratory; 20 Alzheimer cases and 20 control cases from our neuropathology files; 1907 Washington State Vital Statistics; 1920 U.S. Vital Statistics; and the Collman and Stoller (1962) data on Down's Syndrome for comparison. The age distribution of the 1907 Washington State data parallels the 1920 U.S. data. The peak of the age distribution of the mothers of the Alzheimer cases falls between the mothers of the controls and the Down's cases (Cohen and Eisdorfer, 1983).

At least one other laboratory (Whalley et al., 1981) has reported a slight but significant increase in both maternal (p=0.005) and paternal (p=0.01) age in 69 autopsy validated cases of Alzheimer's disease compared to 207 controls. There was no correlation with order of birth.

Recent studies suggest that Alzheimer's disease or perhaps one form, may be an HLA-associated disease. In four out of five studies HLA B7 was increased, and Walford (1983) has argued that individuals with B7 have a 50 percent greater chance of developing Alzheimer's disease. The accuracy of an HLA association requires a large population of patients to be studied, a project ongoing in our laboratory.

Our laboratory is also attempting to replicate a finding

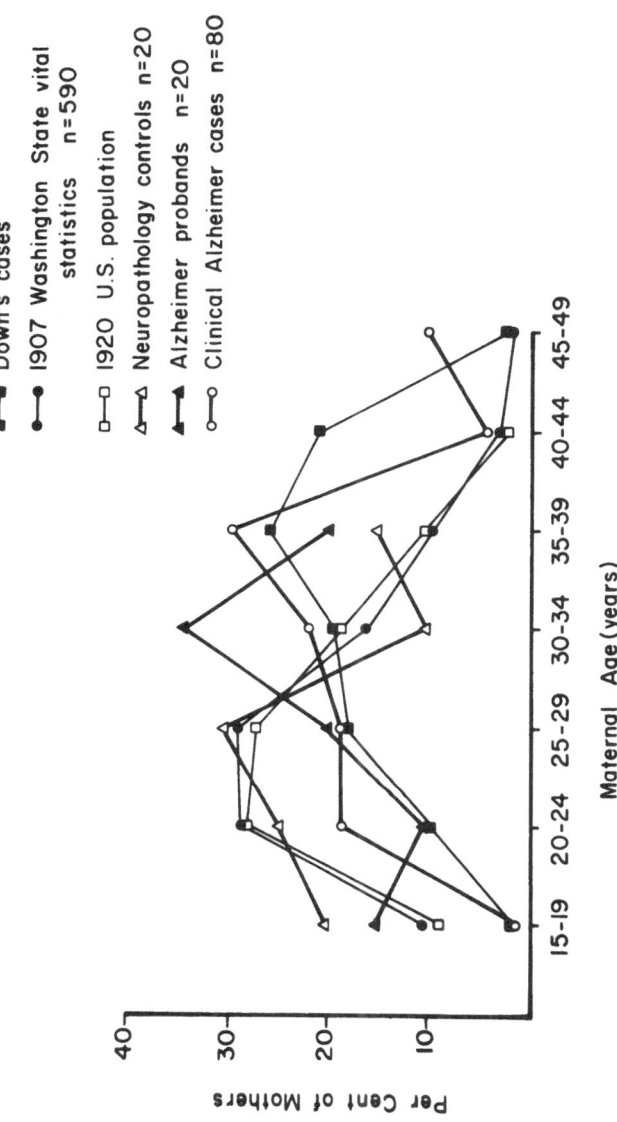

Figure 1. Age distribution of matters at childbirth by 5-year age groupings for Alzheimer probands, Down's cases, and U.S. vital statistics.

reported in 1981, that Alzheimer patients with HLA B7 have a selective attention deficit which is not observed in patients without the B7 (Cohen, Eisdorfer, and Walford, 1981). These findings have led us to postulate that there may be more than one form of Alzheimer's disease.

Although there have been many reports of direct and indirect evidence of immunological abnormalities in dementia of the Alzheimer type (Table 2), our laboratory has begun a systematic study of immunologic parameters in patients with Alzheimer's disease to identify whether this disorder, or forms of this disorder, can be classified as an immunodeficiency disease or an autoimmune disease.

The integrity of the immune system is essential to health and survival. Alterations in immune functions accompany the normal aging process, and several lines of evidence suggest that infectious and immunological factors (or both) may be involved in

Table 2. Immunological Aspects of Primary Neuronal Degeneration of the Alzheimer Type

- Patients appear to have reduced life expectancy.

- Patients are prone to infections in the later stages of illness.

- Death is usually due to pneumonia or other infections.

- Serum immunoglobulins (IgG + IgA) are elevated in early stage patients compared to controls.

- Serum IgG correlates positively with duration of illness.

- Serum IgG and IgM correlate positively with cognitive performance scores.

- Delayed skin hypersensitivity responses suggest immuno-deficiency.

- HLA B7 has been associated with Alzheimer's in 4 of 5 published studies.

- Alzheimer patients with HLA B7 have more impaired attentional skills compared to Alzheimer patients negative for B7.

- Presence of complement in amyloid plaques.

Alzheimer's disease. Improving our understanding of changes in the regulatory mechanisms of the immune system has implications for understanding the pathogenesis of Alzheimer's disease as well as risk factors.

The immune system consists of a complex set of regulatory mechanisms, and our laboratory has begun a series of experiments to identify changes in the number and activity of the immunoregulatory cells. The circulating T-lymphocyte population is composed of several subsets that control most cellular and humoral immune responses (Reinherz and Schlossman, 1980). Using monoclonal antibodies directed against cell surface antigens, two important T-cell subsets can be identified: Inducer/helper T-cells stimulate B-cells to produce immunoglobulins and stimulate lymphocytes to divide; suppressor/cytotoxic T-cells act to inhibit B-cell immunoglobulin production as well as to suppress the proliferation of other T-cells.

Changes in these immunoregulatory cells which control the immune response to self and non-self antigens should be observed if Alzheimer's disease is characterized by immunodeficiency or autoimmunity. Here we report the pilot results of our first experiment where the lymphocytes are analyzed using the fluorescence activated cell sorter (FACS). The FACS is used for the analysis and separation of cells in suspension. It measures the size and fluorescence of individual cells as they flow past a laser illumination system coupled with highly sensitive detectors.

The data presented in Table 3 show the results of our analysis of lymphocytes, T-cells, suppressor/cytotoxic and helper/nuclear T-cells for 12 patients who met research diagnostic criteria for Alzheimer's disease and 10 age-matched controls. The number of T-cells and the cells with cytotoxic/suppressor functions were significantly higher in the patients with Alzheimer's dementia. The suppressor/helper ratio was not higher in the Alzheimer patients which might have been expected if the disease were an autoimmune disease.

Aberrant immunoregulation could affect the prognosis in Alzheimer patients and contribute to the reduced survival in those afflicted. Aberrent immunoregulation is also compatible with the hypothesis of a chronic viral infection. Our results are preliminary and further work is required to identify the activity of suppressor cells in patients with Alzheimer's disease, to characterize the factors which mediate suppression, and to relate the observations more directly to the disease state and its progression.

In part, our research efforts have been attempting to disaggregate dementia, i.e., to examine the hypothesis that there

Table 3. Quantification of Helper/Inducer and Suppressor/
Cytotoxic T-Cells in Patients with Alzheimer's Disease
and Age-Matched Controls.

	CONTROLS n=10	PATIENTS n=12
Lymphocyte Counts	1480 + 121	1881 + 191*
T-Cell Counts	980 + 79	1352 + 152*
T-Cells (%)	66.6%	72.8%
Helper/Inducer T-Cells	645 + 49	846 + 114
%	44.4%	45.7%
Suppressor/Cytotoxic T-Cells	187 + 47	433 + 59*
%	20.2%	23.8%
Ratio	2.76	2.08

*$p \leq 0.05$ (Wilcoxon)

are several types of Alzheimer's disease. Our present line of
experiments may help us to classify and define subclasses of
Alzheimer's disease, if they exist. T- and B-cell quantification
studies demonstrated that there were four classes of acute
lymphocytic leukemia. As we are able to study larger populations
of Alzheimer patients, we may begin to understand the
immunoregulatory changes which characterize the disease(s).

The risk factors or antecedents for Alzheimer's disease and
related disorders are a fertile area for research. Little is
known about the intrinsic and extrinsic factors which increase an
individual's vulnerability for a major brain disease in later
life. As we learn more about risk factors, insights into
etiologic agents, treatment strategies, and even disease
prevention may emerge. Conversely, if indeed there are various
forms of dementia, our knowledge about risk factors should also
improve and lead to further knowledge of the psychopathology of
aging.

REFERENCES

Cohen, D., and Eisdorfer, C., 1983, Risk factors in late life
dementia, in: "Senile Dementias in the 21st Century,"
M. Marois, ed., Alan Liss, New York.
Cohen, D., Eisdorfer, C., and Leverenz, C., 1982, A hypothesis:

Maternal age and Alzheimer's disease, J Am Ger Soc., 30:656-659.

Cohen, D., Eisdorfer, C., and Walford, R.L., 1982, Histocompatibility antigens (HCA) and patterns of cognitive loss in dementia of the Alzheimer type, Neurobiol Aging., 2:277-280.

Collman, R.D., and Stoller, A., 1962, A survey of mongolism and congenital anomalies of the central nervous system in Victoria, N Z Med J., 61:24-32.

Heston, L.L., Mastri, A.R., Anderson, V.E., and White, J., 1981, Dementia of the Alzheimer type: Clinical genetics, natural history and associated conditions, Arch Gen Psychiat., 38:1085-1090.

Kramer, M., 1980, The rising pandemic of mental disorders and associated chronic diseases and disabilities, Acta Psychiat Second Suppl., 62:382-397.

Larsson, T., Sjogren, T., and Jacobson, G., 1963, A clinical, sociomedical and genetic study, Acta Psychiat Second Suppl., 167:1-259.

Reinherz, E., and Schlossman, S.F., 1980, Current concepts in immunology: Regulation of the immune response-inducer and suppressor T-lymphocyte subsets in human beings, N E J Med., 303:370-373.

Sinex, E.M., and Merrill, C.R., 1982, "Alzheimer's Disease, Down's Syndrome, and Aging," New York Academy of Science, New York.

Sluss, T.K., 1980, "A method for investigating a risk factor for senile dementia-Alzheimer type in the Baltimore longitudinal study," unpublished doctoral thesis, The Johns Hopkins University, Baltimore.

Walford, R.F., 1982, Immunological studies of Down's syndrome and Alzheimer's disease, in: "Alzheimer's Disease, Down's Syndrome, and Aging," E.M. Sinex, C.R. Merril, eds, New York Academy of Sciences, New York.

Whalley, L.J., Carothers, S., Collyer, S., DeMey, R., and Frackiewicz, A., 1982, A study of familial factors in Alzheimer's disease, Br J Psychiat., 140:249-256.

PREDICTIVE FACTORS IN SENILE DEMENTIA

A CLINICAL AND CT SCAN STUDY

M. Naguib, and R. Levy

Bethlem Royal and The Maudsley Hospitals and the
Institute of Psychiatry
Denmark Hill, London SE5 8AF, England

The substance of this paper has been reported in two recent publications, Naguib, M. & Levy, R. (1982) and Naguib, M. & Levy R., (1982).

The prediction of outcome and life expectancy in patients with senile dementia is an increasingly important part of our assessment to those patients. Not only does it allow for separation of categories with different clinical developments but it also has greater implications for the planning of the services for the elderly.

We followed up a group of forty patients suffering from senile dementia who had been subjected to detailed clinical and psychological assessment and computed tomography (Jacoby & Levy, 1980). The mean period of follow-up was 28.78 months. All subjects but one were traced. The deceased (27) were compared with the survivors (12).

Table I shows comparison between the deceased and survivors on various psychological tests:

Table I

	Deceased (n = 27) Mean ± SD	Survivors (n = 12) Mean ± SD	Significance level
Age	79.2 ± 7.4	77.2 ± 4.85	Not significant*
Mental Test Score (MTS)	9.69 ± 6.88	15.23 ± 5.69	P < 0.01*
Digit Copying Test (DCT)	22.61 ± 27.81	36.20 ± 25.34	P < 0.05**
Digit Symbol Sub-stitution Test (DST)	0.80 ± 3.16	3.61 ± 5.83	Not significant
Parieto-Temporal Dysfunction Score (PTS) (dysphasia, dysgraphia and dyspraxia)	14.52 ± 4.3	9.75 ± 6.06	P < 0.01*

* t-test (two-tailed)
** Mann-Whitney U Test (two-tailed)

At follow-up all males had died. Almost 25% of the group had died within 6 months and 70% within two years. Although the earlier figure compares favourably with the 60% given by Roth (1955). The 2 years death rate is comparable with his figure of 80% and in line with those of others (Kay, 1962; Shah et al, 1969; Thompson & Eastwood, 1981). Thus although improved care in the 1980's from that of the 1950's might have had an effect on short-term survival, this appears to have had no effect on long-term survival. The deceased differred significantly from the survivors in having performed poorly on a number of clinical and psychological tests particularly those involving speech function and constructional ability. This is similar to that obtained by McDonald (1969) and Hare (1978) and in keeping with those of Javik & Blum (1971).

Those who died did not differ significantly from the survivors on CT scan measurements of ventricular size and cortical atrophy. However, when compared on measures of brain density (Hounsfield Units), the deceased scored lower in all regions of the brain and this was statistically significant at level of (P < 0.05) for the right parietal region.

The mean (HU)values did not correlate with age or the approximate length of dementia history in either group. There was also no correlation between the mean (HU) values with either the ventricular size as measured by the planimeter or the radiologist's rating of cerebral atrophy. In view of the clear differences obtained on measures of radio attenuation and their correspondence to the clinical variables, particularly in the case of the parietal lobe, the use of this measure appears to be worth pursuing. Naeser et al (1980) and Naeser et al (1981) employing this technique were able to differentiate pseudo dementia from early dementia. Bondareff, Baldy and Levy (1981) have also demonstrated clear regional differences between patients with senile dementia and normal controls.

This study confirmed that clinical involvement of the parietal lobes was an indication of poor prognosis and reported the first radiological support for this view.

At a further follow-up of the survivors, all patients retained their initial diagnosis of dementia. Nevertheless, two sub-groups could be identified. The first sub-group (5) showed further deterioration in cognitive function. This was paralleled by an increase in ventricular-brain ratio. In the second sub-group (5) patient's cognitive impairment progressed little, if at all, as was their CT scan appearance.

Initially, there was no difference between the two sub-groups on either the psychological tests or measures of ventricular size and sulcal widening. However, at follow-up, sub-group I, who showed greater intellectual deterioration, had decreased attenuation density (HU) in their original scans. Amongst the survivors, although their number was too small for clear statistical differences to emerge, there was a tendency for affective admixture to be a favourable prognostic indicator and low radiological density particularly in the right parietal region to be an unfavourable one.

References

Bondareff, W., Baldy, R. and Levy, R. (1981) Quantitative computed tomography in senile dementia. Archives of General Psychiatry, 38, 1365-8

Hare, M. (1987) Clnical checklist for diagnosis of dementia. British Medical Journal, ii, 266-7

Jacoby, R. and Levy, R. (1980) Computed tomography in the elderly; 2. Senile dementia: Diagnosis and functional impairment. British Journal of Psychiatry, 136, 256-269

Jarvic, L.F. and Blum, J.E. (1971) Cognitive decline as predictors of mortality in twin pairs; A twenty-year longitudinal study of ageing. In Prediction of Life Span (eds. E. Palmore and F.C. Jeffers). Lexington: D.C. Heath.

Kay, D.W.K. (1962) Outcome and cause of death in mental discrders of old age: A long-term follow-up of functional and organic psychoses. Acta Psychiatrica Scandinavica, 38, 249-276

McDonald, C. (1969) Clinical heterogeneity in senile dementia. British Journal of Psychiatry, 115, 267-271

Naeser, M.A., Gebhardt, C. and Levine, H.L. (1980) Decrease computed tomography numbers in patients with presenile dementia. Archives of Neurology, 37, 401-409

Naeser, M.A., Albert, M.S. and Kleefield, J. (1981) New methods in the CT scan diagnosis of Alzheimer's Disease: Examination of white and grey matter mean CT density numbers. Archives of Neurology, (in press)

Naguib, M. and Levy, R. (1982) Prediction of outcome in senile dementia - a computed tomography study. British Journal of Psychiatry, 140, 263-267

Naguib, M. and Levy, R. (1982) CT Scanning in Senile Dementia A follow-up of survivors. British Journal of Psychiatry, 141, 618-620

Roth, M. (1955) The natural history of mental disorders in old age. Journal of Mental Science, 101, 281-301

Shah, K.U., Banks, G.D. and Merskey, H. (1969) Survival in arteriosclerotic and senile dementia. British Journal of Psychiatry, 115, 1283-1286

Thompson, E.G. and Eastwood, M.R. (1981) Survivorship and senile dementia. Age and Ageing, 10, 29-32

CEREBRAL INSUFFICIENCY IN FIRST STAGE DEMENTIA

Kugler, J.E. and Spatz, R.

Psychiatric Clinic of University of Munich
Nussbaumstrasse 7
D 8ooo   Munich 2 , GFR

PROBLEM

In dementia of patients in advanced age with all
diagnostic criteria we look for their origin (multi-
focal or degenerative). On uses the clinical and technical results for differentiating generalized functional
disturbancies and morphological changes of the brain
from localized changes, for applying the adaequate therapy and establishing prognostic criteria.

In first stage dementia it is sometimes difficult
to establish the diagnosis. We rely often solely on
anamnestic data of the patient or his relatives on specific changes of his behaviour, his personality and his
cognitive or mental abilities and of his psychiatric
findings of a first medical examination. The results
of internal investigation of cardiovascular functions,
of metabolism and the radiological examinations of the
brain allow not always a reliable decision of the
first stage dementia of Alzheimer´s type from a multi-
infarct dementia.

Possibly the use of the term dementia in the
english speaking countries has a broader meaning than
by the german psychiatrists. We prefer in such patients
not to speak of a first stage dementia but of a cerebral insufficiency. That means, that the changes of behaviour and personality are very slight and do not imply
social disturbances and that only certain cognitive
abilities are diminished and this must not be a continuous process. The adaption of the patient in his so-

cial milieu can be undisturbed; if the family does not assure the optimal conditions for the patient, then he must earlier attend the outpatients department for medical treatment before he progresses to the next stage where he must be admitted to the hospital or sent to an old people's home. Then it must be decided which diagnostic possibilities for estimating the degree of a cerebral insufficiency can be used and which therapeutic measures can be taken.

DIAGNOSIS

When neurological signs and anamnestic reports of previous transient deficits are absent on must decide on wether radiological or intensive computerized examinations are necessary. The patient is more likely to accept simple explorations and harmless examinations. We surprisingly found that systematically repeated outpatients examinations with simple methods were willingly accepted from many patients in outpatients care. These simple methods along with a doctors therapeutic interviews may help with the patients adaptation in the family and delay the need for his hospitalization. Thereby a pharmacotherapy with homoepathic substances or as inefficient considered geriatrics may become a vehicle for an interview therapy and may be of benefit for the systematic exploration.

1) Psychometry

In the psychometric methods of investigation we found useful the trail making test (Nuremberg inventory by Oswald et al., 1982), the Hachinski ischemic score (Hachinski et al., 1975), the Heinemann screening (Heinemann et al., 1976) and the list of vegetative symptoms by Janke and Lehmann (Janke et Lehmann, 197o). In the follow up of symptoms and of a pharmacotherapy these methods become wellcome occasions for the patients self-control of his abilities. With the Wechsler Adult Intelligence Scale (Wechsler, 1955, 1956) the decrease of performance with advancing age is statistically well documented (Riegel, 1972).

2) Electroencephalographc investigation

Electroencephalographic examinations have been used for the follow-up of treatment. It is statistically proved that the dominant frequency of EEG-activity decreases in the elderly with advancing age

(Matejcek et al., 1979). This decrease of dominant frequency is about 1/s within 20 years. In shorter time
spans from months or half a year on can't notice any
change in normal circumstances. If there is a visually
noticable slowing down of the EEG activity one correspon-
dingly finds also a reduced psychometric performance or
psychophysiologiacal disturbances. We have patients to
demonstrate this.

3) Vigilosomnography

    The age dependent changes of circadian variations
of vigilance or alertness play a rôle in performance.
Vigilance variation can be seen in simple standard EEG-
records, but depends on many enviromental influences,
banal hypersomnia and different conditions of relaxation
during recording. Therefore they are difficult to quantify.

    With the method of vigilosomnography the variable
indices of vigilance in all consecutive epochs of chosen duration (20, 30, 40 or 60 s) of a 40 to 60 minutes
long EEG registration are estimated and graphically
presented, thereby giving a characteristic course of
free fluctuating alertness (Aufdembrinke et al., 1981;
Kugler, 1982). The comparison of the mean of vigilosomnograms of patients in different age groups show often in
advanced age transitions to stages of subvigilance or
reducend alertness with greater vigilance indices than
in younger adults.

4) Electroencephalographic power spectra analysis

    One of the longest systematic treatment studies
of cerebral insufficiency concerned two groups of
people in an old peoples´home with a mean age of 77 years
in which differences in performance and electroencephalographic power spectra could be shown (Kugler et al.,
1978). The higher scores of power of alpha frequency
expresses the fact that more or higher alpha waves
exist than in the lower scores. The higher alpha scores
correlate with fewer vigilance variations, giving a
better protection against disturbing stimuli and assure
a continuing performance in long lasting tasks. The
meaning of vigilance stabilization is up to now partly
ignored.

SUMMARY

The differentiation and quantification of cerebral insufficiency is important for the early diagnosis of the first stage dementia. On one hand it is unnecessary to declare an age dependent decrease in performance without correlation with all the criteria of a brain organic syndrome as dementia and then to burden the patient with all the technical examinations which are available. On the other hand is the Diagnosis of abnormalities of performance in particular areas of cognitive or performative functions important, when one wishes to start early the adaequate behaviour therapy, sociotherapy and pharmacotherapy with the view of success for delaying the advance of more severe disturbances.

As the methods for quantification of cerebral insufficiency we found useful the simple psychomotric testing, systematically applied scoring procedures along with self rating and external observation and EEG-control with the special presentation of vigilosomnograms completed through automatic analysis. Between increased variations of vigilance or alertness in advancing age and reduced performance exist particular correlations.

In the case of additional transient neurological symptoms, persistent signs or progressive fall in performance there have to be applied all the necessary technical investigations for differential diagnosis of generalized degenerative or multiinfarct brain tissue changes.

The combined psychometric and electroencephalographic investigations are useful to differenciate a pharmacodynamic effect of nootropics or brain metabolic enhancers from placebo effects and to estimate the degree and the duration of their effect.

REFERENCES

Aufdembrinke, B., Kugler, J., Laub, M., Rode, C.P., 1981, Die elektroenzephalographisch bestimmte sed. Wirkung (Vigilosomnographie) des neuen Thieno-diazepin-Derivates·Clothiazepam (Trecalmo), EEG-EMG, 12: 148.

Hachinski, V.C., Iliff, L.D., Zilhka, E., Du Boulay, G.H., McAllister, V.L., Marshall, G., Russell,

R. W. R., Simon, L., 1975, Cerebral blood flow in dementia, <u>Arch. Neurol.</u>, 32: 632.

Heinemann, L., Heine, H., Eisenblätter, D., Rossner, H., Stege, S., Stäber, G., Heinemann, G., Norden, C., Müller, B., Scholze, J., 1976, Zur Eignung des Screening-Fragebogens für akute zerebrovaskuläre Krankheit. <u>Dt. Gesundh.Wesen</u>, 31, 1981.

Janke, W. and Lehmann, H., 197o, unpublihed.

Kugler, J., 1982, Vigilosomnographie bei Patienten mit zerebrovaskulärer Insuffizienz, <u>in</u>: "Fortschritte in Pathophysiologie, Diagnostik und Therapie cerebraler Gefässerkrankungen, H. Lechner, ed., Excerpta Medica, Amsterdam.

Kugler, J., Oswald, W.D., Herzfeld , U., Seus, R., Pingel, J., und Welzel, D., 1978, Langzeittherapie altersbedingter Insuffizienzerscheinungen des Gehirns, <u>Dt. med. Wschr.</u>, lo3/11: 456.

Matejcek, M., Knor, K., Piguet, P.V. and Weil, C.,1979, Electroencephalographic and clinical changes as correlated in geriatric patients treated three month[s]with an ergotalcaloid preparation. <u>J. Am. Geriatr. Soc.</u>, 27: 198.

Oswald, W.D., Matejcek, M., Lukaschek, K., Dennler, H. J. und Oswald, P., 1982, Über die Relevanz psychometrisch operationalisierter Therapie-Effekte bei der Behandlung altersbedingter Insuffizienzerscheinungen des Gehirns am Beispiel des Nürnberger Alters-Inventars, <u>Arzneimittelforschung,</u> 32/5: 584.

Riegel, K.F., 1972, Allgemeine Alternspsychologie, <u>in:</u> "Psychiatrie der Gegenwart", K.P. Kisker, J.-E. Meyer, M. Müller, E. Strömgren, ed., Springer-Verlag Berlin

Wechsler, D., 1955, Manual for the Wechsler Adult Intelligence Scale, New York, Psychological Corporation.

Wechsler, D., 1956, Die Messung der Intelligenz Erwachsener, Huber, Bern.

CEREBRAL GLUCOSE METABOLISM IN AGING,

DEMENTIA, AND DOWN SYNDROME

Neal R. Cutler, Ranjan Duara, Cheryl L. Grady
Arthur D. Kay, James V. Haxby, and Stanley I. Rapoport

Section on Brain Aging and Dementia,
Laboratory of Neurosciences, National
Institute on Aging, National Institutes
of Health, Bethesda, MD 20205

Aging in animals and man is accompanied by many changes in morphometric and neurochemical measures of the brain. In pathologic conditions such as Alzheimer's disease and Down syndrome (DS), furthermore, these alterations have been shown to be greatly accelerated; however, the functional significance of these changes remains to be determined.

In this chapter, we will briefly examine the relation in man between functional alterations and brain metabolism in the normal aging process, in primary degenerative dementia (PDD) of the Alzheimer's type, and in DS.

BRAIN METABOLISM AND AGING IN MAN

The literature regarding brain metabolism during aging in man shows mixed findings. Some reports fail to demonstrate age differences in cerebral blood flow (CBF) and the cerebral metabolic rate for oxygen ($CMRO_2$),[1] whereas others do find decrements in these parameters as well as in the cerebral metabolic rate for glucose (CMR_{glc}).[2-5] Using a new technique of positron emission tomography (PET) and ^{18}F-fluoro-2-deoxyglucose (^{18}FDG), we reexamined the question of whether changes in brain metabolism are correlated with age in healthy men. Prior studies with PET have indicated that brain metabolism ($CMRO_2$ and CMR_{glc}) is reduced in the elderly.[5,6,7]

Subjects were accepted into this study only if by history, physical examination, and laboratory screening they were free of medical and neurologic diseases (particularly hypertension and atherosclerotic changes). These criteria for inclusion resulted in the selection of 21 exceptionally healthy men aged 21-83 years (mean age 50.8 years).

The procedure, similar to that used in the rat,[8] involves the intravenous injection of a positron emitting radiotracer, ^{18}FDG; the repeated measurement of plasma radioactivity and glucose concentration in arterialized venous blood; and the determination of brain radioactivity by PET at fixed times after injection. A 4 time-constant operational equation is employed to calculate the regional cerebral metabolic rate for glucose ($rCMR_{glc}$) from the data.[9] To reduce external stimulation during PET, the eyes of the subjects were covered and their ears were plugged with cotton.

The mean value for CMR_{glc}, at the right cerebral hemisphere was 4.41 ± 1.27 (S.D.) mg/100 g/min for our subjects. The correlation coefficients between age and $rCMR_{glc}$ at 59 brain regions which were examined, were statistically insignificant (p>0.05). These initial studies now have been extended to 40 subjects aged 21-83 years, and the results have been extended and confirmed.[10,11]

Our finding, that brain glucose utilization is not correlated significantly with age, is consistent with the finding of Dastur et al,[1] who examined CBF and $CMRO_2$ with the nitrous oxide method, and of Ferris et al[12] using PET with ^{18}FDG. It differs from other reports[5,6,7] and from the report by Dastur et al[1] that CMR_{glc} is reduced in the elderly and of Gottstein et al[3] that $CMRO_2$ is reduced.

Other research groups[2,3,5] may not have screened as carefully for vascular atherosclerotic changes or hypertension, which may have accounted for the age declines they found in cerebral metabolism. In addition, the care taken to prevent sensory stimulation during the procedure minimized the effect that age-related decreases in auditory and visual function[13,14] might produce on cerebral metabolism.[15,16]

BRAIN METABOLISM AND PRIMARY DEGENERATIVE DEMENTIA
OF THE ALZHEIMER'S TYPE

Primary degenerative dementia of the Alzheimer's type is characterized by a gradual, steady course of deterioration of intellect and memory[17] with associated personality changes. Accelerated neuronal loss, brain atrophy, granulovacuolar degeneration, neurofibrillary tangles and senile plaques constitute the characteristic neuropathological feature. PET scanning with [18]FDG offers the opportunity of examining cerebral metabolic function in this disease state and thus has the potential for characterizing and localizing the disease process.

We used PET in examining PDD patients to characterize the extent of cerebral involvement and the severity of the illness. We will present two cases of PDD, one mild (Case 1) and one severe (Case 2). One limitation of these clinical studies is that final confirmation of diagnosis can be made only at autopsy or by cerebral biopsy; we are awaiting confirmation on the two patients presented. We compared their metabolic findings with those from age-matched healthy controls chosen from our normal aging study, characterized earlier.

Case 1

The patient is a 65-year-old, right-handed male, a former naval aviator and high school mathematics teacher with 16 years of education, who retired 4 years prior to admission because of his inability to maintain discipline in his classes. At that time, he noted the onset of memory problems. He was free of all medical diseases except for his primary brain disease.

The patient scored 24 out of a possible 30 on the Folstein Mini Mental State Exam[18] (the higher the score, the less demented the patient). On the Blessed Dementia Scale,[19] he scored 2.5 of 28 (the higher the score, the more demented the patient). His PET scan revealed a right hemisphere CMR_{glc} of 4.31 mg/100 g/min, not significantly different from the mean value of 4.58 + 0.81 (S.D.) mg/100 g/min for 12 age-matched controls (mean age 58.3 years). The regional cerebral metabolic rates also were not significantly different from those of controls, except for a small reduction at the left medial temporal region.

Case 2

The patient is a 73-year-old, right-handed female with a 6-year history of increasing memory dysfunction. The onset of her memory symptoms was characterized by forgetfulness and episodes of becoming lost. Her speech was mainly incoherent. She had no history of medical problems. A neurologic examination revealed multiple abnormal reflexes, such as grasp, snout, and palmomental, but no focal deficits. The CT scan scan revealed moderate cortical and mild lateral ventricular enlargement. The only severity scale that could be administered was the Blessed Dementia Scale,[19] on which her score was 20 of 28, indicating severe dementia.

All regional metabolic rates examined in both hemispheres were reduced. The patient's right hemisphere CMR_{glc}, for example, equaled 0.22 mg/100 g/min and was significantly reduced, compared with the control mean of 4.71 $\pm$ 1.65 (S.D.) mg/100 g/min (mean age 73.1 years, n=8).

As demonstrated by these two extreme cases, cerebral metabolism as measured with PET correlates well with the severity of the dementia. Case 1, a mildly demented patient failed to show a significant reduction in hemispheric CMR_{glc} or $rCMR_{glc}$, except for a reduced $rCMR_{glc}$ in the left inferior medial temporal region. Case 2, an extremely demented subject as assessed by a high Blessed dementia score and the clinical course, had significant reductions of CMR_{glc} and of $rCMR_{glc}$ throughout the brain.

BRAIN METABOLISM AND ADULT DOWN SYNDROME

Previous studies of brain oxidative metabolism and DS have reported mixed results.[20,21] In the first study of its kind, we measured cerebral glucose utilization with PET and [18]FDG in healthy DS subjects. Five DS subjects (three men and one female, mean age 22.5 years, range 19-27 years, and one 51-year-old male), each with trisomy 21 karyotype, were screened in the same manner as our normal controls. Their mental age ranged from 2 years 10 months to 5 years.

Hemispheric CMR_{glc} and many regional values for $rCMR_{glc}$ in young DS subjects were significantly higher, by as much as 40%, than values in age-matched controls. The right hemisphere mean CMR_{glc} for the young DS subjects equaled 6.53 $\pm$ 0.33 (S.E.) mg/100 g/min, compared with 4.89 $\pm$ 0.24 (S.E.) for the control group (mean age 22.5 years, n=10).[22] CMR_{glc} and $rCMR_{glc}$ in the 51-year-old DS subject did not differ from the mean in middle-aged controls, but was significantly less than the mean for the young DS subjects, particularly in regions of the frontal and parietal lobe.

Although many $rCMR_{glc}$ values in the 51-year-old DS subject were lower than those in the young DS group, they were not as reduced as were values seen in our severely demented PDD patients. Brains of DS subjects above 35 years of age demonstrate neuropathology similar to that found in brains of patients with Alzheimer's disease,[23] and some older DS subjects show signs of dementia.[24] Thus, the relation between dementia and neuropathology in DS remains to be examined. Our 51-year-old Down's subject was not demented.

SUMMARY

Brain glucose utilization, as measured with PET and the 2-deoxyglucose technique, was not correlated with age in 40 healthy men 21-83 years old. Significant metabolic reductions were shown throughout the brain of a patient with late severe PDD, suggesting that the reduction in brain metabolism and severe clinical dysfunction are related. In young adults with DS, on the other hand, cerebral metabolism was elevated as compared to age-matched controls. The complete relations among cerebral metabolism, clinical dysfunction, and neuropathology remain to be determined.

REFERENCES

1. D. K. Dastur, M. H. Lane, D. B. Hansen, S. S. Kety, R. N. Butler, S. Perlin and L. Sokoloff, in: "Human Aging, A Biological and Behavioral Study," edited by J. E. Birren, R. N. Butler, S. W. Greenhouse, L. Sokoloff, and M. R. Yarrow, USPHS Publ. 986, U.S. Govt. Printing Office, pp. 57-76, Washington, D.C. (1963).

2. J. F. Fazekas, R. W. Alman and A. M. Bessman, Am. J. Med. Sci. 223:245-257 (1952).

3. U. Gottstein and K. Held, Acta Neurol. Scand. (Suppl. 72), 60:54-55 (1979).

4. H. A. Shenkin, P. Novak, B. Goluboff, A. M. Soffe and L. Bortin, J. Clin. Invest. 32:459-465 (1953).

5. D. E. Kuhl, E. J. Metter, W. H. Riege and M. E. Phelps, J. Cereb. Blood Flow Metab. 2:163-171 (1982).

6. R. S. J. Frackowiak, G. Z. Lenzi and J. D. Heather, J. Comput. Assist. Tomogr. 4:727-736 (1980).

7. A. A. Lammertsma, R. S. J. Frackowiak, G. L. Lenzi, J. D. Heather, C. Pozzilli and T. Jones, J. Cereb. Blood Flow and Metab. 1(Suppl. 1):S3-S4 (1981).

8. L. Sokoloff, M. Reivich, C. Kennedy, M. H. Des Rosiers, C. S. Patlak, K. D. Pettigrew, O. Sakurada and M. Shinohara, J. Neurochem. 28:897-916 (1977).

9. S. C. Huang, M. E. Phelps, E. J. Hoffman, K. Sideris, C. J. Selin and D. E. Kuhl, Am. J. Physiol. 238:E69-E82 (1980).

10. R. Duara, R. A. Margolin, E. A. Robertson-Tchabo, E. D. London, M. Schwartz, J. W. Renfrew, R. Kessler, L. Sokoloff, D. H. Ingvar and S. I. Rapoport, Neurology. 32:A166-A167 (1982).

11. R. Duara, R. A. Margolin, E. A. Robertson-Tchabo, E. D. London, M. Schwartz, J. W. Renfrew, B. J. Koziarz, C. Grady, A. M. Moore, D. H. Ingvar, L. Sokoloff, H. Weingartner, R. A. Kessler, R. Manning, R. Channing, N. R. Cutler and S. I. Rapoport, Brain. 106:761-775 (1983).

12. S. H. Ferris, M. J. DeLeon, A. P. Wolf, T. Farkas, D. R. Christman, B. Reisberg, J. S. Fowler, R. MacGregor, A. Goldman, A. E. George and S. Rampal, Neurobiol. Aging. 1:127-131 (1980).

13. C. L. Grady, A. Pikus, A. M. Grimes, M. Schwartz, N. R. Cutler, S. I. Rapoport, Cortex (in press).

14. A. D. Weiss, in: "Human Aging: A Biological and Behavioral Study," edited by J. E. Birren, R. N. Butler, S. W. Greenhouse, L. Sokoloff and M. R. Yarrow, U.S. Dept. HEW, PHS Publ. No. 986, U.S. Govt. Printing Office, pp. 111-140, Washington, D.C. (1963).

15. M. E. Phelps, D. E. Kuhl and J. C. Mazziotta, Science. 211:1445-8 (1981).

16. J. C. Mazziotta, M. E. Phelps, R. E. Carson, D. E. Kuhl, Neurology. 32:921-937 (1982).

17. M. Sim, I. Sussman, J. Nerv Ment Dis. 135:489-499 (1962).

18. M. F. Folstein, S. E. Folstein and P. R. McHugh, J. Psychiatry Res. 12:189-198 (1975).

19. G. Blessed, B. E. Tomlinson and M. Roth, Br. J. Psychiatry. 114:797-811 (1968).

20. J. F. Fazekas, W. R. Ehrmantraut, J. G. Shea and J. Kleh, Neurology. 8:558-560 (1958)

21. N. A. Lassen, S. H. Cristensen, K. G. Rasmussen, B. M. Steward, Arch. Neurol. 15:595 (1966).

22. M. Schwartz, R. Duara, J. Haxby, C. L. Grady, B. J. White, R. M. Kessler, A. D. Kay, N. R. Cutler, S. I. Rapoport, Science. 221:781-783 (1983).

23. S. S. Schochet, P. W. Lampert, W. F. McCormick, Acta Neuropathol. 23:342-346 (1973).

24. G. A. Jervis, Am J Psychiatry. 105:102-106 (1948).

PSYCHOPHYSIOLOGIC DISORDERS OF THE ELDERLY

Charles M. Gaitz

Gerontology Center,
Texas Research Institute of Mental Sciences and
Baylor College of Medicine
Houston, Texas

Even more than is true for younger people, the health of elderly persons represents an interplay of psychological and physiological factors. Older persons are more likely to have physical impairments and, though inherently incapacitating, these will affect their emotional state.

Bachrach (1982) distinguishes between psychosomatic and psychofunctional or psychophysiological symptoms. Symptoms associated with an identifiable ("organic") lesion presumed to be the result of psychological factors are called psychosomatic. Symptoms for which no anatomical basis can be discovered and that occur in an environment of emotional stress, are psychophysiological. Because effective treatment is available for many psychosomatic conditions, such as achalasia and peptic ulcer, Bachrach contends that we need not be concerned about identifying precipitating emotional factors, characteristic personality patterns, or unconscious conflicts. Because less specific treatment is available for such "functional" disorders as irritable bowel syndrome, more attention should be given to identifying and dealing with psychological problems.

Clear differentiation between psychosomatic and psychophysiologic symptoms may be of some value, but we rarely are able to do this for elderly patients. Consequently, I shall define one concept of psychophysiologic disorders as including those in which there seems to be an interaction of social, psychological, and morphological elements (Gaitz 1982). Isolating disorders on the basis of their having demonstrable lesions or not has many implications we cannot explore here. I should mention, however, that the attempt at categorization often leads to rigid treatment approaches and limits opportunities for developing a regimen applicable to a specific patient. I do not share the opinion that the presence or absence of a lesion is an overriding factor in determining how a patient should be treated.

Superficially, the interaction of psychological and organic problems in a patient may look like social withdrawal and depression. On investigation, however, one often learns that the patient has a physical impairment that has become more troublesome and is restricting his or her movement and social contacts--or that, because of an elderly person's social isolation, a physiologic disability has gone unnoticed and untreated. The interrelationship of psychic and somatic aspects of illness is especially clear in elderly patients. A comprehensive evaluation will almost always show that psychologic, physiologic, and social factors contribute to the clinical picture.

Any organ system may show manifestations that we could characterize as psychophysiologic disorders of the elderly. Most of my remarks relate to an approach to diagnosis and treatment, with an emphasis on the central nervous system. The next speakers will discuss some examples of the involvement of other systems.

Consequently, I find it extremely useful to consider both psychologic and physiologic aspects when treating patients of all ages, but especially the elderly, who are more likely to have both reduced mental capacity and physical disorders. It is helpful at times to include a life-stage approach in diagnosis and treatment, although by itself such an approach may be negative and defective.

One must remember that there is much heterogeneity among the elderly and that physical and mental capacities do not correlate highly with chronological age. One cannot use age per se to identify physical or emotional problems. Certainly, elderly persons tend to tire faster than younger persons. Even normally, and without brain disease, their memory for medical instructions, for example, is shorter. But as diagnosticians and therapists, we must determine whether their complaints are caused by depression, by a physical disorder, or by processes we think of as normal aging.

We are still struggling with concepts of normal and abnormal aging. Eventually we may be able to distinguish processes attributable to stages of aging and discover correlations. At our present state of knowledge, however, it seems more reasonable to examine our elderly patients with only minimal attention to chronological age. We must continue to use age as only one parameter in understanding function and be aware that it may be important in the outcome of treatment.

But we must avoid value judgments that may result in denying treatment to persons because of their advanced chronological age. Culturally determined attitudes influence both therapists and patients. We must strive for objective appraisal and rational intervention, using chronological age as one, but not an overriding indicator.

We can help our elderly patients to expand their social and support networks. We can help patients gain insight into their emotional disorders, and we can help them improve their physical condition by better nutrituion and medications that correct metabolic disorders. One could continue with a long list of interventions: each professional discipline and medical specialty has much to offer. To be most effective for elderly patients, we must work in concert.

A social worker obviously is unable to treat a patient for congestive heart failure. A specialist in internal medicine cannot prescribe insulin and a special diet for a diabetic patient, without knowing also that the patient is demented and does not understand how much insulin to take or how to follow the diet. Similarly, a psychiatrist who treats a depressed person has to take into account not only the patient's psychological stresses but his or her physical disorders.

Physical illnesses that occur in old age sometimes present an atypical clinical picture: the early signs of a malignancy may, for example, appear to be psychological rather than physiological. A frail, elderly person who has an infection may not have an elevated temperature.

An adequate diagnostic evaluation is essential to determine whether or not the complaint of an elderly patient is caused by a remediable condition. Lack of energy and fatigue may be symptomatic of depression, of a physical disorder, or what might be called normal aging. Some elderly people tend to disengage willingly from an active social schedule, but their disengagement may also be a sign of depression. Confusion and disorientation may be signs of primary degenerative dementia, or they may be related to an electrolyte imbalance or drug toxicity.

Although the explanation is by no means clear, clinicians are likely to agree that many older persons have diminished emotional and physical capacities to adjust to stress. Accepting this concept should not, however, lead us to a nihilistic approach to treatment. Elderly persons are survivors, people who have dealt with many problems in the past and may require only minimal inter-

vention in old age. A careful diagnostic appraisal and treatment
plan, which mobilizes the patient's social and community supports,
often results in a favorable outcome.

DIAGNOSIS OF MENTAL DISORDERS

The latest revision of the Diagnostic and Statistical Manual
(DSM-III) (1978) developed by the American Psychiatric Association
has two categories that are useful in identifying psychophysiologic disorders in elderly persons: adjustment disorders and psychological factors affecting physical disorders. Adjustment disorders are described as maladaptive reactions to identifiable life
events or circumstances. Maladaption is indicated by impaired social or occupational functioning, or by symptoms or other behaviors that are in excess of the normal and expectable reaction to a
stressor. Stressors--single or multiple, social, psychological,
and physical, in various settings and possibly associated with
specific developmental stages--may be implicated. The associated
features of adjustment disorders vary; physical symptoms and such
behavioral manifestations as withdrawal, aggression, excessive
drinking, depression, and anxiety are mentioned. The second category, psychological factors affecting physical disorders, is not
considered a diagnosis in itself, but is a category that helps measure the certainty with which a clinician judges psychological factors to be contributing to the onset or exacerbation of a patient's physical disorder. The diagnosis requires that the onset
or worsening of the physical disorder be related temporally to psychologically important environmental stimuli.

Most elderly persons referred to a psychiatrist because their
symptoms suggest dementia are likely to have what is labeled in
DSM-III as primary degenerative dementia. Alzheimer's disease has
become a popular label, and sometimes the condition is referred to
as senile dementia of the Alzheimer type. A smaller number of referred patients have multi-infarct dementia. Occasionally we see
patients who have a delirium, etiologically related to one or more
factors, but the typical patient has primary degenerative dementia. While advances in our knowledge of neurophysiology and morphology have led to a better understanding of the etiology of organic brain syndrome and a more precise diagnosis, specific treatment based on diagnosis is rarely applied.

DEMENTIA AS A PSYCHOPHYSIOLOGIC DISORDER

Geschwind (1975), writing about the borderland of neurology
and psychiatry, said, "This common ground unfortunately bears more
resemblance to no-man's-land than an open border." The existence
of an area of overlap between neurology and psychiatry is acknowl-
edged, but we have much to learn about it. Errors include not

only failures to diagnose neurologic diseases that cause psychiatric symptoms, but also mistaken diagnoses of untreatable neurologic disorders in patients who actually have reversible psychiatric diseases.

Most of these patients probably do not have reversible conditions, but careful evaluation sometimes reveals that patients have brain tumors, infections, systemic diseases, diseases of other organ systems, head trauma, metabolic disorders, or other conditions that may be associated with symptoms difficult to distinguish from other causes of organic mental disorder.

Appropriate and specific treatment for these other conditions, however, often reverses the mental disorder. An elderly person with uremia or coronary insufficiency may, for example, present symptoms also associated with primary central nervous system degeneration. A history of impaired cognitive function may be attributed too quickly to senile dementia and differential diagnoses scarcely considered. Social and psychological factors must also be taken into account. Social isolation, changes in social roles, losses by death of significant persons, losses of self-esteem, income, prestige, and other stresses may be implicated in the onset and progression of cognitive changes in some of our patients. Not surprisingly, environmental manipulation and psychotherapy may alleviate the severity of such stresses, and thus the behavioral manifestations of cognitive impairment may change.

IMPLICATIONS FOR TREATMENT

If we acknowledge that it is all but impossible to isolate the organic and functional aspects of what we label organic brain syndrome or organic mental disorder, it becomes clear that, rationally, we should treat our patients as having a psychophysiologic disorder. It is impossible to treat them adequately by using only an organ system-disease approach. It also is impossible to treat elderly persons who have psychiatric disorders without giving attention to their physical health status. Age-related changes in metabolism that may affect drug reactions deserve attention, and it is only by using a comprehensive diagnostic treatment approach that we are able to address a variety of stressors likely to affect a given patient. Obviously, specific treatment should be administered when needed, but general measures based on the premise that aging processes represent stresses are also useful. The timing of intervention is important. When life is at stake, we hardly have time to worry about interpersonal relationships and housing problems, but ultimately these become important issues. Morphologic changes may not be noted, but persons with dementia can be helped by environmental manipulation, relieving external stresses by assisting family members. Treatment of depression may have to be deferred when a patient has pneumonia or congestive heart failure, but rehabilitation of persons with physical impairments may require attention to the patients' motivation and willingness to proceed with therapy. Combining treatment for psychological and physical health problems is logical, and it is an especially valuable approach to treating elderly persons. The treatment may be concurrent or sequential, depending on the circumstances.

SUMMARY

Elderly persons are prone to have a combination of physical, social and psychological problems. It is beneficial to patients and caregivers to consider these ailments, including dementia, as constituting psychophysiologic disorders. This provides a rationale for comprehensive treatment that addresses multiple problems and often utilizes a multidisciplinary team approach.

REFERENCES

American Psychiatric Association, 1978, "Diagnostic and Statistical Manual (DSM-III)," (3rd. ed.), American Psychiatric Assn., Washington, D. C.

Bachrach, W. H, 1982, Psychological elements of gastrointestinal disorders, in: "Phenomenology and treatment of psychophysiological disorders," W. E. Fann, I. Karacan, A. D. Pokorny, and R. L. Williams, eds., Spectrum, Jamaica, N. Y.

Gaitz, C. M., 1982, Some psychophysiological problems of the elderly, in: "Phenomenology and Treatment of Psychophysiological disorders," W. E. Fann, I. Karacan, A. D. Pokorny, and R. L. Williams, eds., Spectrum, Jamaica, N. Y.

Geschwind, N, 1975, The borderland of neurology and psychiatry: Some common misconceptions, in: "Psychiatric Aspects of Neurologic Disease," D. F. Benson, and D. Blumer, eds., Grune & Stratton, New York.

HYPERTENSION IN THE ELDERLY:

A SLEEPING DOG?

A.H. Mann

Royal Free Hospital, Pond Street, N.W.3

1) Introduction

Hypertension in old age is common, sufficiently so for us to
think of it as normal. Taking the W.H.O. criteria that a diastolic blood pressure of 90-94 mm Hg refers to borderline hypertension and one of 95 mg or more to definite hypertension, then,
in a U.K. population 7% of men under 35 have borderline hypertension, 18% under 45, 20% under 55 and 25% of those over 55.
Further illustration of blood pressure levels in older age groups
has come from community based research (e.g. Miall and Chinn 1973).

In a Welsh population mean blood pressure levels was shown to
rise in men, until the age of 70 and in women until the age of.75.
After these ages there is a fall in mean pressure. This fall is
accompanied by a dimunition in scatter around the mean level.
Very low levels appear to be no longer recorded, nor do the very
high ones. The loss of the high readings is not surprising, the
demise of sub-ects with low level readings being explained by the
fact that they tend to be poor risk survivors with a previous
history of stroke or myocardial infact.

In the over 60s mean systolic pressure levels can be seen to
increase at a greater rate than do the Mean diastolic pressures
until very old age. This difference is explained by two conditions being recorded (i) of classical hypertension meeting W.H.O.
criteria of 160 mm systolic and greater than 95 mm diastolic and
(ii) isolated systolic hypertension characterised by a systolic
blood pressure level greater or more than 160 mm and a diastolic
level of less than 95 mm. The prevalence rate of classical hypertension probably remains after middle life.

295

2) Risks of Hypertension

Evidence from all longitudinal studies indicate that not only does cardiovascular morbidity increase with age but that the additional risks, arising from the presence of hypertension, also magnify with age, (Kannel et. al. 1971). The increased mortality from stroke and cardiovascular disease associated with increased systolic or diastolic pressure in old age was also shown in the Welsh population.

Apart from these cardiovascular episodes, there also is the possibility of a relationship between hypertension and multi-infarct dementia. However post mortem surveys of patients with dementia such as those of Corsellis (1969) showed that clear cut arteriosclerosis in the brain was only reliably predicted by severe hypertension in life ($<$110 mm Hg diastolic).

3) Aetiology of Hypertension

Hypertension therefore in old age is a prevalent and potentially dangerous condition. However the aetiology of hypertension remains unknown. A current view of the hypertensive state is as the final pathway for more than one aetiological process, thereby explaining the lack of any conclusive findings in hypertension research in attempting to highlight one aetiological process at work for a group of hypertensive subjects. Promising avenues are (1) the demonstration of a familial pattern of blood pressure levels (2) that for some hypertensives there is salt intolerance. These two factors may well be linked (Clegg et. al. 1982). A different avenue, and of more concern for psychiatrists, has been the demonstration of the hyperkinetic stage in some hypertensives particularly with those with borderline elevation of pressure characterised by increased catecholamic excretion- Manuck et. al. (1975) have demonstrated that Type A behaviour is associated with an exaggerated and prolonged blood pressure and catecholamine response to experiments designed to provoke hostility in experiments (Glass 1980). The relationship of stress to hypertension is inconclusive. Variables such as crowding, unemployment, poverty and crime levels have been studied in relation to blood pressure levels in the population. The lack of conclusion may be reflecting the fact that only certain individuals have a propensity to react to such stress by an abnormal cardiovascular response.

Most hypertension research has concerned hypertension in the younger adult. With reference to old age the question arises as to whether hypertension in old age is common because hypertension is in fact part of the ageing process. This is not the case for all. Studies among Kenyan tribes (Shaper 1969) and in the Solomon Islanders (Page et. at. 1974) have shown that there are societies where there is no age related rise in blood pressure at all. Studies from Western cultures, however, suggest that there is a slight upward gradient of blood pressure over time, but most of the age related rise is probably due to 'tracking'. Certain

individuals, beginning with higher than average pressures, have
an accelerated rise with age. One explanation of the isolated
raised systolic pressure seen in the elderly is that it is a
secondary change from underlying arterial damage, in particular
loss of elasticity. This arterial damage being commoner with age
in all Western cultures, but not inevitable. Relevant for the
elderly too is the observation that obesity has virtually no
relationship with blood pressure level in old age. Quite in
contrast to the younger adult, weight loss may occur with increasing blood pressure in old age. Ambient temperature affects the
blood pressure, the elderly being particularly sensitive to
temperature change. The fall in mean pressure levels, in an over
60 population, with a 10°c rise in ambient temperature would be
that hoped after treatment of that population by antihypertensive
drugs.

Cerebral Blood Flow Studies

Radioactive labelling techniques have enabled some knowledge of
cerebral blood flow to be obtained. Cerebral blood flow appears
to be constant at 55 ml per 100 gm of brain tissue to all mean
arterial pressures between 60 mm and 170 mm in the adult. There
is therefore successful aut-regulation, be it mediated by the
automatic nervous system or directly by arterial muscle wall.
Very low levels of blood pressure lead to impairment of cerebral
blood flow, whereas a hypertensive level overrides the protection
for the capillaries by the arterioles and can result in haemorr-
hage. Chronic hypertension, however, does lead to a change in
auto regulation, so that cerebral blood flow is maintained
despite higher levels of blood pressure.

There is evidence that the auto regulation is less effective in
old age, perhaps because of impaired autonomic nervous system
function. Lower perfusion pressures therefore can occur more
readily. The effect of impaired cerebral blood flow is never
even, presumably because of the differential damage in the
cerebral vascular tree. Transient ischaemic attacks result from
lower perfusion pressure and are said to clear if the blood pressure is raised. Multi-infarct dementia is characterised by uneven
cerebral blood flow in the brain but as dementia proceeds,
cerebral flow tends to diminish. It could therefore be concluded
that hypertension may have a protective effect in maintaining
cerebral blood flow in the damaged cerebrovascular tree in old
age. Evidence for this is scanty however. Wilkie (1971) studied
47 elderly provided data and showed that, over 10 years, psychometric test performance was maximal among those subjects with
mild hypertension compared to those normotensive or severely
hypertensive.

Treatment

The advantage of treatment of both classical and systolic
hypertension in the elderly is now in need of re-examination.

The risks of the hypertensive state are now much more clearly
stated and they need placing against the potential hazards of
blood pressure reduction - namely short-term ones resulting from
episodes of postural hypertension leading to transient ischaemia
and toxicity from the antihypertensive drugs, particularly beta-
blocking agents. Longer term risks, too, may be an acceleration
of cognitive impairment from poor perfusion of the cerebrovascular
tree. There are no scientific studies setting the advantage of
treatment in the reduction of blood pressure against potential
hazards. However, three studies of hypertension in the elderly
are underway. Two are assessing psychological effects of
treatment, one in the U.S. (Systolic hypertension in the elderly
project), one in the U.K. (MRC treatment trial of the elderly).
Both studies aim to assess psychological effects of blood pressure
reduction, both immediate and over a five year period. Psychological effects being considered are cognitive change and
psychiatric morbidity. Their results should provide information
not only on the when and which elderly patients should be treated
for hypertension but how serious is the hazard of doing so.

REFERENCES

MIALL W.E., CHINN S.(1973)
  Blood pressure and Ageing. Clinical Science and Molecular
  Medicine. 45 23-33.

KANNEL W.B., GORDON T., SCHWARTZ M.J.(1971)
  Systolic vs Diastolic Blood Pressure and Risk of Coronary Heart
  Disease. American Journal Cardiology 27 336-346.

CORSELLIS J.A.
  The Pathology of the Ageing Brain. British Journal Hospital
  Medicine 2 695-702.

CLEGG G., MORGAN D.G., DAVIDSON C.(1982)
  Heterogeneity of Essential Hypertension. Lancet ii, 891-893.

MANUCK S.B., CRAFT R., GOLA K.J.(1978)
  Coronary Prone Behaviour and Cardiovascular Response.
  Psychophysiology 15 403-411.

GLASS D.C.(1977)
  Stress and Coronary Disease, Behaviour Patterns. American
  Scientist 65, 177-187.

PAGE L.B., DAMON A., MOELLERING R.C.(1974)
  Antecedents of Cardiovascular Disease in Six Solomon Island
  Societies. Circulation 45 1102-11146.

SHAPER A.G., WRIGHT D.H., KYOBE J.(1969)
Blook pressure, body build in three nomadic tribes of northern
Kenya. East African Medical Journal 46 272-1981.

BRENNAN P.J., GREENBERG G.A., MIALL W.E., THOMPSON S.G.(1982)
Seasonal variation in Arterial Blood Pressure. British Medical
Journal (in press).

QUANTITATIVE COMPUTED TOMOGRAPHY IN ELDERLY DEPRESSED PATIENTS

R. Jacoby, R. Dolan, R. Levy and R. Baldy

The Maudsley Hospital and Institute of Psychiatry
London, SE5
England

A detailed account of this investigation is published in the British Journal of Psychiatry 1983, volume 143. An extended summary is given here.

INTRODUCTION

In earlier studies using computed tomography (CT) we identified a sub-group of nine elderly depressed patients with enlarged cerebral ventricles, all bar one of whom had experienced their first depression after the age of 60, who were less anxious and showed a more 'endogenous' clinical picture than the other depressed patients with whom they were studied (Jacoby and Levy, 1980). At follow-up this sub-group showed a significantly higher two-year mortality than their fellow depressives (5 out of 9 cf. 4 out of 31, $p < 0.03$); death being due to a variety of mostly non-cerebral causes (Jacoby et al, 1981). The present investigation employed a new technique for measuring CT numbers or Hounsfield Units (HU) to obtain an index of brain tissue density in an attempt to seek further evidence for cerebral organic change in old age depression.

METHOD

The original numerical CT data were stored on magnetic tape. Data of sufficient quality, i.e. free of movement artefact, were available for 37 patients with affective disorder. Comparisons were made with 36 healthy, age-matched, elderly, community residents and 23 patients with a clinical diagnosis of senile dementia of the Alzheimer type.

Scans were displayed in the familiar picture form on the visual display unit of an independent viewing centre. 12 predetermined brain sites were located with a tracker ball which covered an area of 129 pixels. These sites were left and right: anterior frontal, posterior frontal, temporal, thalamus, parietal and occipital. Mean HU were measured for each 129-pixel area by a single observer. In order to test inter-rater reliability 78 measurements from tomograms chosen at random from all three groups of subjects were made on a separate occasion by a second observer. The mean of the differences and the correlation coefficient between the two sets of observations were calculated.

RESULTS

Inter-rater reliability was high, $p < 0.001$. There were no significant differences in mean HU for individual brain areas on separate t-tests between demented and depressed patients, whereas some differences were found between the healthy controls and both patient groups. Analysis of variance showed a significant separation of all three groups, dements showing the lowest mean HU, controls the highest, with the depressives intermediate between them, F 11.45, $p < 0.001$.

Most of the variance between the controls and the depressed patients was accounted for by the sub-group of nine with global ventricular enlargement, who showed lower mean HU in every brain area than their fellow depressives with normal sized ventricles, F 18.86, $p < 0.001$. By contrast those healthy control subjects who had been found to have enlarged ventricles in the original study had higher mean HU than controls with normal ventricles.

HU were not correlated with age in any group, nor with a history of ECT in the depressives. In the latter, low HU were correlated with sulcal dilatation in several brain areas, but once again this was mainly due to the nine patients with ventricular enlargement.

COMMENT

With respect to an index of brain density the depressed patients were found to occupy an intermediate position vis à vis dements and controls, a finding due mostly to a sub-group with late-onset depression and ventricular enlargement. At follow-up none of this sub-group was considered to be a misdiagnosed case of senile dementia. Low density was probably not an artefact of ventricular dilatation, since controls with enlarged ventricles showed higher mean HU than controls with normal ventricles. Furthermore, membership of this sub-group of depressives predicted an earlier mortality not found in the controls. It seems likely, therefore, that the finding reflected a real organic cerebral change, the nature and cause of which remain obscure, but which may also be of importance in facilitating the emergence and affecting the prognosis of at least some cases of depression in late life.

REFERENCES

Jacoby, R. J., and Levy, R., 1980, Computed tomography in the elderly: 3 affective disorder, <u>Brit. J. Psychiat.</u>, 136:270.

Jacoby, R. J., Levy, R., and Bird, J. M., 1981, Computed tomography and the outcome of affective disorder: a follow-up study of elderly patients, <u>Brit. J. Psychiat.</u>, 139:288.

SEIZURE DISORDERS IN THE AGED

Nurhan Avman, and Ali O. Taşçıoğlu

Department of Neurosurgery
Ankara University, School of Medicine
Ankara, Turkey

Seizure disorders in the aged are mainly due to cerebrovascular diseases and intracerebral tumors[1].

Among cerebrovascular diseases arteriovenous malformations take the leed with 29 % insidance. Other causes are cerebral thrombosis, TIA, and RIND. These three constitutes approximately 3.4 % of seizures in the aged. Insidance of seizures among the various tumors in the aged is shown in table 1.

TABLE 1 : INSIDANCE OF SEIZURES AMONG TUMORS IN THE AGED

	TOTAL	WITH SEIZURE	%
GLIAL TUMORS	: 1296	370	28.0
MENENGIOMAS	: 331	108	32.6
PTUITARY ADENOMAS (254 MACRO—GIANT)	: 394	3	0.8
SCHWANNOMAS	: 54	–	–
TUBERCULOMAS	: 22	7	32.0

As can be seen from the table, glial tumors and especially glioblastoma multiforme type, and menengiomas are the main epileptigenic sources in the aged. While menengiomas result in a higher insidance of seizures, pituitary adenomas and schwannomas due to their locations, produce less seizure disorders. As a result we can say that if an aged person has focal seizures his chance of having a brain tumor is approximately 30 %.

Cranial trauma is an other entity in the aged that will be the cause of seizures. Insidance of early and late seizures in patients with cranial trauma is shown in table 2.

TABLE 2 : INSIDANCE OF EARLY AND LATE SEIZURES IN CRANIAL TRAUMA[2]

	TOTAL	EARLY SEIZURES	LATE SEIZURES
NUMBER OF CASES :	2428	74	157
OVER 50 YEARS	323	5	11

Although cranial trauma patients have an overall insidance of 2.9 % seizures, in the cases where the trauma is severe enough for the patient to be hospitalised insidance of seizures rises up to 4.5 %.

Chronic subdural hematomas which may develop following a trivalant head injury, is rarely the cause of seizures in the aged.

DIAGNOSTIC WORKUP

In any patient with a seizure diagnostic workup starts with an EEG. In recent years neuroradiology has made impressive improvements. These diagnostic advances are summarised in table 3. They are trully indispensable for a rational workup.

TABLE 3 : DIAGNOSTIC ADVANCES

ANGIOGRAPHY
      AORTIC ARC STUDIES—4VESSEL ANGIOGRAPHY
      DIGITAL SUBTRACTION ANGIOGRAPHY
      RADIONUCLIDE ANGIOGRAPHY
COMPUTERISED TOMOGRAPHY
ULTRASONOGRAPHY
DOPPLER SONOGRAPHY
REGIONAL BLOOD FLOW STUDIES
POSITRON EMITTING TOMOGRAPHY
NUCLEAR MAGNETIC RESONANCE

Total cerebral angiography is mandatory for the surgery of cerebrovascular diseases. Aortic arc studies with visualisation of extracranial and intracranial vascularisation are prerequisite for carotid endarterectomy and shunt operations. Newly developed digiüal subtraction angiography enabled us to see extracranial and intracranial vessels without an arterial puncture and with the use of less contrast material.

Radionuclide angiography proved to be helpful in the differentiation of perfussion disturbances from intracranial tumors.

Doppler sonography,gray scale ultrasonography and regional blood flow studies are all nonpenetrating tecnics that give vital information on the flow characteristics and morphology of cerebral vesseles.

Computerised tomography is a fascinating tool that can show lesions as small as 10 mms with accuracy. With this machine we can easly detect intracerebral hematomas, tumors, infarction areas, aneurysms and pituitary microadenomas.

PET and NMR are the new wonders of the market. Though mainly in the experimental stage it has been used in some centers with success. They seem to compete with CT and they may take the upper hand in soon future. They are especially useful in demonstrating the methabolic activities of the brain.

RECENT ADVANCES IN TREATMENT

Brain Tumors

In the recent years the most striking for the treatment of brain tumors is the introduction of microtecnic. With magnification, coaxial illumination, microinstruments and bipolar coagulation many of the so called inoperable tumors, can be totally removed. Advances are particularly striking in benign lesions like menengiomas and acoustic neurinomas. Menengiomas of olfactory groove, planum sphenoidale, tuberculum sella, sphenoidal wing and clivus – once accepter as difficult lesions for total removal – now can be totally removed with low mortality and morbidity. With the menengiomas of convexities epileptic seizures has been cured in 50 % of the cases and in the remaning 35 % they were controlled by medication.

Glial tumors of the brain, unfortunately resists any form of treatment. Eventhough the results are controversial radical resection seems to be the best treatment. It can be supported with radiation theraphy and chemotheraphy. These measures may contribute to a more usefull life, but they have no effect on survival.

Metastatic intracranial tumors – if they are single and if

the condition of the patient is good – can be resected. Quality of survival depends on the treatment of the primary focus also.

Postoperative seizures due to scarr tissue may be an additional nusiance. Laser surgery and ultrasonic aspirators are additional tools that can enable total tumor removal with less brain traction and less scar tissue formation.

Vascular Lesions

Surgical treatment of cerebral ischemic lesions have shown considerable improvement in the last decade. Since 70 % of stenotic or thrombotic lesions occure at the extracranial portion of the carotid and vertebral arteries, endarterectomy operations are now the best form of treatment. Stenosis of the internal carotid artery at the bifurcation point is the most common one and also the one that gives the best results in treatment. Induction of controlled hypertension saved the use of internal and external shunts and simplified the surgical procedure.

Cerebral bypass operation – introduced by Donaghy and Yaşargil in 1967 – to increase the flow in the proximally ocluded cerebral vessels, gives good results in TIA and RIND patients[3]. With this tecnic anastomosis of vessels of 1 mm diameter is possible and 1 to 2 mm increase in the diameter increases the flow 4 – 16 times. An anastomosis patency of 90 % is possible in experienced hands. For anterior circulatory insufficiency superficial temporal artery is anastomosed to one of the distal branches of midle cerebral artery. For posterior circulatory insufficiency occipital artery is anastomosed to PICA.

If a patient starts to have TIAs his chance of having a compleated stroke within two years is 20 – 40 %. In well selected cases bypass operation reduces this risk to 2 %. While TIA and RIND patients benefit from bypass and endarterectomy operations, patients with compleated stroke showe no improvement.

Encephalomyosynangiosis has been used in few instancess where anastomosis was not possible due to small diametered STA or MCA branches. For brances under 0.8 mm preclude useful bypass. We do not have enough cases to evaluate this tecnic statistically.

With the introduction of microtecnic the operability criteria of the arteriovenous malformations has improved. At present, large malformations with multiple feeders and deep seated malformations can be removed with a considerably low mortality and morbidity. Total removal of an arteriovenous malformation either completely eliminates the epileptogenic focus or makes it supressable by medication. But, some arteriovenous malformations are not suitable for surgical resection. In such malformations radiosurgery or embolisation tecnics may be tried.

Introduction of microtecnic has dropped the surgical mortality of intracranial aneurysms significantly. In The Cooperative Study of Intracranial Aneurysms[4], surgical mortality has been reported as 30 %. Selection of low grade patients, hypotensive anesthesia and microtecnic has dropped the mortality to 5 % in experienced hands[5]. If we can exclude vasospasm, which still awaits solution, than we can say that the results are gratifying for aneurysm patients.

REFERENCES

1. G. E. Solomon and F. Plum, Clinical Management of Seizures: A Guide for the Physician. W. B. Saunders Company, Philadelphia, 1976.
2. A. Erdem, Evaluation of patients with cranial trauma: Results of 2428 cases seen in Ankara University, School of Medicine, Department of Neurosurgery. Clinical Study. 1983.
3. M. G. Yaşargil, Microsurgery: Applied to Neurosurgery., Georg Thieme Verlag, Stuttgart, 1969.
4. E. B. Boldrey, ... W. H. Sweet, Report on the Cooperative Study of Intracranial Aneurysms and Subarachnoid Hemorrhage., J. Neurosurg 25:683, 1966.
5. M. G. Yaşargil, and J. L. Fox, The orerative approach to aneurysms of the anterior comminicating artery. In Advances and Tecnical Standarts in Neurosurgery. Edited by H. Krayenbühl, Vol 2 pp. 113-170, Springer-Verlag, New York, 1975.

THE DOPAMINERGIC AND NORADRENERGIC SYSTEMS IN ALZHEIMER-TYPE DEMENTIA

C.M.Yates, I.M.Ritchie, A.Urquhart, A.F.J.Maloney +*
and A.Gordon+
MRC Brain Metabolism Unit
1 George Square, Edinburgh EH8 9JZ and +Western
General Hospital, Edinburgh   *Deceased May 1982

Whilst previous studies point to a loss of noradrenergic neurons in Alzheimer-type dementia (ATD) (Bondareff et al., 1981; Yates et al., 1981; Cross et al., 1981) there are conflicting reports of normal (Mann et al., 1980) and reduced (Adolfsson et al., 1979) dopamine function in this disease. Observations that ATD patients who die below the age of 80 years have a greater loss of choline acetyltransferase activity from the cerebral cortex (Rossor et al., 1981) and of neurons from the locus coeruleus (Bondareff et al , 1981; Tomlinson et al., 1981) suggest that early onset (pre-senile) ATD may differ biochemically from late onset (senile) ATD. We have examined this possibility by measuring dopamine, its metabolite homovanillic acid (HVA) and noradrenaline in brains from cases of pre-senile ATD, senile ATD and Down syndrome. All values are means $\pm$ S.D.

TISSUES AND METHODS

Brains were obtained from cases of ATD (n = 13), Down syndrome (trisomy 21 anomaly, n = 5) and controls (n = 13) with no clinical signs of a central nervous system disorder. The ATD cases were divided into 8 pre-senile cases with onset before 65 and aged less than 70 years at death (59 $\pm$ 9 years) and 5 senile cases with onset after 65 and aged over 70 years at death (82 $\pm$ 6 years). The controls were similarly divided into 7 young cases (57 $\pm$ 8 years) and 6 old cases (76 $\pm$ 4 years). Three of the four cases of Down syndrome aged 53-57 years had changes in personality and behaviour indicative of dementia; there was no convincing evidence of dementia in the fourth case. The fifth case of Down syndrome, aged 27 years, showed no signs of dementia. The major causes of death were bronchopneumonia (18 cases) and myocardial infarction (7 cases). Drugs administered orally within two weeks of death included morphine-type analgesics (10 cases), diazepam/nitrazepam (9 cases) and phenothiazines (7 cases). The cadavers were refrigerated at 4°C within 4 hours and the post-mortem done within 42 hours of death (21 ± 11 hours). The right half-brain from the ATD and Down's cases was fixed for neuropathological examination. The caudate nucleus, olfactory tubercle, hypothalamus and mamillary body, which contain aminergic nerve terminals, were dissected from the left half-brain (Mackay et al., 1978a) and stored at -70°C until radio-enzymatic assay of noradrenaline and dopamine (Mackay et al., 1978b) and fluorimetric assay of HVA (Ashcroft et al., 1976).

RESULTS

All cases of ATD and of Down syndrome in their 50s showed cortical gyral atrophy and large numbers of plaques and tangles in the cerebral cortex. Plaques and tangles were more numerous in pre-senile ATD and Down syndrome than in senile ATD. In 3 cases of ATD and two of Down syndrome the substantia innominata was examined and 'finger-print' tangles observed in large neurons. The 27 year old case of Down syndrome had a low brain weight but no cortical gyral atrophy and no plaques and tangles. Perivascular atrophy was present in the basal ganglia in 5 cases of ATD and 3 cases of Down syndrome (including the 27 year old). The substantia nigra was normally pigmented in all cases.

Post mortem interval was not significantly correlated with the concentration of noradrenaline, dopamine or HVA. A significant decrease with age was observed for noradrenaline in control hypothalamus ($r = -0.61$, $p < 0.05$) and mamillary body ($r = -0.77$, $p < 0.02$) but for neither amine nor HVA in the caudate nucleus. Noradrenaline levels were more markedly reduced in the hypothalamus in pre-senile ATD ($p < 0.01$) and Down syndrome ($p < 0.001$) than in senile ATD ($p < 0.05$) and were reduced in the mamillary body in pre-senile ($p < 0.01$), but not senile, ATD. The 27 year old case of Down syndrome had a very low level of hypothalamic noradrenaline which resembled levels in the older Down's cases (Table 1). Dopamine and HVA in the caudate nucleus and hypothalamus were unaltered in pre-senile or senile ATD. Dopamine was decreased ($p < 0.01$) in the cases of Down syndrome in their 50s but dopamine and HVA were within the control range in the 27 year old Down's case (Table 2). HVA in the olfactory tubercle from 5 (pre-senile and senile) ATD cases ($2.59 \pm 0.29 \mu g/g$ wet wt) did not differ from 7 controls ($3.38 \pm 0.95 \mu g/g$ wet wt). Significantly lower ($p < 0.05$) HVA levels were found in 3 controls ($1.58 \pm 0.75 \mu g/g$ wet wt) in which the anterior perforated substance was included in the olfactory tubercle sample suggesting that the olfactory tubercle in man, as in rat, receives a discrete dopaminergic innervation (Moore et al., 1978). Dopamine and HVA levels in 3 control and 4 ATD cases who had received oral phenothiazines were not significantly different from levels in cases who had not been given these drugs.

DISCUSSION

The observed decrease with age of noradrenaline in hypothalamus and mamillary body may reflect the age-related loss of neurons from human locus coeruleus (Tomlinson et al., 1981). The greater decrease of noradrenaline in pre-senile ATD and Down syndrome than in senile ATD is in accord with the greater loss of neurons from the locus coeruleus in younger, severe, than in older, less severe, ATD (Bondareff et al., 1981; Tomlinson et al. 1981). The low hypothalamic noradrenaline in the 27 year old case of Down syndrome who had no clinical or neuropathological signs of dementia provides further evidence that reduced noradrenergic activity in ATD may not be directly related to dementia (Perry et al., 1981). The unaltered levels of dopamine and HVA in the caudate nucleus and of HVA in the olfactory tubercle, together with normal pigmentation of the substantia nigra, suggests that dopamine neurons are not decreased in number or activity in ATD. Cases of Down syndrome might represent a later stage of the ATD disease process, in which removal of inhibitory cholinergic synapses (De Belleroche and Bradford, 1978) produces an increased dopamine turnover and loss of dopamine from the caudate nucleus. The normal levels of dopamine and HVA in the present 27 year old case and of dopamine in two cases aged 15 and 35 years with no clinical signs of dementia (Nyberg et al., 1982) suggest that the dopamine changes seen in older cases of Down syndrome were related to aging and/or dementia rather than to the syndrome itself.

The present and previous studies indicate that loss of noradrenergic neurons is much more pronounced in pre-senile ATD and Down syndrome than in senile ATD. We found no evidence that dopamine neurons are affected in neuropathologically confirmed cases of ATD although dopaminergic activity does appear to be altered in cases of Down syndrome with the neuropathological and clinical characteristics of ATD.

We are indebted to Pathology Department staff and clinicians of hospitals in Edinburgh, West Lothian and Dundee for the supply of post-mortem material and clinical assessments.

TABLE 1   Noradrenaline concentrations in hypothalamus, mamillary body and caudate nucleus in pre-senile and senile ATD and Down syndrome, ug/g wet wt., mean ± S.D. (no. of cases)

Group	Hypothalamus	Mamillary body	Caudate Nucleus
< 70 yr			
Young Controls	$1.74 \pm 0.40(7)$	$0.18 \pm 0.04(4)$	$0.06 \pm 0.03(6)$
Pre-senile ATD	$0.71 \pm 0.38(5)$*	$0.04 \pm 0.01(3)$*	$0.10 \pm 0.05(8)$
Down syndrome	$0.28 \pm 0.24(3)$**	$0.06, 0.04(2)$	$0.05 \pm 0.01(4)$
" " (27 yr)	$0.2(1)$	not done	$0.08(1)$
> 70 yr			
Old Controls	$0.78 \pm 0.16(6)$**	$0.08 \pm 0.03(5)$	$0.06 \pm 0.03(6)$
Senile ATD	$0.37 \pm 0.24(4)$[+]	$0.11 \pm 0.07(4)$	$0.12 \pm 0.08(5)$

*p < 0.01 } compared to young controls
**p < 0.001 }

+p < 0.05) compared to old controls

Analysis of variance

TABLE 2 Dopamine and HVA concentrations in caudate nucleus and
dopamine concentrations in hypothalamus in pre-senile
and senile ATD and Down syndrome
ug/g wet wt., mean ± S.D. (no. of cases)

| Group | Caudate Nucleus | | Hypothalamus |
	Dopamine	HVA	Dopamine
≤70 yr			
Young Controls	2.84 ± 0.71(6)	3.80 ± 1.21(6)	0.16 ± 0.10(6)
Pre-senile ATD	3.02 ± 1.13(8)	3.46 ± 0.65(7)	0.12 ± 0.10(5)
Down syndrome	1.46 ± 0.09(4)*	5.50 ± 0.84(3)	0.03, 0.11(2)
" " (27 yr)	2.65(1)	3.55(1)	0.05(1)
≥70 yr			
Old Controls	1.86 ± 0.96(6)	3.87 ± 1.74(5)	0.07 ± 0.04(6)
Senile ATD	2.95 ± 1.07(5)	4.10 ± 0.79(4)	0.11 ± 0.10(3)

* p <0.01 compared to young controls.   Analysis of variance

315

REFERENCES

Adolfsson, R., Gottfries, C.-G., Roos, B.-E. and Winblad, B., 1979, Changes in the brain catecholamines in patients with dementia of Alzheimer type, Brit. J. Psychiat., 135: 216.

Ashcroft, G.W., Dow, R.C., Yates, C.M. and Pullar, I.A., 1976, Significance of lumbar CSF metabolite measurements in affective illness, in: Proceedings of the Sixth International Congress of Pharmacology, J. Tuomisto and M.K. Paasonen, eds., Pergamon Press, Oxford.

Bondareff, W., Mountjoy, C.Q. and Roth, M., 1981, Selective loss of neurons of origin of adrenergic projection to cerebral cortex (nucleus locus coeruleus) in senile dementia, Lancet, i: 783.

Cross, A.J., Crow, T.J., Perry, E.K., Perry, R.H., Blessed, G. and Tomlinson, B.E., 1981, Reduced dopamine-β-hydroxylase activity in Alzheimer's disease, Brit. Med. J., 282: 93.

De Belleroche, J. and Bradford, H.F., 1978, Biochemical evidence for the presence of presynaptic receptors on dopaminergic nerve terminals, Brain Res., 142: 53.

Mackay, A.V.P., Davies, P., Dewar, A.J. and Yates, C.M., 1978a, Regional distribution of enzymes associated with neurotransmission by monoamines, acetylcholine and GABA in the human brain, J. Neurochem., 30: 827.

Mackay, A.V.P., Yates, C.M., Wright, A., Hamilton, P. and Davies, P., 1978b, Regional distribution of monoamines and their metabolites in the human brain, J. Neurochem., 30: 841.

Mann, D.M.A., Lincoln, J., Yates, P.O., Stamp, J.E. and Toper, S., 1980, Changes in the monoamine containing neurones of the human CNS in senile dementia, Br. J. Psychiatry, 136: 533.

Moore, R.Y. and Bloom, F.E., 1978, Central catecholamine neuron systems: Anatomy and physiology of the dopamine systems, Ann.Rev. Neurosci. 1: 129.

Nyberg, P., Carlsson, A. and Winblad, B., 1982, Brain monoamines in cases with Down's syndrome with and without dementia, J. Neural Transm., 55: 289.

Perry, E.K., Tomlinson, B.E., Blessed, G., Perry, R.H., Cross, A.J., and Crow, T.J., 1981, Neuropathological and biochemical observations on the noradrenergic system in Alzheimer's disease, J Neurol. Sci., 51: 279.

Rossor, M.N., Iversen, L.L., Johnson, A.J., Mountjoy, C.Q., and Roth, M., 1981, Cholinergic deficit in frontal cerebral cortex in Alzheimer's disease is age dependent, Lancet ii: 1422.

Tomlinson, B.E., Irving, D., and Blessed, G., 1981, Cell loss in the locus coeruleus in senile dementia of Alzheimer type, J. Neurol. Sci., 49: 419.

Yates, C.M., Ritchie, I.M., Simpson, J., Maloney, A.F.J., and Gordon, A. 1981, Noradrenaline in Alzheimer-type dementia and Down syndrome, Lancet ii: 39.

DEMENTIA IN PATIENTS WITH PARKINSON'S DISEASE:

REVIEW OF BIOCHEMICAL DATA

Merle Ruberg, Bruno Dubois, France Javoy-Agid
Jacques Epelbaum, Bernard Scatton, and Yves Agid

Centre hospitalo-universitaire
Hôpital Pitié-Salpêtrière
Paris 75010, France

It is estimated that at least one third of patients with Parkinson's disease suffer from intellectual deterioration.[1] A figure of 33% was advanced on the basis of an anatomopathological study[2] showing that the stigmata normally associated with Alzheimer's disease (neurofibrillary tangles, senile plaques, granulovacuolar degeneration) are found on autopsy in the cortex and hippocampus of Parkinsonian subjects, especially those who are demented. These figures are considerably higher than those given for the prevalence of dementia in elderly persons in general (10% of those over 65; up to 20% in those over 80).[3] It should also be kept in mind that subjects with Alzheimer's disease may develop extrapyramidal symptoms (about 60% of the cases according to one estimate[4]) and that Lewy bodies, the neuropathological criterion for Parkinson's disease, are found in 10% of these patients.[5]

Although the neuropathological data would seem to comfort the notion that Parkinsonian subjects often develop Alzheimer's disease as well, clinicians tend rather to distinguish the types of intellectual deterioration observed in these diseases. The concept of "subcortical dementia" has been defended by several authors.[6,7] The principal characteristics of this form of dementia are considered to be "some form of memory defect, alterations in personality, impaired ability to manipulate acquired knowledge and a slowing down of all mental activity," with the striking absence of aphasias, agnosias and apraxias."[6] It should be added that depression is also prevelent in Parkinsonians and has been related to impaired intellectual performance.[8]

A number of biochemical parameters have been studied, postmortem, in patients with Alzheimer's disease (references for the following brief summary may be found in the review by Rossor[9]). The major finding is that choline acetyltransferase (CAT) activity is decreased in the cerebral cortex of these subjects. This is due to degeneration of the cholinergic pathway from the substantia innominata to the cortex which has been confirmed by cell counts and biochemical assay. The septo-hippocampal cholinergic pathway is also damaged. Noradrenergic projections to the cortex from the locus coeruleus are also lesioned in many patients and serotoninergic projections to the cortex from the raphé nuclei may be damaged as well. The only neurons intrinsic to the cortex which have been found, to date, to be lesioned in patients with Alzheimer's disease are somatostatin containing cells. While the cholinergic lesion has been correlated both with the degree of dementia in patients with Alzheimer's disease and with the neuropathological stigma associated with the disease [10,11] and most probably has something to do with memory defects, [12] there is, as yet no indication of the functional significance of the other biochemical deficiencies that have been detected in these patients.

In subjects with Parkinson's disease, cell counts have shown that the innominato-cortical cholinergic neurons degenerate in these

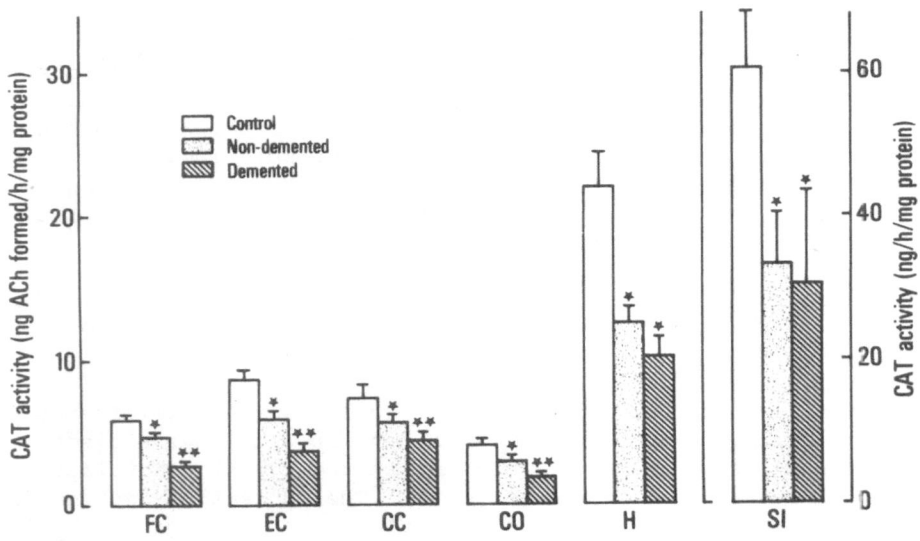

Fig. 1.   Choline acetyltransferase activity in demented and non-demented Parkinsonian subjects. FC: Frontal cortex; EC: Entorhinal cortex; CC: Cingulate cortex; OC: Occipital cortex; H: Hippocampus; SI: Substantia innominata.
Significantly different than controls (p 0.05).
Significantly different than controls and non-demented Parkinsonian subjects (p 0.05).

patients as well as in those with Alzheimer's disease.[13,14] Biochemical studies on a population of Parkinsonian subjects, demented and non-demented (for characteristics of the patients, see reference 15), have shown that CAT activity was significantly lower in all Parkinsonians than in controls, and significantly lower in demented Parkinsonians than in non-demented subjects, in all the cortical regions examined Fig. 1). CAT activity was correlated with the degree of intellectual deterioration observed in the patients.[15] In the hippocampus and the substantia innominata, CAT activity was also significantly decreased in Parkinsonians compared to controls, but there was no difference between demented and non-demented patients, perhaps because these structures are affected precociously by the degenerative process. The decrease in CAT activity in non-demented Parkinsonians suggests that the degenerative process is underway before clinical symptoms become evident. Not all cholinergic systems are affected in Parkinsonians, and the observed decreases in CAT activity are not secondary to lesion of the dopaminergic systems. Indeed, CAT activity is normal in the caudate nucleus although the cholinergic cells in this structure are innervated by the nigrostratal dopamine neurons which degenerate 85-95% in Parkinsonian subjects.[16]

Somatostatin concentrations were assayed in the same subjects[17] and were significantly lower than controls in some cortical regions and the hippocampus of demented Parkinsonians but not in non-demented patients (Fig. 2).

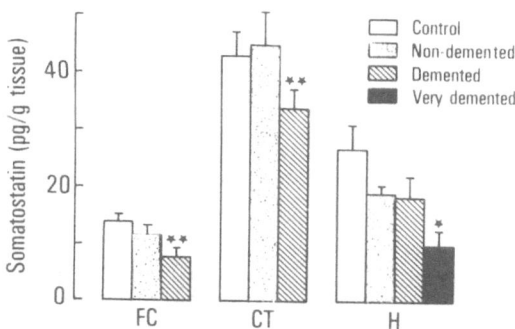

Fig. 2. Somatostatin concentrations in demented and non-demented Parkinsonian subjects. For symbols, see legend Fig. 1.

Several other neuropeptides were assayed as well: met-enkephalin, leu-enkephalin, substance P, cholecystokinin-8. [18] All were found in normal concentrations in cortical regions of Parkinsonian subjects whether or not they were demented.

Noradrenalin (Fig. 3) and serotonin (Fig. 4) levels were also decreased compared to controls in these Parkinsonian subjects.[19] The decreases were not specific to demented subjects, however.

As this data shows, all the biochemical deficiencies related to neurotransmitter systems detected thus far in subjects with Alzheimer type dementia are also found in patients with Parkinson's disease. While the decreases in CAT activity and somatostatin concentrations concern more particularly demented Parkinsonians, the significance of the noradrenergic and serotoninergic lesions, which are found to the same degree in demented and non-demented Parkinsonians, remains to be determined and suggests that prudence should be exercised in the interpretation of similar lesions in the brains of patients with Alzheimer's disease.

In addition to the lesions which Parkinsonian patients have in common with subjects with Alzheimer's disease, Parkinsonians also have lesions of the mesocortical and mesolimbic dopaminergic pathways.[19,20] Lesion of these neurons, which project to the cortex, nucleus accumbens and anterior caudate nucleus where dopamine-sensitive cortico-

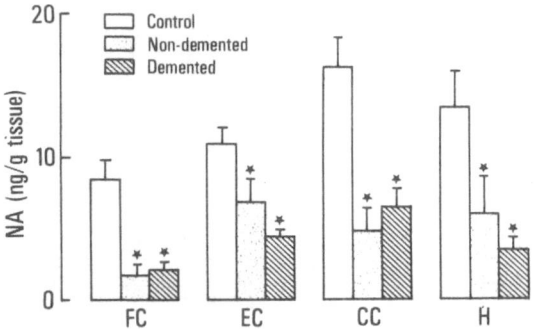

Fig. 3. Noradrenaline concentrations in demented and non-demented Parkinsonian subjects. For symbols, see legend Fig. 1.

striate projections terminate,[21] must certainly have an effect on the intellectual performance of Parkinsonians. Dopamine concentrations were reduced in the nucleus accumbens[16] and cortical regions[19] of the Parkinsonian subjects studied (Fig. 5). The reduction in the cortex seems to be more severe in demented patients, but the effects of levodopa therapy on dopamine concentrations in these patients renders this data difficult to interpret. There are some indications that these lesions may be implicated in the psychic akinesia or "frontal" type behavior observed in Parkinsonians and characterized by slowness of mental activity, disturbed attention and a tendency to perseveration?[22] In animal studies, selective lesions of the mesocorticolimbic dopamine neurons produce the same effects as lesions of the frontal cortex and nucleus accumbens (see review in reference 23). The result is a perturbation of selective attention leading to disorganization of vital

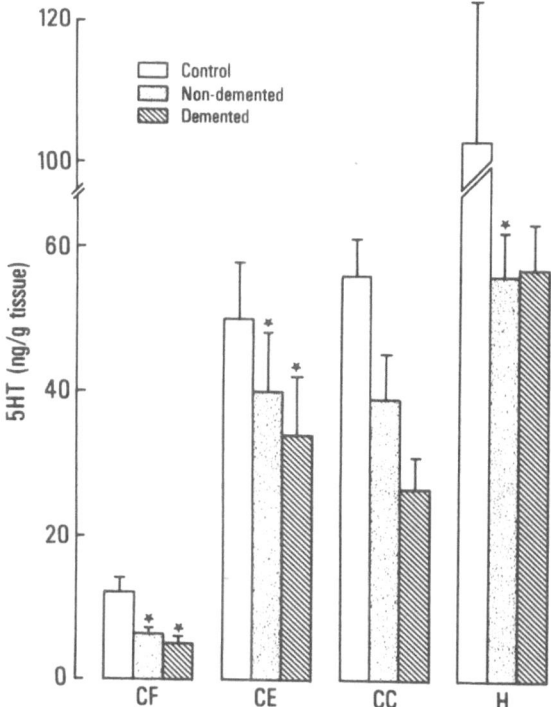

Fig. 4. Serotonin concentrations in demented and non-demented Parkinsonian subjects. For symbols, see legend Fig. 1.

behaviors and disturbances of learning processes which may be akin to frontal syndrome and subcortical dementia. The terms "frontal system dementia" and "frontosubcortical dementia" have, in fact, been suggested.[6]

The functional implications of the lesions already detected in subjects with Alzheimer's and Parkinson's disease remain to be elucidated. It is, furthermore, probable that other lesions in addition to those described will be detected. It is, therefore, perhaps premature to ask if some Parkinsonians may have Alzheimer's disease as well. Neither disease is sufficiently well defined at the present time. Clinically, we must learn to distinguish clearly between intellectual deterioration per se and deficiencies such as bradyphrenia or depression which may interfere with adequate intellectual performance but do not damage innate capacity. The relationship between cell degeneration and the anatomopathological stigmata considered to be essential to the definition of Alzheimer's disease must also be elucidated. A number of clinically demented subjects without these histological alterations have been reported.[2,24,25] There were several such subjects among the Parkinsonians we have studied.[14] In these patients, cell counts showed severe loss of cholinergic neurons in the substantia innominata, and CAT activity in both the substantia innominata and the cerebral cortex were reduced to the same degree as in demented

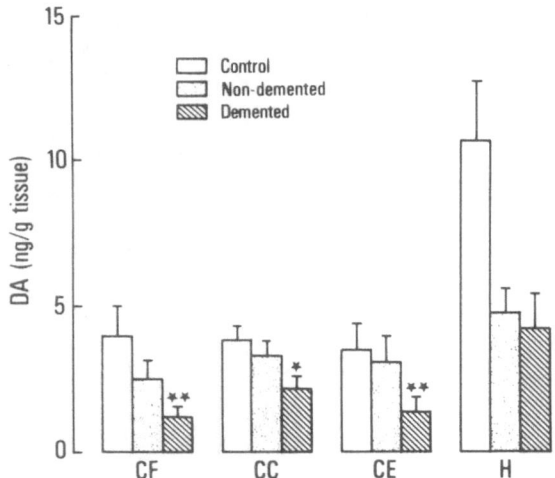

Fig. 5. Dopamine concentrations in demented and non-demented Parkinsonian subjects. For symbols, see legend Fig. 1.

patients with histological alternations. This raises questions about the significance of these signs of dementia. The formation of senile plaques or neurofibrillary tangles may be an epiphenomenon of cell degeneration and depend on factors which are independent of the disease process and which remain to be determined. Finally, the reason why certain neuronal pathways degenerate in these diseases is completely unknown, and must be known before any conclusions relating these diseases can be drawn.

According to our present knowledge, Parkinsonian patients have the same lesions as patients with Alzheimer's disease, and have as well dopaminergic lesions which are not found in the latter. In both diseases, except for the somatostatin containing cells which are intrinsic to the cortex, the other known lesions affect cell nuclei in subcortical structures which send projections to the cortex. Although the additional lesions in Parkinsonians may be related to the symptoms of a frontosubcortical syndrome, the absence of certain symptoms in demented Parkinsonians - aphasia, apraxia, agnosia - is paradoxical. In order to resolve this paradox as well as other puzzling questions concerning the relationship between Parkinson's disease and Alzheimer's disease, more information about the etiology and the pathophysiology of the diseases is required. The hypothesis which points to a fragility of the isodendritic neurons[26,27] is, in this sense, intriguing.

REFERENCES

1. A. Lieberman, A. Dziatolowski, M. Kupersmith, M. Serby, A. Greengold, J. Korein and M. Goldstein, Dementia in Parkinson's disease, Ann. Neurol. 6:355 (1974).
2. F. Boller, T. Mizutani, U. Roessmann and P. Gambetti, Parkinson disease, dementia and Alzheimer disease: clinicopathological correlations, Ann. Neurol. 7:329 (1980).
3. D. W. Kay, K. Bergmann, E. M. Foster, A. A. McKechnie and M. Roth, Mental illness and hospital usage in the elderly: a random sample followed up, Compr. Psychiatr. 11:26 (1970).
4. J. Pearce, Mental changes in Parkinsonism, Brit. Med. J. 1:445 (1974).
5. L. S. Forno, Pathology of Parkinson's disease, in: "Movement Disorders," C. D. Marsden, S. Fahn, eds., Butterworth, London (1982).
6. M. L. Albert, Subcortical dementia, in: "Alzheimer's Disease: Senile Dementia and Related Disorders," R. Katzman, R. D. Terry and K. L. Bick, eds., Raven Press, New York (1978).
7. R. Mayeux, Y. Stern, J. Rosen and D. F. Benson, Subcortical dementia: a recognizable clinical syndrome, Ann. Neurol. 10:100 (1981).
8. R. Mayeux, Y. Stern, J. Rosen, J. Leventhal, Depression, intellectual impairment and Parkinson disease, Neurology 31:645 (1981).

9. M. Rossor, Dementia, Lancet 2: 1200 (1982).

10. E. K. Perry, B. E. Tomlinson, G. Blessed, K. Bergmann, P. H. Gibson and R. H. Perry, Correlation of cholinergic abnormalities with senile plaques and mental test scores in senile dementia, Brit. Med. J. 2:1457 (1978).

11. G. K. Wilcock, M. M. Esriri, D. M. Bowen and C. C. T. Smith, Alzheimer's disease: Correlation of cortical choline acetyltransferase activity with the severity of dementia and histological abnormalities, J. Neurol. Sci. 57: 407 (1982).

12. D. A. Drachman, Memory and cognitive function in man: does the cholinergic system have a specific role? Neurology 27:783 (1977).

13. P. J. Whitehouse, J. C. Haldreen, C. L. White and D. L. Price, Basal forebrain neurons in the dementia of Parkinson's disease, Ann. Neurol. 13:243 (1983).

14. F. Gray, P. Gaspar, M. Ruberg, B. Dubois, F. Agid, R. Escourolle and Y. Agid, Neuropathology and biochemistry of demented and non-demented Parkinsonian subjects, Acta Neuropath., submitted for publication.

15. B. Dubois, M. Ruberg, F. Javoy-Agid, A. Ploska and Y. Agid, A subcorticocortical cholinergic system is affected in Parkinson's disease, Brain Res., in press.

16. B. Bokobsa, M. Ruberg, B. Scatton, F. Javoy-Agid and Y. Agid, 3H-Spiperone binding, dopamine and HVA concentrations in Parkinson's disease and supranuclear palsy, Eur. J. Pharmacol., submitted for publication.

17. J. Epelbaum, M. Ruberg, E. Moyse, F. Javoy-Agid, B. Dubois and Y. Agid, Somatostatin and dementia in Parkinson's disease, Brain Res., in press.

18. F. Javoy-Agid, H. Taquet, F. Cesselin, J. Epelbaum, D. Grouselle, A. Mauborgne, J. M. Studler and Y. Agid, Neuropeptides in Parkinson's disease, Proceedings, Fifth International Catecholameine Symposium, Alain Liss Inc., New York, in press.

19. B. Scatton, F. Javoy-Agid, L. Rouquier, B. Dubois and Y. Agid, Reduction of cortical dopamine, noradrenaline, serotonin and their metabolites in Parkinson's disease, Brain Res. in press.

20. F. Javoy-Agid and Y. Agid, Is the mesocortical dopaminergic system involved in Parkinson disease, Neurol. 30:1326 (1980).

21. J. P. Tassin, A. Cheramy, G. Blanc, A. M. Thierry and J. Glowinski, Topographical distribution of dopaminergic innervation and of dopaminergic receptors in the rat striatum. I. Microestimation of 3H-dopamine uptake and dopamine content in microdiscs, Brain Res. 107:291 (1976).

22. J. de Ajuriaguerra, Etude psychopathologique des parkinsoniens, in: "Monoamines, Noyaux Gris Centraux et Syndrome de Parkinson," J. de Ajuriaguerra and G. Gautier, eds., Georg et Cie., Geneva (1971).

23. H. Simon, Neurones dopaminergiques A10 et système frontal, J. Physiol. (Paris) 77:81 (1981).

24. M. N. Rossor, N. J. Garrett, A. J. Johnson, C. Q. Mountjoy, M. Roth and L. L. Iversen, A post-mortem study of the cholinergic and GABA systems in senile dementia, Brain 105:313 (1982).
25. D. M. N. Mann and P. O. Yates, Pathological basis for neurotransmitter changes in Parkinson's disease, Neuropath. and Appl. Neurobiol. 9:3 (1983).
26. M. N. Rossor, Parkinson's disease and Alzheimer's disease as disorders of the isodendritic core, Brit. Med. J. 283:1588 (1981).

VASOPRESSIN AND COGNITIVE PERFORMANCE IN MAN

Jellemer Jolles

Psychiatric University Clinic
Nicolaas Beetsstraat 24
3511 HG Utrecht, The Netherlands

INTRODUCTION

In recent years, interest has been aroused in neuropeptides as potentially useful in the treatment of cognitive deficits in man. This interest is based primarily on animal experiments, in which peptides derived from the pituitary hormones ACTH and vasopressin appeared to improve the performance in several behavioral paradigms[1,2] Unfortunately, the results obtained in clinical trials with vasopressin, are difficult to evaluate because of differences in treatment parameters (nature of the vasopressin-congener used; dosage, route and duration of administration etcetera), in patient population, and in methods for treatment evaluation[3,4].

The present paper is written from the viewpoint that vasopressin peptides have in fact acted as tools in the study of memory processes: the studies performed until now yield information on the mechanism of action of the peptide. This information will be discussed, with an emphasis on vasopressin in aging/dementia. The reader is referred to other papers for a more thorough evaluation of the clinical studies with vasopressin[3], the pharmacology of memory[4,5] and animal studies with vasopressin[2].

BEHAVIORAL EFFECTS OF VASOPRESSIN-LIKE PEPTIDES IN ANIMALS

Vasopressin - like peptides have been found to improve aspects of learning in normal aminals and in animals which are characterised by inferior learning, such as after hypophysectomy[1] and after treatment with CO_2, protein synthesis inhibitors or electroconvulsive shock[2]. Treatment effects have also been noted in vasopressin-deficient animals such as the Brattlebaro strain, or rats treated with vasopressin-antiserum. Vasopressin fragments exist -such as Desgly-cinamide-Arginine[8]-Vasopressin (DGAVP)- which are devoid of peripheral endocrine activity (on blood pressure and water retention), yet retain the behavioral activity. Several arguments favor the notion of a direct action on the CNS: For instance, vasopressinergic neurons exist in the brain[6], and much less of the peptide is needed after central- than after peripheral application (de Wied, 1976 in[3]). However, alternative interpretations are possible[7].

Vasopressin has been found to have an action on memory processes such as consolidation and retrieval, or a process common to both. It has a longterm effect which lasts for days after a single administration. Its neurochemical mechanism of action seems to involve the dorsal noradrenergic bundle[2]. The hypothesis has been raised that the peptide acts as a neuromodulator, that is by altering the efficiency of other (eg noradrenergic) synapses: A brain state is thereby created which is optimal for the selection of relevant information from the environment[3].

CLINICAL TRIALS IN AGING AND DEMENTIA PATIENTS

The first study that aimed at assessing the potential clinical usefulness of vasopressin was performed by Legros and coworkers[9]. These investigators have used Lysine[8]-Vasopressin (LVP), applied intranasally, in treating twelve aging patients (aged 50-64 years) that were hospitalised with somatic complaints. These patients performed better than control subjects on certain tests of attention and memory. Effects of LVP were also found in senile dementia patients: a single administration of LVP improved the performance of nine out of ten patients on a word list retention task, and these effects were still present after 48 h[10]. Others have used DDAVP (Desamino-D-Arginine[8]-Vasopressin; effects water retention and behavior but not bloodpressure). They found that a single administration of DDAVP can improve the memory for semantic structures (i.e. word memory) in patients suffering from progressive dementia[11]. This was also found in a later study in which seven patients suffering from primary degenerative dementia were treated with gradually increasing doses of DDAVP for 10 days. The demented patients were better able to generate appropriate words to verbal stimuli, and the authors suggested that the peptide helps facilitate access to semantic memory[12]. In addition, they noted that these patients showed enhanced arousal with increased motor and speech activity. In another recent study on patients suffering from mild to moderate dementia (n=20) LVP appeared to have small but consistent improvements in memory tests (Ferris and Reisberg, 1982, cited in[13]). The observation that speed factors are involved in the peptide effects[12] has been made by several authors; In a study in which carefully diagnosed Alzheimer patients were treated with LVP, no effects were noted on tests of memory, learning and visual perception. The only measurable effect concerned an improved performance in a reaction time test. These authors concluded on a "non-specific effect"[14],[15]. Likewise, preliminary data are mentioned, which would show that LVP alters auditory and visual evoked responses, in a manner suggestive of greater alerting[17]. A similar suggestion was made by Tinklenberg et al.[13], who treated patients suffering from a primary degenerative dementia (Alzheimer). Neither DDAVP nor DGAVP had measurable effects on the tests used. Their impression was that some patients might have more energy and less depression. This was especially the case in patients with comparatively mild dysfunctions. We did similar observations in our studies on the effects of DGAVP in patients with cognitive deficits (Jolles and Verhoeven, unpublished): In a mixed population of patients with memory complaints (n=25) four elderly subjects (which were in a very early stage of dementia associated with vascular insufficiency) reported to work and think in a faster way and to have more energy and initiative. These patients mentioned the changes only in the period of active drug treatment (in a double blind cross over study). It appears from these studies that the methods to evaluate the treatment effect are of utmost importance. The methods used may not be sensitive enough, or they measure the wrong aspects of the cognitive functions which are affected. This may be the case in several negative studies. Jenkins and coworkers[16] treated three patients suffering from 'early dementia of the Alzheimer type' (aged 58-65 years) with DDAVP. They stated that none of their patients showed significant improvement with DDAVP for any of the testprocedures used. Similarly, Franceschi et al.[17] did not find statistically significant changes in a mixed population of patients suffering from Alzheimer's disease (n=10) and multi-infarct dementia (n=8). These patients had been treated with intranasal LVP for 7 days. The importance of both test- and pharmacological parameters, and the severity of the disease process in determining any treatment effect is discussed more fully in[3].

CLINICAL TRIALS IN OTHER PATIENTS

The following account is a brief exerpt of a recent review on clinical effects of vasopressin. The references will be found there[3]. Clinical trials employing vasopressin-like peptides in *brain trauma patients* have been largely unsuccesful. Several studies did report an improved performance. However, no treatment effects were seen in patients with more serious head injuries. Our own studies suggest that patients suffering from a (light) concussion may benefit more from the treatment than those having a more serious head trauma. The findings with *alcoholic patients* are similarly unpromising. Again, the data indicate that patients suffering from a serious amnesic syndrome do not benefit from peptide treatment. A beneficial effect has been reported in the treatment of *depression, diabetes insipidus,* in children with *attention deficits or Lesch Nyhan disease* and in *healthy volunteers*.

Some interesting results have been obtained in *schizophrenic subjects*. Several authors described a treatment effect in chronic patients.

This resulted in the reappearance of positive symptoms, and eventually a more social and interested attitude; a decrease in thinking disorder accompanied by an increase in energy and activity; and a beneficial effect on blunted affect and emotional withdrawal. These studies are of importance as they point -again- to a vasopressin-effect on the cognitive functions associated with energy/activity/interest. The same applies to our study with DGAVP in a mixed population of patients (n=25). More than half of the times that these patients spontaneously reported to feel better, they mentioned an increased speed, more energy, more activity, etcetera (Jolles and Verhoeven, unpublished).

Many studies in which the peptide was ineffective were performed on patients with a complex pattern of neuropsychological deficits or other symptoms of a profound brain degeneration. This should not be surprising, because degeneration of the relevant brain structures may well destroy the sites of action of the peptide: When animals were treated with vasopressin after lesioning thalamic nuclei, septum or hippocampus, no effects were noted[2,3]. The studies referred to, do indicate that the treatment effects are too small to be of clinical usefulness, but they do yield relevant information on the aspects of memory affected. It may be that the effects on speed factors, energy, activity and mood, which have been seen in demented patients, depressives and schizophrenics, depend on a similar cerebral substrate.

ON MEMORY PROCESSES AND VASOPRESSIN

Careful neuropsychological research in patients with subjective complaints of failing memory has shown that virtually any kind of lesion in the brain can give rise to memory deficits[19]. These deficits can reflect a 'real' memory disorder, or they can be secondary to another deficit, such as an attention deficit, a planning deficit, or slowness. In other words, a memory complaint does not necessarily reflect a memory disorder. Likewise, the performance of animals in tests designed to assess 'learning' and 'memory' depends in part of other cognitive functions such as attention, and the state of arousal of the animal.

In man, many different kinds or aspects of memory exist with their own anatomical localisation. For instance, posterior neocortical areas are essential for material/modalityspecific memory (e.g. memory for faces and memory for words): the frontal neocortex has a role in the encoding of new information and the retrieval of old memories; the ascending fibre system plays its part in attention and arousal and diencephalic structures and the hippocampus are important for memory consolidation[18]. Recent neurobiological research on memory-processes discerns 'intrinsic' from 'extrinsic' systems. It is in the intrinsic system that the informationrepresentation develops, probably as a permanent change in synaptic efficiency in large neuronal networks. The extrinsic pathway is the system of pathways that can influence, modulate or express the information storage but which do not contain memory themselves[5]. All existing information suggests that the neuropeptides may primarily affect performance in these more or less 'aspecific', or extrinsic aspects of memory. It is important to mention the role of the stress-hormones in this respect: These peripheral hormones and the pituitary hormones vasopressin, ACTH and their central counterparts are physiologically involved in the adaptation of an organism to a changing environment. Important aspects of this 'adaptation' can be described in terms of 'learning' and 'memory'. As a stress component can be found in many different task situations, the cerebral mechanisms underlying stress (eg arousal) seem to play a crucial role in mediating the behavioral effects of the neuropeptides. The finding in animal experiments, that vasopressin might effect consolidation, retrieval or a process common to both is in line with the notion that extrinsic mechanisms are involved and not memory per se (intrinsic). Neuropsychologically, subcortical structures (ascending fibres, diencephalon) are involved more than cortical structures. Yet, in the clinical trials performed until now, the focus has been on tasks of pure memory (intrinsic): This may explain the lack of cleancut peptide effects obtained with *objective* tests in patients who did report a *subjective* improvement. Clearly, other tasks may have to be designed, which have their emphasis on other aspects of memory (attention, activity, energy, rate of information processing).

SUMMARY

It is clear that 'memory' per se does not exist. Intrinsic and extrinsic mechanisms of memory exist, and the different aspects of memory depend upon a different cerebral substrate. Vasopressin may exert its effect by modulating the effects of other (eg noradrenergic) neurotransmitters, and thereby affect extrinsic mechanisms[3,4]. The data from animal and human studies, generally, point in the same direction. Generally, the clinical trials performed until now do not favor the notion that the presently available vasopressins are a potent and useful drug. However, they do provide information on the mode of action of these substances; on memory processes; and on the strategies to follow for a more efficient development of drugs for treatment of cognitive deficits in the future.

REFERENCES

1. de Wied, D. Effects of peptide hormones on behavior. (In: W.F. Ganong and L. Martini, eds.). Frontiers in Neuroendocrinology, Oxford Univ. Press, London pp. 97-140 (1969).
2. de Wied, D. Central actions of neurohypophyseal hormones. In: Progr. Brain Res. (B.A. Cross and G. Leng, eds.). Elsevier, pp. 155-167 (1983).
3. Jolles, J. Vasopressin-like peptides and the treatment of memory

disorders in man. In: Progr. Brain Res. (B.A. Cross and G. Leng, eds.). Elsevier, pp. 169-182 (1983).

4. Jolles, J. The Pharmacology of memory. International Medicine, in press (1983).

5. Squire, L.R. and H.P. Davis. The pharmacology of memory: a neurobiological perspective. Ann. Rev. Pharmacol. Toxicol. 21: 323-356 (1981).

6. Buys, R.M. Intra- and extrahypothalamic vasopressin and oxytocin pathways in the rat: Pathways to the limbic system, medulla oblongata and spinal cord. Cell. Tiss. Res. 192: 423-435 (1978).

7. Gash, D.M. and G.J. Thomas. What is the importance of vasopressin in memory processes? Trends Neurosci. 6: 198-199 (1983).

8. de Wied, D. and J. Jolles. Neuropeptides derived from pro-opiomelanocortin: behavioral, physiological and neurochemical effects. Physiol. Rev. 62: 976-1059 (1983).

9. Legros, J.J., P. Gilot, X. Seron, J. Claessens, A. Adams, J.M. Moeglen, A. Audibert and P. Bechier. Influence of vasopressin on learning and memory. Lancet I: 41-42 (1978).

10. Delwaide P.J., J.M. Devoitille and M. Ylieff. Acute effects of drugs upon memory of patients with senile dementia. Acta Psychiat. Belg. 80: 748-754 (1980).

11. Weingartner, H., W. Kaye, P. Gold, S. Smallberg, R. Peterson, J.C. Gillin and M. Ebert. Vasopressin treatment of cognitive dysfunction in progressive dementia. Life Sci. 29: 2721-2726 (1981).

12. Kaye, W.H., H. Weingartner, P. Gold, M.H. Ebert, J.C. Gillin, N. Sitaram and S. Smallberg. Cognitive effects of cholinergic and vasopressin - like agents in patients with primary degenerative dementia. In: Alzheimer's disease: a report of progress (S. Corkin et al. eds). Raven Press, New York, pp. 433-442 (1982).

13. Tinklenberg, J.R., R. Pigache, A. Pfefferbaum and P.A. Berger. Vasopressin peptides and dementia. In: Alzheimer's disease: a report of progress in research. (S. Corkin et al., eds). Raven Press, New York, pp. 463-469 (1982).

14. Durso, R., P. Fedio, P. Brouwers, C. Cox, A.J. Martin, S.A. Ruggieri, C.A. Tamminga and T.N. Chase. Lysine vasopressin in Alzheimer's disease. Neurology 32: 674-677 (1982).

15. Chase, T.N., R. Durso, P. Fedio and C.A. Tamminga. Vasopressin treatment of cognitive deficits in Alzheimer's disease. In: Alzheimer's disease, a report of progress. (S. Corkin et al., eds.). Raven Press, New York pp. 457-461 (1982).

16. Jenkins, J.S., H.M. Mather and A.K. Coughlan. Effect of desmopressin in normal and impaired memory. J. Neurol. Neurosurg. and Psychiat. 45: 830-831 (1982).

17. Franceschi, M., O. Tancredi, G. Savio and S. Smirne. Vasopressin and physostigmine in the treatment of amnesia. Eur. Neurol. 21: 388-391 (1982).

18. Luria, A.R. The neuropsychology of memory. Winston, Washington D.C. (1976).

CLINICAL ASSESSMENT OF COGNITIVE DECLINE IN NORMAL AGING AND

PRIMARY DEGENERATIVE DEMENTIA: CONCORDANT ORDINAL MEASURES

Barry Reisberg, Steven H. Ferris, Ravi Anand
Mony J. de Leon, Micheal K. Schneck, and Thomas Crook*

New York University Medical Center, New York, NY 10016
*National Institute of Mental Health, Rockville, MD 20857

Primary degenerative dementia (PDD), assumed to be equivalent to neuropathologically defined Alzheimer's disease, is now recognized to be a major cause of morbidity and mortality in our elderly population. Increasing recognition and study of this illness and attempts to ameliorate the symptomatology with pharmacologic agents, have necessitated the development of clinical instruments for the assessment and staging of the disorder. One such instrument, the Global Deterioration Scale (GDS) for PDD, has recently been described.[1] The GDS is based upon our increasing understanding of the characteristic clinical symptomatology and course of age-associated cognitive decline and PDD.[1-3]

In addition to global assessments, clinical assessments are necessary which can be utilized to quantify the progression of deficit in greater detail. Ideally, these should be relatively brief as well as accurately reflecting the characteristic clinical symptomatology of progressive cognitive deficit in the aged. On the basis of our observations of hundreds of elderly patients over the past five years, we have developed concordant, multi-axial clinical assessments, which are designed to accurately reflect progressive cognitive deterioration in normal aging and PPD.

The magnitude of cognitive impairment is assessed on five clinical axes, using specified criteria (see Table 1). Items are scored from information obtained during a structured clinical interview conducted in the presence of a spouse or caretaker whenever possible. This interview procedure is particularly important because of the denial which frequently accompanies moderate to severe memory loss.[4]

Table 1. Concordant, ordinal clinical assesments in normal aging and primary degenerate dementia

Axis	Rating	Item
Axis I:	(Circle Highest Score)	
Concentration and Calculating Ability	1	No objective or subjective evidence of deficit in concentration.
	2	Subjective decrement in concentration ability.
	3	Minor objective signs of poor concentration (e.g., on subtraction of serial 7s from 100).
	4	Definite concentration deficit for persons of their background (e.g., marked deficit on serial 7s; frequent deficit in subtraction of serial 4s from 40).
	5	Marked concentration deficit (e.g., giving months backwards or serial 2s from 20).
	6	Forgets the concentration task. Frequently begins to count forward when asked to count backwards from 10 by 1s.
	7	Marked difficulty counting forward to 10 by 1s.
Axis II: Recent Memory	1	No objective or subjective evidence of deficit in recent memory.
	2	Subjective impairment only (e.g., forgetting names more than formerly).
	3	Deficit in recall of specific events evident upon detailed questioning. No deficit in the recall of major recent events.
	4	Cannot recall major events of previous weekend or week. Scanty knowledge (not detailed) of current events, favorite TV shows, etc.
	5	Unsure of weather; may not know current president or current address.
	6	Occasional knowledge of some recent events. Little or no idea of current address, weather, etc.
	7	No knowledge of any recent events.
Axis III: Past Memory	1	No subjective or objective impairment in past memory.
	2	Subjective impairment only. Can recall two or more primary school teachers.
	3	Some gaps in past memory upon detailed questioning. Able to recall at least one childhood teacher and/or one childhood friend.
	4	Clear-cut deficit. The spouse recalls more of the patient's past than the patient. Cannot recall childhood friends and/or teachers but knows the names of most schools attended. Confuses chronology in reciting personal history.
	5	Major past events sometimes not recalled (e.g., names of schools attended).
	6	Some residual memory of past (e.g., may recall country of birth or former occupation).
	7	No memory of past.
Axis IV: Orientation	1	No deficit in memory for time, place, identity of self or others.
	2	Subjective impairment only. Knows time to nearest hour, location.
	3	Any mistake in time > 2 hrs; day of week > 1 day; date > 3 days.
	4	Mistakes in month > 10 days or year > one month.
	5	Unsure of month and/or year and/or season; unsure of locale.
	6	No idea of date. Identifies spouse but may not recall name. Knows own name.
	7	Cannot identify spouse. May be unsure of personal identity.
Axis V: Functioning and Self-Care	1	No difficulty, either subjectively or objectively.
	2	Complains of forgetting location of objects. Subjective work difficulties.
	3	Decreased job functioning evident to co-workers. Difficulty in traveling to new locations.
	4	Decreased ability to perform complex tasks (e.g., planning dinner for guests, handling finances, marketing, etc.).
	5	Requires assistance in choosing proper clothing.
	6	Requires assistance in feeding, and/or toileting, and/or bathing, and/or ambulating.
	7	Requires constant assistance in all activities of daily life.

Each axis utilizes seven rating points which correspond to seven definable and distinguishable stages of cognitive functioning within each axis. The axes were designed so that patients with normal aging or PDD show a fairly uniform magnitude of cognitive and functional ability on each of the concordant axes. The clinical characteristics of the ratings on each axis are also designed to coincide with each corresponding GDS stage. We have attempted to assess the validity of these assumptions with respect to the design of the clinical axes and to also obtain information on the validity of the axes utilizing the procedures described below.

METHOD

Fifty consecutive outpatients were studied, 25 men and 25 women. The mean age was 71.2 ± 7.01 years. These subjects consisted of controls (GDS = 1) with average or superior cognitive function for their ages who demonstrated neither subjective nor objective evidence of cognitive deterioration (N = 9), subjects with very mild impairment (GDS = 2) consistent with the generally benign symptomatology of normal aging (N = 21), subjects with mild cognitive deterioration (GDS = 3) consistent with either age-associated decline or PDD (N = 4), and subjects with moderate to severe cognitive deterioration (GDS = 4-6) consistent with PDD (N = 16). Patient evaluations were conducted by experienced geriatric clinicians (R.A. and M.K.S.), who were not involved in the development of the clinical rating instruments. All subjects received extensive medical, psychiatric, neurologic, and neuroradiologic examinations prior to entry into the study. Subjects with factors which might contribute to cognitive impairment other than normal aging or PDD were excluded from participation.

All study subjects received psychometric and mental status evaluations as well as clinical assessments. The psychometric evaluations were conducted by psychologists independently of the clinical assessments. The specific evaluations utilized can be seen in Table 2.

To evaluate the validity of the clinical axes, Pearson correlation coefficients were computed between scores on each of the clinical axes and performance on the psychometric tests and Mental Status Questionnaire. In order to evaluate the concordance of deficit across the five clinical axes, the intercorrelations among the axis scores were examined.

RESULTS

The relationships obtained between clinical assessments and the independently obtained psychometric and mental status evaluations can be seen in Table 2. All correlations were statistically significant (p's < .001) and ranged from .51 to .84. The correlations

Table 2. Concordant, Ordinal Clinical Assessments: Pearson
Correlations* with Independent Psychometric and
Mental status questionnaire evaluations (N = 50)

	Axis I	Axis II	Axis III	Axis IV	Axis V	Axis I-V Total Score
Guild Test Battery						
(a) Paragraph, initial recall	.69	.74	.64	.69	.67	.72
(b) Paragraph, delayed recall	.68	.70	.61	.69	.68	.71
(c) Paired associate recall, initial	.60	.63	.51	.62	.62	.63
(d) Paired associate recall, delayed	.57	.60	.48	.56	.59	.59
(e) Designs	.65	.71	.59	.66	.69	.70
Combined Guild Score	.72	.76	.64	.72	.72	.75
WAIS Vocabulary (raw scores)	.72	.78	.74	.68	.69	.76
Digit Symbol Substitution Test	.76	.78	.71	.71	.73	.78
Digit Span, forward	.64	.71	.71	.68	.66	.72
Digit Span, backward	.69	.77	.71	.71	.65	.74
Total	.73	.84	.78	.77	.68	.79
Mental Status Questionnaire Scores	.72	.75	.68	.78	.72	.77

*P < .001

Table 3. Pearson Intercorrelations* of Clinical Axes (N = 50)

	Axis I	Axis II	Axis III	Axis IV	Axis V
Axis I		.91	.89	.91	.88
Axis II			.88	.94	.90
Axis III				.88	.83
Axis IV					.94
BCRS Total Scores	.96	.97	.94	.97	.95
GDS Scores	.90	.94	.87	.94	.91

*P < .001

Table 4. Axis V; Functioning and self-care; Ordinal staging in
severe primary Degenerative Dementia

6 - (a) Difficulty putting on clothing properly
(b) Unable to bathe properly; may develop fear of bathing
(c) Inability to handle mechanics of toileting
(d) Urinary incontinence
(e) Fecal incontinence

7 - (a) Ability to speak limited to one to five words
(b) All intelligible vocabulary lost
(c) All motoric abilities lost
(d) Stuporous
(e) Comatose

with the combined psychometric assessments (total Guild scores and digit span total scores) tended to be higher than the correlations with any individual psychometric assessment measures. Similarly, the correlations obtained for the WAIS vocabulary scores, the digit symbol substitution test scores, and the Mental Status Questionnaire scores were of comparable magnitude to the combined psychometric assessments. Hence, the clinical axes correlated most strongly with combined memory test scores, general assessment of language ability, coupled psychomotor interaction, and global mental status.

Interrelationships among the five clinical axes ranged between .83 and .94 (see Table 3). All individual clinical axis correlations with total clinical scores were $\geq$ .94.

DISCUSSION

These findings indicate that each of the clinical axes is consistently and significantly correlated with the magnitude of psychometrically determined cognitive impairment in subjects with age-associated cognitive decline and PDD. These correlations appear to be particularly strong for combined and relatively "global" psychometric assessments. Furthermore, as intended in the design of the clinical assessments, the clinical axes do indeed show strong concordance over the range of normal aging and PDD. The magnitude of these interrelationships is sufficiently great as to raise the question of redundancy and whether multiple clinical modalities (or axes) are needed.

There are several reasons why multiple clinical assessments are desirable. These include the utility of such measures in (1) confirming the diagnosis and in differential diagnosis of these disorders; (2) the utility of detailed assessments in sensitively and accurately guaging the value of putative treatment interventions; and (3) the utility of detailed assessments as research tools in increasing our understanding of the clinical characteristics and evolution of the disorder.

The ordinal clinical assessments may also be useful in the succinct staging of age-associated cognitive decline and PDD. With respect to succinct staging, Axis V, reflecting "Functioning and Self-Care" may be particularly useful. Recent observations indicate that ten distinct ordinal stages of functional disability can be subsumed under the ratings of "6" and "7," respectively, on this axis (see Table 4). Hence, with respect to functioning, fifteen ordinal stages from normal aging to severe PDD are identifiable. These fifteen ordinal functional assessments may prove especially useful to clinicians in the staging of PDD and in exploring the prognostic concomitants of the ordinal stages.

Since patients with a particular level of cognitive impairment, tend to score relatively uniformly across the five clinical axes, each rating point on each of the five axes can be utilized to provide a succinct description of a particular stage of cognitive impairment. The etiologic, prognostic, and therapeutic implications of discordance across axes have not been well worked out, but may eventually assist investigators in the identification of subgroups of PDD patients who might, for example, respond differentially to treatment interventions.

CONCLUSION

We have described five concordant, ordinal clinical assessment axes of progressive cognitive decrement in normal aging and PDD. The axes were designed so as to show relatively uniform scores for a given level of deterioration in patients with age-associated cognitive decline and PDD. Data from 50 patients indicate that the axes do indeed appear to be concordant in this patient population. The axes also relate strongly to psychometric evaluations of cognitive change. These results provide evidence for the validity of the concordant, ordinal clinical assessments. Hence, these assessments as defined in Table 1 and 4, may be useful to clinicians and investigators as a clinical cognitive assessment scale. The terminology "Brief Cognitive Rating Scale (BCRS)," has previously been proposed for this instrument.[2]

ACKNOWLEDGMENT

This study was supported in part by U.S. Public Health Service grants AG 03051 and MH 29590.

REFERENCES

1. B. Reisberg, S.H. Ferris, M.J. de Leon, and T. Crook, The global deterioration scale (GDS): an instrument for the assessment of promary degenerative dementia (PDD). Am. J. Psychiatry 139:1136 (1982).
2. B. Reisberg and S.H. Ferris, Diagnosis and assessment of the older patient. Hosp. and Community Psychiatry 33:104 (1982).
3. B. Reisberg, E. Shulman, S.H. Ferris, M.J. de Leon, and V. Geibel, Clinical assessments of age-associated cognitive decline and primary degenerative dementia: Prognostic concomitants. Psychopharm. Bull. 19:4 (1983), in press.
4. B. Reisberg, B. Gordon, M. McCarthy, and S.H. Ferris, Insight and denial accompanying progressive cognitive decline in the aged, in: "Senile Dementia of the Alzheimer's Type and Related Disorders: Ethical and Legal Issues Related to Informed Consent," V.L. Melnick and N. Dubler, eds. (1984), in press.

PRE-DEMENTIA AND PSYCHOTROPIC DRUG TREATMENT

WITH CEREBRAL SPECIFIC PHOSPHOLIPIDS

Harry S. Feldmann

Outpatient Clinic
15, avenue Krieg
CH - 1208 Geneva, Switzerland

INTRODUCTION

There have been many treatments for the pre-senile dementias, Alzheimer type, with questionable results or at best temporary improvement because of largely unknown factors influencing the progression of these illnesses (Schneck, Reisberg and Ferris, 1982). Choline (Thal, Rosen et al., 1981), Lecithin (Peters and Levin, 1979), Physostigmine (Denber, 1982; Wettstein, 1983), Piracetam (Stegink, 1972), Méthylphenidate (Crook, Ferris et al., 1977), Neuropeptides (Pigache, 1982), vaso-dilatators and cerebral phospholipids (Feldmann et Crétallaz, 1969).

Our own major approach has been with the total purified phospholipids extracted from young calves by physico-chemical methods and standardized (Feldmann, 1969)

CEREBRAL PHOSPHOLIPIDS

Phospholipids are key elements in the construction of all cell membranes and living elements. Essentially, they contain one molecule of glycerine, two of fatty acid and one of phosphoric acid. Phospholipids are built up into the brain cells. For many years, phospholipids were held as static components of the brain tissular structure.

Studies by Green and Fleischer (1963) and Burton (1964) show a considerable functional role of these lipid complexes. Green (1961) has proved that each elementary particle of mitochondria has a complete respiratory chain and that the four enzymatic complexe inside

339

the elementary particle are separated by a structural protein, which forms lipid-protein complexes with the phospholipids. If phospholipids are removed from these elementary particles, respiratory activity of the chains disappear. If solubilized phospholipids are associated to the elementary particles, the respiratory activity of mitochondria is reestablished.

Vignais and Lehninger (1964) have isolated phosphatidylinositol, a thermolabile phospholipid from mitocondria, required for their contractility, and essential for the respiratory process as for the oxidative phosphorylation of cells (ATP cycle). Larrabee and Leight (1965) have discovered the track of synaptic transmission when stimulating the pre-ganglionic nerve: this long-term memory track after a fugacious electrical phenomenon is registred in a phospholipid. Memory of behaviour is directly bound to phospholipids.

In biological systems, phospholipids organize themselves in a three-dimensional association of several molecules. These micelles are indispensable for the functioning of all biological membranes and cellular systems in which energy transformations take place. The cellular system ensures continuity in all membranes, enabling an absorbed molecule to travel into the territory of a membrane without leaving the phospholipid phase, that is to say in a unimolecular layer.

When phospholipids are extracted from membrane system, all the fundamental membranal characteristics disappear, whereas they can be restored by re-introducing the phospholipid-extract mix. Ansell and Hawthorne (1964) have described the essential role of phospholipids in selective membrane permeability.

Burton (1964), Hokin and Hokin (1963) have demonstrated the very important functional role of phospholipids, capable of dissolving non-miscible substances in water and transporting them through membranes; they are responsible for transportation of sodium, potassium, acetylcholine, coenzyme Q, etc.

Himwich (1962) has stated that there is a close relationship between phospholipids and central nervous system activity. It is known that the proportion of phospholipids increases during childhood, remaining unchanged through middle age and decreasing in older age. Balakrishnan and Goodwin (1961), Le Baron, Mc Donald and Ramarao (1963), Suzuki (1965), Torwik and Sindman (1965) have demonstrated that the decrease in proportion of CNS phospholipids coincides with the decrease in nervous and mental activities. Any CNS injury will disturb phospholipid synthesis. For instance, Curri (1967), producing experimental cranial traumata in animals, put in evidence a decrease in rate of phospholipid formation in the injured zones, reaching as much as 30 to 40 %.

340

In man, phospholipid synthesis may diminish in pathologic conditions of the central nervous system. In senile dementia with cerebral atrophy, Bunge and Chevalier (1967) have found a considerable diminution of the amount of phospholipids in the areas of neuronal degeneration. Any decrease in intra-cranial circulation, any trauma, intoxication, chronic psychoses or even a simple excess in physical effort with emotional and mental overload are accompanied by marked decrease in synthesis of phospholipids [Clarenburg, Chaikoff and Morus (1963), Knauff and Bock (1961), Ropp and Snedeker (1961), Miani (1963)].

The very importance of protein and phospholipids synthesis into neurons is well known. Studies of Weiss and Taylor (1965) on protein metabolism in brain cells have demonstrated that axoplasmic flow runs regularly in a distal direction, whether the animal be awake or sleepy, working or quiet. Most of the neuronal energy is used to maintain functioning of the "sodium pump", through which the cell-membrane can permit passage and transmission of the nerve impulse.

Rosenzweig, Krech, Bennet and Diamond (1962) studied the biochemical synthesis in brains of trained rats in a stimulus enriched environment compared to a stimulus poor, static situation, as in tiny cages. There were significant differences indicating that experience, training etc. increase the amount of the phospholipids tremendously, independently of age.

Meldrum (1966) has shown that phospholipids, like polypeptides, provoke facilitation or blocking of the action of psychotropic drugs on neuronal synapses.

Cerebral metabolism is highly complex and it is the entire phospholipid complex which functions in the brain. Curri, Vecchio and Mursia (1961) have experimentally shown that specific heterogenous brain phospholipids may cross the blood brain barrier and aim at suplementing the insufficiency CNS phospholipid synthesis. Knowles (cited in Bovet, 1970) has demonstrated that intensity of protein and phospholipid metabolism is common to the brain, liver and pancreas.

Gaillard and Infante (1971) have emphasized the specificity of action of various phospholipids by introducing liver and brain phospholipids marked with P 32 through a gastric sound into rats. He has demonstrated that cerebral phospholipids are distributed in the proportion of 60 % in the brain, the remaining 40 % being disseminated through all the other organs. Liver phospholipids remain in the liver in a proportion of 65 %, with 35 % being distributed to other parts of the organism. An equivalent dose of radioactive phosphorus is uniformly distributed in the entire body, but not as specifically as phospholipids. The intestinal resorption of phospholipids was shown by Baruk, Liteanu, Cretallaz and Lasalle (1967) by measuring blood levels of phospholipids before and after administration of coated pills of phospholipids.

CLINICAL RESEARCH

We have examined the action of phospholipids derived from young calves brain, which supply elaborated elements capable of participating directly in the essential functions of brain tissues without requiring re-synthesis by neurons.

This total phospholipidic extract from cerebral cortex of young calves by physico-chemical techniques and biologically standardised * contains : Phosphatidylcholine, Phosphatidylethanolamine, Phosphatidylserine, Plasmalogeno-choline, Plasmalogeno-ethanolamine, Plasmalogeno-serine, Phosphatidic acid, Diphosphoinositide, Sphingosylphosphorylcholine; and each coated tablet = 20 mg.

Clinically, the most evident effect of phospholipids lies in increasing cerebral oxidation-reduction reactions and improving the electro-encephalographic tracing. Symptomatology of geriatric patients is really improved, with improved memory, attentiveness, concentration and attention, as well as diminished fatigue. The higher intellectual functions slowly improve, attention set and alertness are increased.

Among a series of 350 patients treated with Gricertin, we gave this drug to 61 geriatric patients with advanced memory disorders at a dosage of 60 mg/day, alone in fourty cases, but associated with different vaso-dilatator agents in 21 other patients. The age range was 68 to 87 years, with a mean of 73. Memory deficits before and after 60 days of treatment were measured by means of Rey's 15 words acquisition and retention (Rey, 1958) and the test of associative recall (Rey, 1968)

See next page the results after 60 days of treatment.

54 % of patients were greatly improved (memory recovered within the normal average range) and 23 % of the others improved and were capable of quasi normal every-day behavior. The ratio of much improved with drug versus drug plus vaso-dilatators was about 2:1. The intra-group ratios were about the same. The considerable functional action of phospholipids described above (see introduction) can easily

---

* Gricertin "Chemedica" (Vouvry, Switzerland)

explain the good results with this drug, as long as memory is not totally lost as in the terminal dementias.

TABLE 1. RESULTS AFTER 60 DAYS OF TREATMENT

Memory disorders in :	N of cases	GRICERTIN alone					GRICERTIN + vaso-dilatator agents				
	N	N	++	+	0	–	N	++	+	0	–
Senile involution	18	12	6	3	3	–	6	4	1	1	–
Prae-senile dementia (Binswanger)	6	5	2	1	2	–	1	–	1	–	–
Senile vasculopathia	16	10	6	2	2	–	6	4	1	1	–
Arteriosclerotic dementia	6	3	1	1	1	–	3	1	1	1	–
Pseudo-bulbar palsy	3	2	–	–	2	–	1	–	–	1	–
Advanced chronic cerebral alcoholism	12	8	6	2	–	–	4	3	1	–	–
Total	61	40	21	9	10	–	21	12	5	4	–

++ means recovering of memory within the normal average range

+ means improvement of memory giving to the patient the ability to behave "normally" in every day life.

0 means no significant change in the results.

Side effects were rarely observed : headaches in one case; excitation with irritability in 3 cases at the outset and disappearing after decrease to 40 mg/day.

CASE HISTORY

U.R., male, 68, manager. Senile vasculopathy. Hypertension discovered at 45 during an episode of stress. At 67, ictus, left hemi-paresia. Retired since then.

Physical examination on Jan.19th,1981 (age 68) : Blood pressure 190/100 mm Hg. The reflexes were hyperactive on the left with a left Babinski, normal on the right side. Romberg positive, festinating gait, but without other signs of pseudo-bulbar palsy. EEG-alpha activity was normal, although the tracing was desynchronized on both frontal areas and some sporadic maximally frontal delta waves at 3,5 c/s were seen. There was numerous rapid rythms 22 c/s activity.

Psychological findings : Very poor memory; remote memory recall good, but deficient in short term recall : serial numbers, words (15 words of Rey) and association recall test (Centile 0 in all tests).
Treatment : The patient received 60 mgr Gricertin per day, b.i.d. (40 mgr in the morning and 20 mgr before lunch) for 60 days.
Results : Recall of 15 words, Centile 70. Association recall test, Centile 97, although while this test has a visual aspect which helps the patient to memorize.

CONCLUSIONS

Cerebral phsopholipids given to 61 aged people with memory disorders between 68 and 87 years of age, during 60 days, gave very good improvement of brain function in 54% of patients, improving 23% allowing a quasi normal existence.

This improvement is noticeable as long as memory is not completely distroyed as in terminal dementia. It is obvious that the administration of phospholipids should be regularly carried on in order to avoid any drop of the improved results.

We are going now to investigate the value of specific cerebral phospholipids in a double blind study with Piracetam and Centrophenoxine.

REFERENCES

Ansell, G.B., and Hawthorne, J., 1964, "Phospholipids : chemistry, metabolism and function", Elsevier Publishing Co New York
Balakrishnan , S., and Goodwin, F., 1961, The Distribution of Phosphorus Containing Lipid Compounds in the Human Brain. J. Neurochem. 8, 276.
Baruk, H., Liteanu, D., Cretallaz J.C. et Lasalle, 1967, Premiers résultats d'essais cliniques d'un complexe phospholipidique de cerveaux de bovidés dans les syndromes mentaux. Ann. Méd.-Psych, 2,788-796
Blonstrand, J., and Nakayama, 1961, Neurochem.,8, 230
Bloom, B.S., 1964, Stability and change in human characteristics.Wiley ed., New York.
Bovet, D., 1970, Approche biochimique et biopsychologique de la mémoire et de l'apprentissage in La Mémoire, symposium de l'Association de Psychologie scientifique de langue française (1968), Presses Universitaires de France, Edit., p.7.
Bunge, A. et Chevalier, B., 1967, Démences organiques de l'adulte. Feuill. Prat. 271, 464.
Burton R.M., 1964, Int. J. Neuropharmacol., 3, 13.
Clarenburg, R., Chaikoff, I.L., and Morus, M.D., 1963, J. Neurochem. 10, 135-143.

Cretallaz, J.C. et Gaillard, J.P., 1967, Les phospholipides cérébraux sélectionnés en thérapeutique humaine. C.R.L., cahier 2.

Crook, T., Ferris, S., Sathananthan, G., Raskin, A. and Gershon S., 1977, The Effect of Methylphenidate on Test Performance in the Cognitively Impaired Aged, Psychoparmacology, 52, 251-255.

Curri, S.B, Vecchia, P. and Mursia, V., 1961, Distribuzione quantitativa dei Fosfolipidi nel Sistema nervoso centrale, Biochem. Biol. Sper., 2, 202.

Denber, H.C.B., 1982, Physostigmine in the Treatment of Memory Disorders : A case Report, Psychiatr. J. of Univ. of Ottawa, 7, 1:8-12.

Feldmann, H., 1971, Les phospholipides cérébraux et leur utilisation en neuro-psychiatrie. Observations cliniques sur 200 cas, Revue Méd. Fonctionnelle, Paris, 1: 1-38

Feldmann, H., 1979, Present Drug Treatments for Mental Retardation, Cytobiologische Revue, 2 : 1-15

Feldmann, H. et Cretallaz, J.C., 1969, Essai thérapeutique d'un complexe de phospholipides cérébraux, Médecine et Hygiène, 27 : 209-210.

Feldmann, H. et Cretallaz, J.C., 1969, Les phospholipides cérébraux en neuro-psychiatrie. Etude de 100 cas, Praxis, 58, 46:1504-1516.

Gaillard, J.P. et Infante, R., 1971, Absorption intestinale et métabolisme des phospholipides extraits du foie et du cerveau, C.R. Journées d'Etudes sur le métabolisme des lipides, (3.4.1969) ITERG, Paris.

Green, D.E., 1961, Funktionelle und morphologische Organisation der Zelle, p. 76, Springer-Verlag, Berlin-Göttingen-Heidelberg.

Green, D.E., and Fleischer, S., 1963, Biochem. and Biophys. Acta, 7 554.

Himwich, W.A., 1962, Biochemical and Neurophysiological Development, in the Prenatal Period. Int. Rev. Neurobiol., 4: 117-158.

Hokin, L.E. and Hokin, M.R., 1963, The Role of Phosphatides in Active Transport with particular Reference to Sodium Transport. Int. Drugs and Membranes, Pergamon Press, Oxford, 4 : 23-40.

Knauff, H.C., and Bock, F., 1961, Ueber die freien Gehirnaminosaüren und das Aethanolamin der normalen Ratte, sowie über das Verhalten dieser Stoffe nach experimenteller Insulinhypoglykämie. J. Neurochem., 6 : 171-182.

Knowles : see Bovet, D., 1970, in loc. cit.

Laborit, H., 1965,, Les régulations métaboliques, Masson éd., Paris.

Larrabee, M.G., and Leight, W.S., 1965, Metabolism of Phosphatidyl-Inositol and Other Lipids in Active Neurones of Sympathetic Ganglia and Peripheral Nervous Tissues. The site of the Inositide Effect. J. Neurochem., 12 : 1-13.

Le Baron, F.N., Mc Donald, C.P., and Ramarao, B.S.S., 1963, Amounts and distribution of Free Inositol and Free and Proteinbound Phosphoinositides in Brain Tissues, J. Neurochem., 10, 677.

Lehninger, A.L., 1964, The Mytochondrion. W.A. Ed. Benjamin, New
     York, Amsterdam.
Meldrum, B.S., 1966, Electrical Signals in the Brain and the Cellular
     Mechanism of Learning, in Richter, D., ed. Aspects of Learning
     and Memory, Heinemann, London.
Miani, N., 1963, Analysis of the Somato-Axonal Movement of Phospholi-
     pids in the Vagus and Hypoglossal nerves. J. Neurochem,10,859-874.
Peters, B.H. and Levin, H.S., 1979, Effects of physostigmine and Leci-
     thine on memory in Alzheimer disease. Ann. Neurol, 6, 215-221.
Pigache, R.M., 1982, A peptide for the Aged ? Basic and clinical Stu-
     dies, in Psychopharmacology of Old Age. D. Wheatley Ed., Oxford
     Univ. Press, Oxford, 67-96.
Rey,A., 1958, Mémorisation d'une série de 15 mots en 5 répétitions, in
     L'examen clinique en psychologie, Presses Univ. de France, ed.,
     141-193.
Rey,A., 1968, Profil de Rendement Mnésique (P.R.M.), in Les Troubles
     de la Mémoire et leur examen psychométrique, Dessart Ed.
Ropp, R.S. (de) and Snedeker, E.H., 1961, J. Neurochem., 7, 128
Rosenzweig, M., 1966, Environmental Complexity, Cerebral Change and
     Behavior, Amer. Psychologist, 21, 321-332.
Rosenzweig, M., 1968, Effects of Experience on Brain Chemistry and
     Brain Anatomy, in Bovet, D., Bovet-Nitti, F. et Oliverio, A., éd.,
     Attuali orientamenti della ricerca sull'apprendimento e la memoria
     Acc. maz. Lincei. Roma. Quad. 109.
Rosenzweig, M., Krech, D. Bennet, E.L., Diamond, M.C.,1962, Effects
     of Environmental Complexity and Training on Brain Chemistry and
     Anatomy.J. Comp. Physiol. Psychol, 55 : 429-437.
Schneck, M.K., Reisberg, B., and Ferris, S.H., 1982, An overwiew of
     Current Concepts of Alzheimer's Disease, Am. J. Psychiatry, 139:2.
Stegink, A.J., 1972, Die Behandlung der Symptome seniler Involution mit
     Piracetam, Arzneimittel-Forsch, 22 : 975-977.
Suzuki, K., 1965, J. Neurochem., 12 : 969-979
Thal L.J., Rosen W., Sharpless, N.S. and Urgstal, H., 1981, Choline
     Chloride in Alzheimer disease, Ann. Neurol, 10, 580.
Torwik, A. et Sindman, R.L., 1965, Autoradiographic Studies on Lipids
     Synthesis in the Mouse Brain During Postnatal Development,
     J. Neurochem., 12 : 555-565.
Vignais, P.V. et Vignais, P.M. and Lehninger, A.L., 1964, J. Biol.
     Chem., 239, 2011.
Weiss, P.A., 1952, Patterns of Organization in the Central Nervous
     System. Res. Publ. Ass. nerv. ment. Dis., 30 : 3-23.
Weiss, P., and Taylor, A.C., 1965, Synthesis and Flow of Neuroplasm.
     Science, 148 : 669-670
Wettstein, A., 1983, Effectless double blind trial of physostigmine
     and lecithin in Alzheimer disease, Ann. Neurol., 13 : 210-212.

PROGRESSIVE BRAIN FAILURE -

A HOME ASSESSMENT AND TREATMENT PROGRAM

H. F. Reichenfeld

Department of Psychiatry
University of Ottawa
Ottawa, Canada

INTRODUCTION

It is widely recognized that in view of the higher incidence of the dementing disorders among the elderly an increase in the proportion of the elderly in the population will bring about a concomitant rise in the number of individuals suffering from progressive brain failure. Though other diseases can be responsible for gradual and progressive deterioration of mental functioning, such as Korsakoff's psychosis, Pick's disease, Huntington's chorea, multi-infarct dementia, and permanent disability can be the result of a head injury, the most common cause of progressive brain failure is recognized to be due to Senile Dementia, Alzheimer Type, commonly referred to as Alzheimer's disease. The overall prevalence of definite dementia among the elderly living in the community varies in different studies and partly depends on the criteria used for identifying affected individuals. It ranges from a low of 1.6% reported by Bollerup[1] to a high of over 9% in the study by Hagnell.[2] Mild cases are reported to range between 2.6%[3] and 24.7%[4] depending on the investigator whereas total prevalence peaked at 31.8%[4] in North Carolina compared with a Chinese study reporting a mere 0.5%[5] A recently carried out study on a representative community sample in London and New York[6] showed a point prevalence rate of 4.9% of pervasive dementia for New York City and 2.3% for London. In both cities most of these were due to Senile Dementia, Alzheimer Type. By widening the criteria to include a "latent class" the respective point prevalence rates were 10.6% for New York

and 4.3% for London. On the other hand, about 40% of the
residents of long term care facilities were found to be
suffering from dementia in both London and New York giving
a total point prevalence of between 5% - 7.5% in the 65
plus age group. An Ontario study [7] into the institutionalized elderly using a different instrument, the Multidimensional Observation Scale for Elderly Subjects (MOSES),
gave similar results for different types of long term care
facilities taking care of the elderly. A demonstrable
degree of disoriented behaviour ranged from 9% in residential beds of Homes for the Aged to 66% in geriatric beds
of psychiatric hospitals. In extended care beds of Homes
for the Aged, extended care hospitals and nursing homes,
the respective figures were 49%, 60% and 47%. (Table I)

TABLE I

CUMULATIVE PERCENTILES FOR DISORIENTED BEHAVIOUR

MOSES SCORE	Homes for the Aged Residential	Homes for the Aged Extended Care	Extended Care Hospitals	Nurs-ing Homes	Psych.Hos. Geriatric Beds
8	68	20	15	24	12
9	76	23	18	29	17
10	81	29	21	33	21
11	84	34	25	37	22
12	82	37	27	41	24
13	88	40	30	46	27
14	88	43	34	47	29
15	89	47	35	50	31
16	91	51	40	53	34
17	91	52	42	56	35
18	92	55	45	59	38
19	94	57	48	63	40
20	94	61	50	65	46
21	95	65	54	68	50
22	95	68	57	71	52
23	95	70	60	73	54
24	96	76	68	78	63
25	96	79	70	80	66
26	98	82	71	83	69
27	98	86	77	87	75
28	99	90	80	90	81
29	99	93	87	94	86
30	99	95	90	96	90
31	99	96	90	96	92
32	100	100	100	100	100

In making the assumption that the overall prevalence in
the Ottawa-Carleton region was comparable to the total
Ontario sample as well as to the reported prevalence in
other studies it was concluded that in an estimated population of 51,000 elderly in the region, of whom 4,656
or approximately 9% were in various types of institutions,
(Table II)

TABLE II

REGIONAL MUNICIPALITY OF OTTAWA-CARLETON

Number of Institutionalized Elderly with
Progressive Brain Failure

	TOTAL	PERCENTAGE WITH PROGRESSIVE BRAIN FAILURE	TOTAL WITH PROGRESSIVE BRAIN FAILURE
Homes for the Aged Residential Beds	1500	9	135
Psychiatric Hospitals Geriatric Beds	180	66	119
Homes for the Aged Extended Care Beds	593	49	290
Extended Care Hospital	910	60	546
Nursing Homes	1473	47	692
Total	4656		1782

TABLE III

Estimated Population
    Ottawa-Carleton, 1982   Total   560,000

                              Over 65 51,000

Assumed Overall Prevalence
of Progressive Brain Failure   7.5%

Assumed Total Number with
Progressive Brain Failure 51,000 x 7.5%   3,825

Less   Estimated Total with Progressive
       Brain Failure in Institutions   1,782

       Estimated Total with Progressive
       Brain Failure in the Community   2,043

2,043 individuals with progressive brain failure were living in the community. The proposal to develop the Alzheimer Home Assistance (AHA) program was based on the need to provide domiciliary help for this population.

SERVICES FOR THE ELDERLY

As part of its mandate to plan health services for the region, the Ottawa-Carleton Regional District Health Council decided late in 1979 to carry out a study on mental health care of the elderly. In December 1981, through the Mental Health Operational Plan Sub Committee, it published its report on the Mental Health Care of the Elderly, 1981 - 1991. [8] Its conclusions about the need of mental health services for the elderly were succinct and definite. It recommended "that when preventative measures are inadequate or simply ineffective, services for the assessment, treatment and management of mental disorders in the elderly should strive to recognize, support, and make the most effective possible use of the capacities of all persons and resources concerned with the care of the afflicted person, beginning with that person, and including family, care givers and professional personnel. That these services be provided in the communitywhenever possible" and "That these services be provided as economically as possible..." The report particularly emphasized "that domiciliary assessment and consultation be available for the elderly with mental disorders.." and that "methods of increasing family responsibility for the care of the elderly, whether psychogeriatric or not, must be developed," and that "self-help groups for families caring for the elderly at home...should be promoted." However, in assessing the availability of these services the report concluded "that there are no community services which are designated as mental health services for the elderly or which apparently specifically recognize such services as part of their mandate even though they carry them out". The lack of such mental health services for the elderly is in marked contrast to expressed government policy of encouraging comprehensive and co-ordinated community care programs.[9] In view of the slow pace at which government agencies are proceeding to carry out expressed policy, consumer groups have sprung up in relation to different disorders. On the one hand they exert pressure on behalf of their members to have their needs met while, on the other hand, they encourage self-help activities to assist the afflicted individuals and their families. The Alzheimer Society has become one of the best organized and goal oriented groups in respect of catering to the needs of individuals suffering from progressive brain failure. Its goals are:

  1. Continuing family and patient support
  2. Information and education
  3. Advocacy on behalf of the patient
  4. Research

The following proposal[6] which was submitted on behalf of the Society to the Regional District Health Council developed as a result of discussions between members of the Society and a number of professionals from different disciplines with experience and interest in patients with progressive brain failure.

THE PROPOSAL

The aims of the program were as follows:

1. To provide functional domiciliary assessment in the Ottawa-Carleton region for patients with progressive brain failure.
2. To develop methods which will delay the rate of deterioration in individuals suffering from progressive brain failure.
3. To develop management programs enabling such individuals to remain in their own homes with community support.
4. To assist families in coping with the distress

related to the illness of one of their members.
5. To provide significant data to other agencies, in particular institutions considered for eventual placement.
6. To participate with other agencies in the development of a comprehensive network of services.

The program was designed to consist of 5 parts which include: assessment, management, counselling for families, integration with community support services and assistance with related research.

The proposed team, which would be responsible for the program, would consist of: 1) a physician for assessment and drug management, medical consultation and liaison, and co-ordination of the program through weekly team meetings; 2) a nurse for counselling, teaching and follow-up particularly in relation to personal care; 3) a registered nursing assistant for practical help in the home; 4) a social worker for assisting with assessment, follow-up and family counselling, and 5)an occupational therapist to undertake the development of a program of activities related to the capabilities of the patient and also for teaching activities related to daily living adaptations.

The program was submitted to the District Health Council but although accepted, received a low rating in priority for its implementation, and remains a proposal. It nevertheless demonstrated that collaborative effort involving interested professionals, representatives of consumer groups as well as responsible government agencies can be expected to lead to significant developments in the planning for comprehensive health services.

References

1. Bollerup, T.R.: Prevalence of Mental Illness Among 70-year olds domiciled in Nine Copenhagen Suburbs. Acta Psychiatr., Scand., 51: 327-339 (1975)
2. Hagnell, O.: Disease Expectancy and Incidence of Mental Illness Among the Aged. Acta Psychiatr. Scand., (Suppl.), 219: 83-89. (1970)
3. Kay, D.W.K.: Epidemiological Aspects of Organic Brain Disease in the Aged. In: Aging and the Brain; C.M. Gaitz (Ed.), Plenum Press, New York. (1972)
4. Pfeiffer, E.: A Short Portable Mental Status Questionnaire for the Assessment of Organic Brain Deficit in Elderly Patients. J. Am. Geriatr. Soc., 23: 433-441 (1975)
5. Lin, A.Y.: A Study of the Incidence of Mental Disorder in Chinese and Other Cultures. Psychiatry

(Minneap.)., 16: 313-336. (1953)

6. Gurland, B., Copeland, J., Kuriansky, J., Kelleher, M., Sharpe, L., and Dean, L.L.: The Mind and Mood of Aging; Haworth Press, New York (1983)

7. Csapo, K. G.,Short, J., and Reichenfeld, H. F.: Development of a Functional Rating Scale for Institutionalized Elderly. Paper presented at XII International Congress of Gerontology, Hamburg. (1981)

8. Ottawa-Carleton Regional District Health Council: Final Report of the Mental Health Operational Plan Subcommittee on Mental Health Care of the Elderly, 1981-1991. (1981)

9. Government of Canada: Care of the Aging. (1982)

10. Alzheimer Society, Ottawa-Hull: Program Proposal - Alzheimer Home Assistance (AHA) Program (1983)

DIAGNOSTIC PROBLEMS WITH AGED PEOPLE,

SHOWING DEMENTIAL BEHAVIOUR

Frederik van 't Hooft

Christelijk Sanatorium voor Neurosen en Psychosen
Postbus 20
3700 AA Zeist, The Netherlands

The chairman of this symposium asked me to speak about Dementias as multistage Processes. Frankly speaking, in my opinion we cannot find clearly discernable stages in the course of the syndrome dementia. I have to emphasize, that dementia is not a separate disease, but a syndrome, caused by different and multiple pathological circumstances. Common is only a global impairment of the functions of the brain.

If we consider the course of an illness as a sequence of clinical states, and if we try to find stages - that means some regularity in this sequence - we have the duty to analyse every state as exactly as possible. In my opinion we can discern the following psychopathological and psychological components in every state of an old person, showing the behaviour which we call demential behaviour.
1. The results and consequences of the impaired functions of the brain, not only impairment of memory, orientation, judgement, and other neuropsychological disturbances, but also disturbances of concentration, attention and of the physical and mental speed. That is what many doctors consider to be the only real symptoms of dementia. But in fact there are more components in the clinical picture.
2. The reactions of the old person to this symptoms and to the changes in his psychosocial situation. Many of these reactions can be considered as defense mechanisms, according to the American psychiatrist Verwoerdt. The old person can try to conceal the impairment behind a facade of unimpairedness, he can also become depressed, apathetic and inactive, or on the contrary he can show

an ineffective overactivity; he can also try to evoke pity, and
so on.
3. The qualities of the former character form a third element of
the clinical state. They give a certain colour to all symptoms.
Mostly the former character is very well discernable.
4. Finally the clinical picture can be complated by other psychiatric symptoms, illusions, paranoid symptoms, and so on.

In the case of dementia, the course of the illness is very
much dependant on the origin, the cause of the impaired brain
functions. By all these circumstances the clinical pictures of
dementia show a caleidoscopic variety. In many cases we observe a
rather slow decline, not rectilinear but with some undulations.
In other cases however we observe a rather rapid decline of the
condition of the patient within a short time, or a rapid increase
of the complaints from the relatives, with some improvement later
on. Mostly it is explained as the result of some intercurrent
physical disease, for instance a cerebrovascular accident. Sometimes that will be correct, but in many cases the explanation has
to be found in a crisis in the patient and in the psychosocial
situation. I call this crisis a decompensation-crisis. I can explain it as follows.

Every old person with demential symptoms tries to cope with
these symptoms, but has to cope also with the slowly changing
psychosocial situation. We can consider these coping mechanisms
as rather succesfull defense mechanisms. But sooner or later the
coping becomes deficient, the defense mechanisms collaps, and the
patient comes into a crisis, a state of decompensation. And that
is what we psychogeriatrists observe very often, because we are
consulted very often in such a crisis.

In such a crisis of decompensation we can discern certain
stages:
- Chaos and negations
- Aggression
- Depression
- Resignation
As you see, these stages are stolen from Mrs. Kübler-Ross.

The first stage is chaos and negation. The old person is
functioning on a much lower level than before; he fails in many
respects and often he is confused. Mostly the patient denies that
there is something wrong and he opposes sensible measures. Nearly
always the relatives must handle the situation, while the patient
does not know and understand what is happening. The decompensation
is at his top, the relatives are upset and the doctor is consulted.

Later on a certain understanding about what is happening
arises in the old person. He notices that certain measures have

been taken without his knowledge and approval. That can lead to aggression, often accompanied by anxiety and paranoid symptoms. The aggression can be understood as a manifestation of beginning insight what is going on, but on the other side it shows the inability to a more normal reaction. That leads to anxiety and acting-out behaviour.

The third stage is called depression. When understanding in the patient is increasing, and anxiety decreasing, the need for acting-out behaviour fades away. But the old person realizes his situation more or less and depression can follow. Depression in the elderly can be very complicated, and in every case we have to find out which kind of depression is present. We can discern the following kinds:
1. A sad mood as the result of realizing the problems of old age, or as a reaction to difficult circumstances of life.
2. A defense mechanisme in beginning dementia, with the unconscious intention to avoid the demands of daily life.
3. A stage in a decompensation crisis, as described before.
4. A manifestation of an endogenous depression.
5. A symptom of physical illness, which has caused tiredness.

After such a decompensation crisis some resignation arises at last. It often implies that the symptoms of demential behaviour improve, and also the coping with the demands of daily life can return. But mostly the level of functioning remains somewhat lower than before the crisis.

The explanation of the whole decompensation crisis as the result of some transitory physical impairment of the brain is too easy. Nearly always a deep psychosocial, and at the same time existential crisis is also existing, often in the first place. During the decompensation crisis there is a need not only for extensive psychiatrc, physical and psychosocial diagnostics, but also for a deep empathy for the old person.

DEMENTIAS AS MULTI-STAGE PROCESSES

(Conceptual semiological approaches)

Meinhardt S. Tropper

Department of Geriatric Psychiatry, Rishon le-Zion
Geriatric Center, and Neuropsychiatric Department
Zamenhof Central Out-patient Clinic, Tel-Aviv, Israel

MATERIAL

Our presentation reflects observations on assessment, follow-up,
treatment and rehabilitation in a sample of 1631 patients (PTS)
during a time axis of 10 years (1973-1983). The PTS characteristics
in accordance with age and sex are presented on Figure 1.

Age (yrs) Sex	50-54 M F T	55-59 M F T	60-64 M F T	65-69 M F T	70-74 M F T	75-79 M F T	80-84 M F T	85+ M F T	TOTAL M F T
N	4 31 35	12 61 73	39 173 212	222 339 561	83 149 232	17 97 114	6 149 155	2 247 249	385 1246 N=1631
(percent)	(2,14)	(4,5)	(13,0)	(34,4)	(14,22)	(6,98)	(9,5)	(15,3)	(23,6)(76,4)

Figure 1 Patients characteristics in accordance with age and sex

As can be seen 19.6 percent of all the PTS were first seen and
assessed before age 70.
Initially all the PTS underwent a thorough geropsychiatric basic
assessment and psychological evaluation, including a special neuropsychological assessment. The patients were followed-up every 3-5
months through out the time axis mentioned. Almost all of them have
undergone an EEG (1439 - 88 percent) and 109 PTS a brain CT scan.
All the PTS presented symptoms as well as the psychopathological
followed-up data, the anamnestic items, the results of paramedical
investigations and especially the course of the disease shows us
that these PTS fit into the diagnostic criteria of Primary Degenerative Dementia (DSM-III) of early or late onset. Many psychiatrists
use to coin these states as Senile or Presenile Dementia, and many
others regard PTS with analogous sympotms and course of disease as
suffering from Alzheimer disease. We excluded from our report PTS

whose symptoms and clinical course of disease did not conform to the diagnostic criteria of the discussed illness.

Dealing with our PTS sample we encountered many problems as medical and social, psychological and legal, moral and management, and others. However, for us the most interesting subject is and remains the clinical course of Dementia, the speed of progress in this crude disease, the clinical stages (STS) through which the patient passes, the duration and transformation of STS and last but not least, the possibilities of intervention.

I will try to show you on the example of 3 cases how deep we often are concerned when we encounter such cases, how uncertain we are in predicting exactly the furhter development of the disease, especially when we are questioned by the patients relatives.

Mrs M., who is now 73 years old, suffers from the disease we are discussing here. Her first clinical signs appeared when she was 65 and after 2 years she was already institutionalized in a geropsychiatric closed department. This lady was in the past a well known personality in society. Two years after the onset of the disease symptoms the only way of communication with the outside world, which she was able to maintain was the drawing of nice pictures. At that time her brain CT scan was characterized by enlargement of ventricles and signs of cortex atrophy. The PT is now at a point of the time axis of the disease which belongs, according to our hypothesis of STS, to a very advanced ST of the disease.

Another woman, Mrs. A., who belonged to the intellectual group of society too, started with her symptoms at age 77, 12 years later than the first case. However, she succeeded in remaining manageable longer and continues to live in her habitual home atmosphere even though she is cognitively compromised.

A third PT, Mrs. N., suffered, contrarily to the first and the second cases, from a very rapid, "galloping" course of Dementia : her transition from ST to ST on the axis of time took less than 1,5 years. The age of onset of symptoms was 68. This was simply a catastrophical course and she very soon reached the ST of "Cognitive Death", soon followed by physical death.

DISCUSSION

Based on these 3 examples we would like to put 3 questions :
1. What are the reasons for such differences in the speed of the the disease progression ?
2. What are the typical stages of this disease ?
3. Do reliable ways of intervention now exist ?

We have thoroughly studied our group of PTS : anamnestical data

and hereditary predisposition, age of onset and kind of symptoms
presented, appearance of new symptoms and sings on the axis of time,
pecularities of the transformation of symptoms and syndromes.
We come to the assumption that there exist STS of develpment and
levels of functioning parallel with the axis of time. Both these
notions - stage and level - are closely connected with a third one
- cognition -, because at the end of the axis of time of our observation period there is practically speaking a ST of "Cognitive
Death".

According to Webster's Dictionary "Cognition is the act or process
of knowing including both awareness and judgement." Consequently,
when both awareness and judgement are absent, the ST can be defined
as "cognitive death".

Let us consider the discussed matter outgoing from 3 premises :
<u>First</u> that normal behaviour reflects the existence of cognitive
        intactness of Homo Sapiens.
<u>Second</u> that cognitive intactness reflects a normal integrative brain
        activity.
<u>Third</u> that normal integrative brain activity is closely connected
        and based on neurochemical processes and chemical substances
        such as acethylcholine and dopamine, serotonin and noradre-
        nalin, and many others.
These 3 premises permit us to improvise the intactness of cognition
as well as the impairment of human cognitive functions in pathological brain ageing in the shape of a chemical structural formula.
This in order to make clearer our assumption concerning the course
and STS of the disease.

On figure 2 this improvised structural formula of Cognitive Intactness is shown resembling the original Benzole formula discovered by
Kekule in 1865. I am fully aware that this represents only a model,
an improvisation. However it seems important when we turn to the
notion of STS in Dementia.

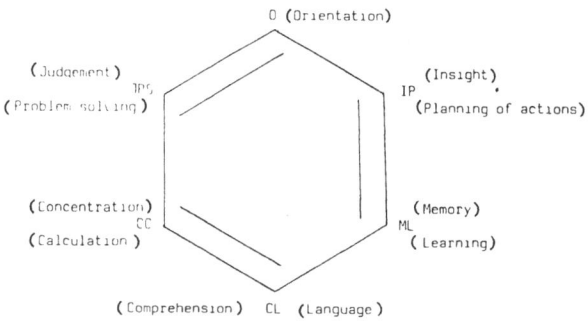

Figure 2   The "Structural Formula" of Cognitive Intactness

As you can see this model of Cognitive Intactness includes such functions as orientation, insight, planning of actions, memory, learning, comprehension, language, concentration, calculation, judgement and problem-solving. The main question is whether Dementias could be classified as multi-stage processes ?

Here we first have to define what the term ST means in developmental concepts in our profession - medicine -, in our speciality - psychiatry - and in our so fast growing nwe speciality - geriatric psychiatry.

The term ST implies some form of progression towards an expected end state. An example of such a situation may be that of a journey with a number of stages form an initial one to a final one, let us imagine from Tel-Aviv by ship to New-York : Tel-Aviv - Naples, Naples - Gibraltar, Gibraltar - New-York. But a succession of stages not only implies a start and an end in terms of temporal duration but also succesive changes along the dimension of time. Consequently, when we speak of STS especially in a biological-medical sense, we intend a typical sequence of segments along the temporal axis, segments each one of which can be characterized by changes, respectively symptoms and syndromes relative to the adjacent ones. This changes expressed in psychopathological items constitutes one step in a progression.

On figure 3 the design of Senile Dementia as a multi-stage process consisting of 5 STS can be seen. The course of this degenerative brain process represents a trajectory of changes, a progress of severity, respectively a regression in the level of cognitive functioning.

SENILE DEMENTIAS (RESP. PRIMARY DEGENERATIVE DEMENTIA) AS MULTI-STAGE PROCESSES

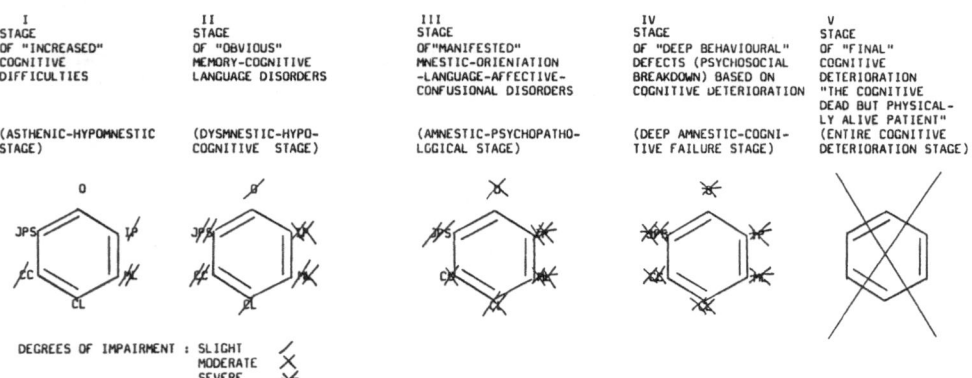

I STAGE OF "INCREASED" COGNITIVE DIFFICULTIES	II STAGE OF "OBVIOUS" MEMORY-COGNITIVE LANGUAGE DISORDERS	III STAGE OF "MANIFESTED" MNESTIC-ORIENTATION -LANGUAGE-AFFECTIVE-CONFUSIONAL DISORDERS	IV STAGE OF "DEEP BEHAVIOURAL" DEFECTS (PSYCHOSOCIAL BREAKDOWN) BASED ON COGNITIVE DETERIORATION	V STAGE OF "FINAL" COGNITIVE DETERIORATION "THE COGNITIVE DEAD BUT PHYSICAL-LY ALIVE PATIENT"
(ASTHENIC-HYPOMNESTIC STAGE)	(DYSMNESTIC-HYPO-COGNITIVE STAGE)	(AMNESTIC-PSYCHOPATHO-LOGICAL STAGE)	(DEEP AMNESTIC-COGNI-TIVE FAILURE STAGE)	(ENTIRE COGNITIVE DETERIORATION STAGE)

DEGREES OF IMPAIRMENT : SLIGHT
MODERATE
SEVERE

Figure 3   What are the characteristical features and symptoms for each of these 5 STS (based on our clinical observations)? This can be seen on the next 5 figures (4-8).

STAGE I
Of "increased" cognitive difficulties
10 principal symptoms (in percents of patients sample)

- Difficulties in finding the proper names   84
- Forgetfulness for placement of objects   81
- Difficulties in planning complex actions   72
- Difficulties in remembering appointments   64
- Decrease in energy, "cerebral asthenia"   63
- Difficulties in work capacity or in house work   62
- Difficulties in understanding logical-grammatical structures   62
- Attentional difficulties   61
- Difficulties in understanding of wits and lessening of sense of
  humour   58
- Hypochondriazation   52

STAGE II

Of "obvious" memory-cognitive-language disorders
10 principal symptoms (in percents of patients sample)

- Obvious forgetfulness   91
- Loss of insight, of interpretation of sensory defects and
  metamemory   86
- Decrease in capitalizing appropriate cues in memory strategies
  and organization   85
- Anxiety during psychological testing and social demand   72
- Disorders in clearly expressing of thoughts   69
- Difficulties in reading of anagrams   63
- Difficulties in understanding metaphors   61
- Expressed mood swings   58
- Mild expressed and evaluated only by special testing language
  disorders   57
- Appearance of prefrontal abnormal reflexes   54

STAGE III

Of "manifested" mnestic-orientation-language-affective-confusional
disorders ; 10 principal symptoms (in percents of patients sample)

- Facial recognition disorders   82
- Topographic memory disorders   80
- Restlessness and psychomotor agitation   67
- Aggression and hostility   63
- Paranoid mood (Wahnstimmung) and the hiding possession symptom   60
- Inability to detect own errors   58
- Inability to perform arithmetical operations   58
- Disorders in verbal fluency   57
- Manifested social withdrawal   55
- Disorders in narrative speech   51

STAGE IV

Of "deep behavioural defects" (psychosocial breakdown) based on
cognitive deterioration ; 10 principal symptoms (in percents of
patients sample)

- Deep spatial disorientation   92
- Significant language deterioration (omission of words, in-
  complete sentences, verbal iteration, stable intrusions of
  coherent kind)   89
- Confabulations   86
- Misidentifications   85
- Total lack of critical attitudes   85
- Total helplessness   84
- Hypersexuality (verbal and in activities)   66
- Disturbances of the diurnal rythm   64
- Delusional behaviour   53
- Diogenes-like syndrome   32

363

STAGE V

The "final" stage of entire cognitive deterioration - "cognitive death"

"The cognitive dead but physically alive patient"

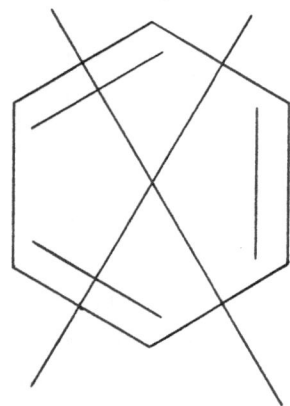

The data of our clinical sample show that the duration of STS (time range) is different between male and female (M=3,9 - 8,8 ; F=5,3 - 10,8). According to our material the whole range for both sexes was 3,9 - 10,8 years.
One thing I would like to emphasize here. Inspite of the difficulties in overcoming this harsh degenerative brain process we have been able in 265 cases (16,2 %) by real efforts of the caregivers, by cooperation with the patients and their relatives, by a more benign course of the disease, to prolong the being of PTS in STS I, II and sometimes even III for 1 - 3 years, and consequently to prolong the period of maintance of cognitive functioning, even when this occured at a lower level.
The interventional approaches used by us were :
1. Pharmacotherapy (Nootropics-Nootropil-UCB; Cholinergics-Lecithin; Phospholipides-Gricertine; Neuropeptides-Diapid)
2. The Classroom-Memory-Cognitive Rehabilitation Therapy, which appears to be halpful in capitalizing strategies (ekphoria ability, sifting out redundancy, using spatial and temporal cues) and training the facial recognition ability.

CONCLUSIONS

1. The developmental concept concerning the course of Dementias allows us to assume that the term clinical stage - as a stretch of time - is characterized by qualitative changes beginning from mnestic-cognitive difficulties and weakness (cerebral asthenia) till the final stage ("cognitive death").

2. The 5 clinical stages which we proposed are : I "increased" cognitive difficulties; II "obvious" memory, cognitive, language disorders; III "manifested" mnestic, orientation, language, affective, confusional disorders; IV "deep behavioural defects" (psychosocial breakdown) based on cognitive deterioration; V "final" cognitive deterioration.
3. There are 3 types of course, resp. speed of cognitive deterioration in Senile Dementia : a) slow, b) gradual, and c) rapid, galloping progress.
4. The taxonomic key approach, the higher brain functions concept and the newest achievements in Neuropharmacology coudl be regarded as important and promising in our search for intervention, which means early detection, prompt pathogenetic treatment and functional rehabilitation.

MENTAL IMPAIRMENT IN THE AGED:

TOWARDS ESTABLISHING A DIFFERENTIAL DIAGNOSIS

Marc A. Schuckit

University of California San Diego
Alcoholism Treatment Program
Veterans Administration Medical Center
3350 La Jolla Village Drive
San Diego, California 92161

INTRODUCTION

I approach this topic as both a clinical researcher and a clinician who regularly treats patients. As my goal is to present information which can be used in daily practice, a few relevant references will be offered to encourage the reader to seek more details but most conclusions offered here represent a synthesis of existing paper and clinical experience.

I begin this discussion of diagnosis by setting forth my biases. First, as clinicians, the most important dictum is "first do no harm". Yet, all interventions are capable of harming patients physically, economically, or psychologically. The dangers of intervention are especially important in the elderly as they may be more ill, may be more sensitive to side effects of medications, and probably show less resiliency in recovering after iatrogenic damage[1].

Second, of equal importance is the danger which accrues when important interventions are withheld. Just as older people react more intensely to improper treatments, they may deteriorate more rapidly than younger individuals when a treatable illness is overlooked or not addressed with enough vigor. Thus, caring clinicians are faced with a physical dilemma: the problem is one of aggressively treating important illness while exposing the patient to as little iatrogenic risk as possible. For me, the key to this quandry rests with proper diagnosis.

I use diagnostic labels to indicate the probable prognosis (i.e., what is likely to happen without treatment) and to select among various therapies (i.e., which treatment has the greatest benefit/risk ratio).[2]   While this may seem obvious to the primary care physician, it is easy to lose sight of these goals in behavioral medicine.

To be useful, diagnosis must be stated in objective terms which are likely to be interpreted similarly in different parts of the world. These relatively objective criteria must have been applied to groups of patients who were then followed up over time to determine probable prognosis and exposed to various forms of treatment to demonstrate the benefit/risk ratio.

Unfortunately, behavioral medicine has few (if any) signs or symptoms which are diagnostic in themselves. This may relate to the limited repertoire of human behavior so that the same symptoms are likely to be seen in a variety of disorders. For instance, serious and incapacitating anxiety with associated panic attacks can be part of a major depressive disorder, might be noted in some cases of schizophrenia, are often observed with misuse of stimulant drugs, or might represent a primary anxiety illness - each diagnosis carrying its own prognosis and proper treatment.[3] Therefore, the proper diagnosis is established by observing the pattern of all signs and symptoms, determining their time course, and taking a number of common sense steps to rule out conditions likely to mimic behavioral problems, especially medical disorders and substance-related problems.

In the sections which follow, I will briefly review the major relevant diagnostic questions which the clinician must address in attempting to establish a psychiatric diagnosis in the elderly. Thus, this paper reviews medical problems as they may mimic emotional disorders (especially cognitive loss or depression), reactions to medications and substance abuse, major affective disorders (i.e., depressive disease), psychosis, and dementia. Each of these topics is raised as part of a logical differential diagnosis and as an introduction to the other papers offered in this symposium.

MEDICAL DISORDERS

As a psychiatrist, I am in danger of mislabeling the behavioral manifestations of a primary medical disorder as if they represent a primary psychiatric problem. It is essential that I recognize the possibility of medical illness in all patients presenting with behavioral or emotional problems and that I take steps to rule out physical disorders before concentrating exclusively on the behavior.

TABLE 1. Physical Disorders Likely to Present with Serious Depression

Cancer (e.g., head of the pancreas)
Anemia
Electrolyte imbalances
Influenza, hepatitis, and other viral infections
Pneumonia
Endocrine imbalances (e.g., thyroid, adrenal)

Clinically, a primary medical disorder is especially likely if the behavioral syndrome is atypical or whenever signs of confusion exist. Many medical disorders can cause malfunction in the central nervous system (CNS) with resulting confusion, a problem of special importance in the elderly. Others cause signs of depression which must be carefully differentiated from primary affective disease.

While medical syndromes associated with confusion are discussed in greater depth in other texts, an example of the diagnostic problems seen for depression might be helpful at this point. Table 1 gives a number of physical disorders which are likely to present with many of the signs and symptoms of major depressive disease. In each of these, proper recognition and treatment of the primary medical problem should result in an alleviation or disappearance of the depressive symptoms. Treating the clinical picture of depression and ignoring the primary medical disorder has little chance of success but exposes the patient to the dangers of possible reactions to improper medications.

Similar illustrative examples can be given for physical disorders causing a confused state resembling a dementia.[4] The bottom line is the necessity for considering physical disorders as an underlying cause for any psychiatric syndrome. A relevant physical examination and laboratory test must be part of the work-up for all individuals, especially the elderly population as they are at elevated risk for medical disorders.

REACTIONS TO DRUGS

No primary psychiatric disorder can be diagnosed without first ruling out the possibility that the symptoms are related to a pharmacological agent. This is an especially important rule with the elderly because they are more likely to be taking medications and may be at higher risk for adverse reactions to all substances.[5] Therefore, all work-ups must include an indepth review of every prescription drug, all over-the-counter medications (including laxatives, aspirin, etc.), and borrowed drugs, and alcohol.

TABLE 2. Drugs Likely to Cause Significant Depression

<u>All CNS depressants</u>

> Prescription hypnotics
> Prescription antianxiety drugs
> Alcohol

<u>CNS stimulants</u>

> Prescription and over-the-counter weight
>   reducing medications
> Amphetamines
> Methylphenidate (Ritalin)
> Cocaine

<u>Many prescription medications including:</u>

> L-Dopa
> Antihypertensives
> Anticonvulsants

Table 2 is a brief list of some substances which must be considered in working up patients presenting with even severe, debilitating signs of depression. In addition to a long list of prescription drugs, two categories of substances of misuse must also be considered. The brain depressants can cause signs of sadness after even acute intoxication and routinely induce signs of depression with heavy chronic use.[6,7] Similarly, all brain stimulants (including all prescription and many over-the-counter weight reducing products) rapidly induce severe depressions and should rarely, if ever, be prescribed for elderly individuals.[8] The brain depressants are also likely to induce states of even severe confusion in the elderly and must be considered as part of the differential diagnosis given here, reactions to prescription and over-the-counter medication and deliberate or inadvertent misuse of brain stimulants and depressants must always be considered early in the differential diagnosis of signs of mental deterioration in the aged.

MAJOR DEPRESSIVE SYNDROMES (PRIMARY AFFECTIVE DISORDER)

Now that you recognize that medical disorders and drug use can produce states of profound sadness, it is time to discuss a primary psychiatric disorder of depression which requires active treatment. The proper diagnosis of primary affective disorder is made by carefully observing the time course of development of symptoms in the absence of major medical disorders or reactions to substances.

TABLE 3.   DSM III – Diagnosis of Affective Disorders[11]

296.2 Major Depression

296.3   A. Dysphoria or loss of interest

               B. At least four symptoms daily for two+ weeks

                    Appetite disturbance
                    Sleep disturbance
                    Psychomotor change
                    Loss of interest
                    Loss of energy
                    Guilt and worthless feelings
                    Decreased ability to think or concentrate
                    Death thoughts or wishes

               C. No pre-existing psychiatric disorders

296.4 Bipolar Disorder.   Mania diagnosed when:
296.5
296.6   A. Prominent elevated, expansive or
                    irritable mood

               B. Last one+ week with three+ symptoms

                    Increased activity
                    Talkative
                    Thoughts racing
                    Inflated self-esteem
                    Decreased sleep need
                    Distractability
                    Poor judgement

               C. No pre-existing psychotic disorder

Table 3 outlines the criteria for major affective disorder given in the Third Diagnostic and Statistical Manual of the American Psychiatric Association.[11] The syndrome involves a persistent mood of depression which interferes both with physical functioning (e.g., insomnia and appetite disturbances) and mental facilities (e.g., loss of interest in activities and problems with concentration). The patient is likely to feel hopeless and worthless.

One important reason to diagnose this syndrome is that with proper treatment the chances for recovery are excellent.[2] Adequate care includes aggressive use of antidepressants, being certain to give the proper amount of medications and if at all possible, monitoring blood levels. In the elderly, untreated depressive disorder carries a serious risk for premature death[12] related to the increased chance of successful suicide with increasing age[13] and the inanition and inactivity which are part and parcel of the affective syndromes.

Establishing this important and potentially life-threatening illness of major affective disorder in the elderly is not always straightforward. First, clinicians may erroneously assume that signs and symptoms of depression are inherent in growing old, ignoring the clinical picture until it is too late. In addition, as briefly presented in Table 4, older men and women with major depressive syndromes may present with some atypical symptoms. These include less obvious changes in mood, somatic preoccupation, or a smiling denial of "depression" while still presenting with a fairly rapid onset of many of the appetite, sleep pattern and energy level changes associated with major affective disorders.

In any age group, one part of a major depressive syndrome is an inability to concentrate and to pay attention to what is happening in one's surroundings. This frequently results in signs and symptoms of memory impairment and confusion.[14] In the elderly, there is the danger that this fairly rapid appearance of a cognitive defect along with depressive symptoms will be mislabeled as a "dementia or senility" and not treated. This could have potentially lethal results. The differential diagnosis between the bonafide dementias (e.g., Senile Dementia of the Alzheimer's Type or SDAT) and major affective disorder with secondary confusion has been discussed in depth elsewhere.[15,16] Briefly, it is important to consider the association of affective disorder with a family history of depressive disease, a past personal history of affective disorder, a rapid onset, a fluctuation in mood, and a clinical picture indicating a more global cognitive defect than is documented on formal psychological testing.

In summary, major affective disorders must be adequately diagnosed and aggressively treated in the elderly. The differential diagnosis includes many medical disorders, reactions to prescription or over-the-counter medication, and either deliberate or inadvertent misuse of substances, especially brain depressants and stimulants. This diagnosis may be more difficult to establish in the elderly than in younger populations because of erroneous stereotypes of normal mood states in the elderly and the higher prevalence of atypical symptoms in older age groups. However, because this illness has

TABLE 4. Atypical Presentation of Affective Disorder in the Elderly

1. Smiling depressions denying feelings of sadness
2. A reluctance to express feelings of guilt
3. Concomitant medical disorders
4. Somatic preoccupation and atypical pain

such a great chance of responding to adequate treatment, affective disorder must always be considered with any behavioural syndrome in elderly groups.

PSYCHOSIS

The term psychosis is not a diagnosis but a description of a clinical picture which can be seen in a variety of illnesses and thus responds to a variety of interventions.[2,17] The clinical picture of hallucinations (usually auditory) and/or delusions (usually paranoid) in the absence of cognitive impairment can be seen in elderly as well as younger populations. As is true of all clinical pictures in older groups, one must first rule out medical problems (e.g., thyroid abnormalities, electrolyte imbalances, pernicious anemia, etc.), misuse of substances (especially stimulants and depressants) and transient psychotic symptoms which often occur in the midst of major cognitive deficits (e.g., SDAT) as well as major depressive disorders.[2,8,17] Each of these carries its own prognosis and proper treatment.

The rapid development of a psychosis in the absence of any of the conditions mentioned above in an older person usually represents Late Onset Paraphrenia.[18] While the cause of this disorder is not known, these patients usually respond to fairly low doses of anti-psychotic medications (e.g., thiaridazine or Mellaril).[2,18] The risk for adverse reactions such as movement disorders with these medications must always be considered, but the judicious use of anti-psychotics is warranted once the diagnosis has been adequately established in light of the good chance of a clinical response.

DEMENTIA: A SUMMARY OF THE APPROACH TO DIFFERENTIAL DIAGNOSIS

The purpose of this paper has been to document some of the steps which must be taken in establishing the proper differential diagnosis of mental deterioration in the aged. The two classical dementias, SDAT and Multi Infarct Dementia, each carry a serious prognosis. The proper diagnosis must be established in order to rule out other more treatable disorders, to help the patient and the family adequately plan for the future, and to highlight behavioral and pharmacological interventions which can be helpful early in the course. Examples of these include prescription of ergot derivatives to help improve cellular metabolism[19] and behavioral manipulations.

Proper prognosis and treatment exposing patients to the most favorable benefit to risk ratio requires adequate diagnosis. Physical disorders must be considered not only in the initial work-up but whenever the patient demonstrates a rapid decline in his cognitive state. All patients must receive a thorough review of medication and substance

intake or the clinician runs the risk of missing a readily treatable
condition which can masquerade as an affective disorder or dementia.
Recognizing its relatively high prevalence in the elderly, the
potential atypicality of symptoms, the bleak prognosis without
treatment, and the probable disappearance of symptoms with adequate
pharmacological interventions, affective disorder must always be
listed as a possible diagnosis in dealing with any patient presenting
with confusion.

REFERENCES

1. D. E. Harrison, The Nature of Aging, in: "Psychopharmacology of Old Age," D. Wheatley, ed., Oxford University
   Press, New York, Toronto (1982).
2. D. W. Goodwin and S. B. Guge,"Psychiatric Diagnosis," Oxford
   University Press, New York (1980).
3. M. A. Schuckit, Current Therapeutic Options in the Management of Typical Anxiety, J Clin Psychiatry 42:11 (1981).
4. M. N. Rossor, Neurotransmitters and CNS Disease, Lancet
   Vol. II (1982).
5. M. Raskind and C. Eisdorfer, Psychopharmacology of the
   Aged, in: "Drug Treatment of Mental Disorders," L. L.
   Simpson, ed., Raven Press, New York (1976).
6. S. Gibson and J. Becker, Changes in Alcoholics' Self-
   Reported Depression, Quart. J. Stud. Alc. 34: 829-836,
   (1973).
7. M. A. Schuckit, Alcoholism and Affective Disorder: Diagnostic Confusion, in: "Alcoholism and Affective Disorders," D. W. Goodwin and C. K. Erickson, ed., Spectrum
   Publications, New York (1979).
8. M. A. Schuckit, "Drug and Alcohol Abuse," Plemum Press,
   New York (1979).
9. M. A. Schuckit and M. A. Moore, Drug Problems in the Elderly,
   in: "Psychopathology of Aging," O. J. Kaplan, ed.,
   Academic Press, New York (1979).
10. D. A. Segal and M. A. Schuckit, Animal Models of Stimulant-
    Induced Psychosis, in: "Stimulants: Neurochemical, Be-
    havioral, and Clinical Perspectives," I. Creese, ed.,
    Raven Press, New York (1983).
11. American Psychiatric Association: Diagnostic and Statistical
    Manual of Mental Disorders (Third Edition), American
    Psychiatric Association, Washington D.C. (1980).
12. M. A. Schuckit et al., A Three Year Follow-Up of Elderly
    Alcoholics, J Clin Psychiatry 41:412-416 (1980).
13. R. H. Gerner, Depression in the Elderly, in: Psycho-
    pathology of Aging," O. J. Kaplan, ed., Academic Press,
    New York (1979).
14. L. R. Squire and P. C. Slater, Electroconvulsive Therapy
    and Complains of Memory Dysfunction: A Prospective Three-
    Year Follow-up Study, Brit. J. Psychiat. 142:1-8 (1983).

15. E. D. Caine, Pseudodementia, <u>Arch Gen Psychiatry</u> Vol. 38 (1981).

16. L. Grunhaus, et al., Depressive Pseudodementia: A Suggested Diagnostic Profile, Biol. Psychiatry. Vol. 18, (1983).

17. D. W. Goodwin, P. Alderson, and R. Rosenthal, Clincial Significance of Hallucinations in Psychiatric Disorders, <u>Arch Gen Psychiat</u>, Vol. 24 (1971).

18. B. Pitt, Paranoid psychosis in the elderly, <u>in</u>: "Psychopharmacology of Old Age," D. Wheatley, ed., Oxford University Press, New York, Toronto (1982).

19. P. Cook, Cerebrovascular Dilators, <u>N Eng J Med</u> 305:1508-1513 (1981).

THE CONTRIBUTION OF BLOOD LEVELS TO THE REVERSIBILITY OF "RESISTANT" DEPRESSION

Mark S. Gold

Fair Oaks Hospital
19 Prospect Street
Summit, NJ 07901

Within the descriptively homogenous endogenous subgroup of depressives, at least 35% of patients fail to respond to treatment with standard dosages of antidepressants (AD). Among many of the "responders" the quality of response is quite variable. Furthermore many "responders" in a research study relapse within six months and some are even included in another study. Others are treated and studied by other physicians. Undoubtedly, some patients are treatment resistant because they have been misdiagnosed and suffer from medical illness (Koranyi, 1979; Gold et al., 1981; Hall et al., 1981; Estroff et al., 1983).

There are several reasons why "non-medical" endogenously depressed patients may fail to respond to standard treatment. Firstly, the subgroup of endogenous depression is a heterogenous group of illnesses. Patients may meet criteria for a major depression but have an undiagnosed medical, neurobiological, endocrinological, drug or substance abuse illness (Gold et al., 1983). Patients may have an endogenous depression but since neither pathophysiology nor prediction of treatment response are considered in the diagnosis, the clinical diagnosis fails to predict who will respond to which treatment, for what duration, at what dose, etc. Demonstrable biochemical differences as indicated by variable patterns of 24 hour urinary 3-methoxy-4-hydroxy phenylglycol (MHPG) (Schildkraut, 1973; Maas, 1975; Hollister et al., 1980; Schatzberg et al., 1982) excretion and CSF 5-hydroxy-indoleacetic acid (HIAA) levels suggest many differences exist between "similar" patients (Maas et al., 1982; Asberg et al., 1973; Appelbaum et al., 1979). Given the probable biochemical heterogeneity of endogenous depression, it is no more reasonable to expect that every individual will respond to a given antidepressant than it is to assume that all sore throats with fever will respond to the same pharmacological treatment. However, another reason why many patients fail to respond to treatment is that they have not received an adequate therapeutic trial of antidepressant drug therapy. Most physicians do not even know the definition of an antidepressant trial. The use of standard dose regimens unrelated to plasma levels has been identified as a major source of antidepressant non-response. The reasons for this fact are numerous but include pharmacokinetic, pharmacodynamic, and other factors. This confusion contributes to nonresponse and undertreatment (Keller et al., 1982). Other, less obvious factors may contribute to inadequate drug treatment and include interpatient pharmacokinetic variability resulting in non-therapeutic blood levels, drug-drug interactions, generic substitution, non-compliance, and inadequate duration of drug treatment. Of these factors since the majority of depressed patients do not seek treatment and those who do seek treatment feel a stigma upon filling a prescription (they may even go to a pharmacy outside their area) compliance must be lower than that reported for hypertension. This chapter will examine these variables and suggest ways in which therapeutic drug monitoring can help the clinician to reduce the failure rate in pharmacological treatment of depressed patients by assuring the adequacy of the therapeutic trial.

Impatience on both the part of the patient and the treating physician can result in premature termination of treatment. Dose adjustments, adding additional medications and so on are made all too often and for no apparent reason. If a trial or dose is not defined by blood levels it is difficult to decide when to raise or lower dose or switch medications. The usual lag time between the initiation of treatment and the onset of therapeutic effect is usually two to three weeks. There does not seem to be any significant evidence that this lag time can be shortened by choice of drug, route of administration, or adjunctive medication treatment (Kessler, 1978). A therapeutic drug trial, then, should consist of a minimum of 21 (post steady-state) consecutive days at a therapeutic blood level of the AD being used, with documented blood level determinations to assure compliance.

It is best to do single medication trials at a time in order to be sure which intervention is having a therapeutic effect. It is important that medication trials be well defined so that they are adequate in dosage and duration in order to assess the efficacy of a medication for a given patient. Equally importantly, a medication which has not been helpful after an adequate trial should be discontinued. Though there are some patients who do better on combinations, such as ADs plus neuroleptics, or ADs plus lithium, it is best to add the second medication in a step-wise fashion. There is little place for medications combining a fixed ratio of two medications (e.g. Trilafon and Elavil are more effectively prescribed individually than as Triavil). If two medications are needed, the dosages are best adjusted independently.

For other tricyclics, other antidepressants and most anticonvulsants, therapeutic levels are best described as thresholds required for therapeutic efficacy (Amsterdam et al., 1980; Risch et al., 1979). For ADs that are metabolized to substances that are themselves antidepressant, these "active metabolites" must be taken into account also. Thus, amitriptyline is metabolized to nortriptyline, and imipramine is metabolized to desipramine. For patients taking either of the parent medications, plasma levels of both parent and active metabolite must be measured.

The best correlation between plasma AD levels and clinical response has been demonstrated for nortriptyline (NT). The majority of studies have been conducted in patients with endogenous depression (major depressive disorder with melancholia, DSM-III). Asberg and associates (1971) reported that a minimum level of 50 ng/ml and an upper level of 150 ng/ml were associated with the maximum probability of therapeutic response in patients treated with NT. The use of the "therapeutic window" has been prospectively shown to be an effective way of monitoring drug response (Kragh-Sorensen et al., 1976). These investigators used a dosage of NT which resulted in plasma levels under 150 ng/ml in one group of patients, and in a second group used dosages which resulted in plasma levels over 180 ng/ml. The results of Lehmann et al. (1982) indicate that a strategy of promptly determining NT plasma concentrations and requiring that the psychiatrist systematically adjust dosage can achieve the goal of bringing plasma concentration into a targeted range resulting in improved clinical response. Additionally, a greater percentage of NT-treated discharged patients had improved at 3 weeks suggests that the dosage adjustment speeded clinical response. This was in contrast to amitriptyline.

Our experience (Gold and Martin, 1982) and the data reported by others (Lehmann et al., 1982; Dawling et al., 1981) suggest that use of the NT window with regular monitoring increases both response time and response rate.

The AD "dose prediction test" has been employed to try to ascertain in advance whether a patient is a rapid or slow metabolizer, and hence the approximate dosage that will be needed to achieve therapeutic levels (Cooper and Simpson, 1978). This test consists of measurement of plasma level 24 hours after administration orally of a test dose of 50 or 100 mgs of a AD. Nomograms have been worked out for NT which relate blood level at 24 hours to optimal daily dosages needed.

Factors which can result in an inadequate therapeutic drug trial include inadequate dosage, interpatient pharmacokinetic variability, drug interactions, noncompliance, and insufficient duration of drug treatment. The use of accurate therapeutic blood level monitoring in documenting the adequacy of drug treatment has been presented. No patient should be considered a nonresponder unless an adequate drug trial with documented therapeutic blood level monitoring has been completed. As seen in the two studies utilizing specific groups of depressed patients, NT with NT level monitoring can improve efficacy (Gold and Martin, 1982). For carefully selected major depressives, response rates to anti-depressants have been reported as low as 50–60% without monitoring of plasma levels, and as high as 70–90% of adolescents and adults with monitoring of levels (Klein et al., 1980; Goodwin, 1977; Baldessarini, 1975; Gold et al., 1980). Early documentation of therapeutic drug levels could save the unnecessary expense of prolonged hospitalization additional outpatient visits, medication costs, and unnecessary patient suffering. Additionally, surprise blood level checks can also maximize compliance and reduce the treatment failure rate.

References

Amsterdam, J., Brunswick, D., and Mendels, J., 1980, The clinical application of tricyclic antidepressant pharmacokinetics and plasma levels, Am J Psychiatry, 137:653.
Appelbaum, P. S., Vasile, R. G., Orsulak, P. J., and Schildkraut, J. J., 1979, Clinical utility of tricyclic antidepressant blood levels: a case report, Am J Psychiatry, 40:58.
Asberg, M., Cronholm, B., Sjoqvist, F., and Tuck, D., 1971, Relationship between plasma level and therapeutic effect of nortriptyline, Br Med J., 3:331.
Asberg, M., Bertilsson, L., Tuck, R., Cronholm, B., and Sjoqvist, F., 1973, Indoleamine metabolites in the cerebrospinal fluid of depressed patients before and during treatment with nortriptyline, Clin Pharmacol Ther., 14:277.
Baldessarini, R. J., 1975, "Chemotherapy in Psychiatry," Harvard University Press, Massachusetts.
Cooper, T. B., and Simpson, G. M., 1978, Prediction of individual dosage of nortriptyline, Am J Psychiatry, 135:333.
Dawling, S., Crome, P., Heyer, E. J., and Lewis, R. R., 1981, Nortriptyline therapy in elderly patients: dosage prediction from plasma concentration at 24 hours after a single 50 mg dose, Brit J Psychiatry, 139:413.
Estroff, T. E., and Gold, M. S., 1983, Psychiatric misdiagnosis, in: "Advances in Psychopharmacology: Predicting and Improving Treatment Response," M. S. Gold, R. B. Lydiard, and J. Carman, eds., CRC Press, Inc., Boca Raton, (in press).

Gold, M. S., Lydiard, R. B., and Carman, J. S., 1983, "Advances in Psychopharmacology: Predicting and Improving Treatment Response," CRC Press, Inc., Boca Raton, (in press).

Gold, M. S., and Martin, D., 1982, Diagnosis and treatment with tricyclic antidepressants, Presented at the 34th Institute on Hospital and Community Psychiatry, Louisville.

Gold, M. S., Pottash, A. L. C., and Extein, I., 1981, Hypothyroidism and depression, JAMA, 245:1919.

Gold, M. S., Pottash, A. L. C., Stoll, A., Martin, D. M., Extein, I., Mueller, E. A., and Finn, L. B., 1980, Nortriptyline plasma levels and clinical response in familial pure unipolar depression and blunted TRH test patients, Int J Psychiatry Med., (in press).

Goodwin, F. K., 1977, Drug treatment of affective disorders: general principles, in: "Psychopharmacology in the Practice of Medicine," M. E. Jarvik, ed., Appleton-Century-Crofts, New York.

Hall, R. C. W., Gardner, E. R., Popkin, M. K., LeCann, A. F., and Stickner, S. K., 1981, Unrecognized physical illness/prompting psychiatric admission: a prospective study, Am J Psychiatry, 138:629.

Hollister, L. E., Davis, K. L., and Berger, P. A., 1980, Subtypes of depression based on excretion of MHPG and response to nortriptyline, Arch Gen Psychiatry, 37:1107.

Keller, M. B., Klerman, G. L., Lavori, P. W., Fawcett, J. A., Coryell, W., and Endicott, J., 1982, Treatment received by depressed patients, J Am Med Assoc., 248:1848.

Kessler, K. A., 1978, Tricyclic antidepressants: mode of action and clinical use, in: "Psychopharmacology: A Generation of Progress," M. A. Lipton, A. DiMascio, and K. F. Killam, eds., Raven Press, New York.

Klein, D. F., Gittelman, R., Quitkin, F., and Rifkin, A., 1980, Diagnosis and drug treatment of psychiatric disorders, Williams and Wilkins, Baltimore.

Koranyi, E. K., 1979, Morbidity and rate of undiagnosed physical illness in a psychiatric clinic population, Arch Gen Psychiatry, 36:414.

Kragh-Sorensen, P., Eggert-Hansen, C., and Baastrup, P. C., 1976, Self-inhibiting action of nortriptyline antidepressive effect at high-plasma levels, Psychopharmacologia, 45:305.

Lehmann, L. S., Bowden, C. L., Redmond, F. C., and Stanton, B. C., 1982, Amitriptyline and nortriptyline response profiles in unipolar depressed patients, Psychopharmacology, 77:193.

Maas, J. W., 1975, Biogenic amines and depression: biochemical and pharmacological separation of two types of depression, Arch Gen Psychiatry, 32:1357.

Maas, J. W., Kocsis, J. H., Bowden, C. L., Davis, J. M., Redmond, D. E., Hanin, L., and Robins, E., 1982, Pre-treatment neurotransmitter metabolites and response to imipramine or amitriptyline, Psychol Med., 12:37.

Risch, S. C., Huey, L. Y., and Janowsky, D. S., 1979, Plasma
        levels of tricyclic antidepressants and clinical efficacy:
        a review of the literature, J Clin Psychiatry, 40:6 & 58.
Schatzberg, A. F., Orsulak, P. J., Rosenbaum, A. H., Maruta, T.,
        Kruger, E. R., Cole, J. O., and Schildkraut, J. J., 1982,
        Toward a biochemical classification of depressive dis-
        orders, V: heterogeneity of unipolar depressions, Am J
        Psychiatry, 139:471.
Schildkraut, J. J., 1973, Norepinephrine metabolites or biochemical
        criteria for classifying depressive disorders and predict-
        ing response to treatment: preliminary findings, Am J
        Psychiatry, 130:695.

PSYCHOGERIATRICS AND THE FAMILY DOCTOR:

COLLABORATION IN THE CARE OF DEMENTIA

Tom Arie

Professor of Health Care of the Elderly
University of Nottingham
Sherwood Hospital, Nottingham NG5 1PD, U.K.

This paper looks briefly at aspects of the relationship between the general practice "primary care team" and special services for the elderly. For both the task is a triple one:

- to make available skill and resources directly to patients
- to support the lay supporters of the demented
- to support each other

The ways in which scarce trained skills and formal resources can be made to go furthest in support of the informal care network is a central question in regard to the demented, who are some 5 per cent to 10 per cent of elderly people, and thus in my country now number between half a million and one million persons; those involved in their support are more numerous still. Dementia therefore touches the lives of millions of people, particularly the middle-aged (or older) lay supporters, who give the bulk of care.

In the British system of care nearly everyone is registered with a general practitioner (GP), who has responsibility for continuing availability and who leads the "primary care team". Alongside the GP are nurses and social workers; the practice manager and the receptionist are also usually of key importance. Remedial staff, psychologists, and others who in the past have worked in hospitals are now more and more available alongside the primary team. Access to the specialist is by referral from the GP, whose responsibility for a patient only partly lapses during the period of specialist treatment, and resumes fully after it. Shared responsibilities with the specialist team - e.g. when the latter is involved in follow-up support, or in providing day care - need particularly sensitive co-ordination.

My comments focus on four topics:

- The growth of specialised psychiatric services for the elderly
- Case-finding, surveillance and prevention
- "Holding the line" between care at home and in institutions
- "Styles" of helping

SPECIALISED PSYCHIATRIC SERVICES FOR THE ELDERLY

A remarkable feature of the British scene, and fast becoming a worldwide movement, is the differentiation within psychiatric services of a component directed particularly to the needs of the elderly. Practically all psychiatric disorders occur in old age, and an old age psychiatric service must deliver good psychiatry across the whole range of these disorders — but dementia poses most of the problems in sharpest focus.

Geriatric psychiatry, or psychogeriatrics, has grown rapidly in the British National Health Service. At the end of 1980 some 120 psychiatrists were specialising in this work,[1] and psycho-geriatric services exist in wel' over one half of all health districts, most of them providing comprehensive psychiatric care for a population defined only by area of residence. These new services are natural partners for the older sister specialty geriatrics.

In Nottingham we combine old age medicine and psychiatry in one department. Services are thus more readily able to respond according to the needs of patients, rather than merely with what is available in that compartment into which the patient happens to have fallen. We are also making progress in preventing patients from falling between services, or from being bounced from one to another, and GPs from having to "shop around" for help. The service is also a prime taching resource in our heavy educational programme.

The principles of organising psychogeriatric services have lately been much reviewed.[2,3,4,5] They form not only an important practical resource for mentally ill old people and their families, but also a focus for interest, for education and for advocacy. Similar developments are taking place in many countries.[6]

CASE-FINDING, SURVEILLANCE AND PREVENTION

Psychogeriatrics begins not with the specialist, but with the primary care team, by early detection, definition of those at risk, and effective programmes of surveillance and support.[7] Williamson had found in the 1960s that of a community sample of old people in Edinburgh, nearly 90 per cent of the demented were unknown to have this condition by their GPs. Things are probably better in the 1980s, but there is evidence that in this preventive role general practice still has much scope for advance. The recent study by Bowling and Cartwright[8] of newly bereaved old people and their GPs raises relevant issues. They found that:

- three fifths of GPs did not feel that it was always appropriate to visit an old person after bereavement
- only one third of old people had seen their GP between the death and the funeral
- one third of all bereaved old people had no contact at all with their GP in the 5 to 6 months after bereavement
- likelihood of contact was not related to the existence of major social problems such as living alone, poor housing, or financial difficulty
- there were big discrepancies between the problems reported by old people, and their GPs' awareness of them

Bereavement is not the same as dementia, but that there are lessons here is obvious, for a similar preventive model applies. There is also good news. The "younger" GPs appeared to perform more favourably: GPs born after 1937 by comparison with those born before 1917

- saw these elderly patients much more often
- visisted them at home much more often
- were more likely to be described as "very sympathetic" (whereas the latter were twice as likely to be described as "not easy to talk to")

These figures are worth quoting for two reasons. First, because I do not know of similar recent data in relation to dementia; second, because behaviour on the part of GPs seems to be changing. As a teacher, I hope this will further be reinforced by now fast improving education about the elderly. In Nottingham we always have 3 or 4 trainee GPs doing a 6-month residency in the care of the elderly alongside trainee specialists; and our undergradute students have a month's full-time course.[9]

The task of case-finding and surveillance in general practice is not insurmountable. Screening for mental disorder in the elderly can be undertaken by other members of the primary care team than just the doctor.[7] An average GP with some 2,000 patients will have in our country about one hundred patients aged over 75. Of these up to about 20 may be demented, and the task in regard to these and other "at risk" old people can be shared between the members of the team. Age/sex registers for each practice are very desirable.

That this is important derives from two essential
characteristics of dementia:

- its tendency to cause crises
- its unparalleled consumption of long term care

Decisions taken in crisis are constrained by those solutions
which happen to be available at the time; plans made early can take
account of what, after cool assessment, appears actually to be
needed.

Similarly, early intervention can palliate disabilities that
might later become irremediable, and can enhance the "morale" of
supporters, for whom a sense that their problem is being shared
from an early stage can greatly extend their capacity to go on
coping. The "snapping" of tolerance leading to demand for
institutional care which is apt to occur after a long period of
unsupported coping, and which often is unmasked only by the
bursting of a crisis, may thus be prevented. Preventive education
can be fully effective only if case-finding is early. A growing
range of publications for laymen may help (one of the best is Mace
and Rabins' "The 36-Hour Day"[10]).

"HOLDING THE LINE" AND THE BALANCE OF CARE

Containment of the growing pressure of dependent very old
people with failing brains depends on "holding the line" between
home care and institutions. The "line" is drawn at very different
levels in different countries. In Britain Emily Grundy and I[11]
recently showed that the rate of statutory residential provision
for the elderly is contracting alarmingly, though community support
services have meanwhile been expanding; but these too show
retraction in recent years.[12,13]

Where the line is drawn depends also on the expectations of a
particular community, its standards of living, its traditional
attitudes to old people; yet everywhere the most demented people
are looked after at home, and those at home include many people
with the most severe disabilities. The trickiest problem is of the
demented who live alone. Inherent in the nature of dementia is
lack of capacity safely and decently to function without round-
the-clock surveillance. Where this is not available through family
or friends, early breakdown is common, regardless of support
offered.[14] Attempts to support by merely episodic interventions
people so disabled that they actually need round-the-clock surveillance, is usually fruitless. The solo dement is an instance where
the GP and his team may sometimes labour too hard to give support,
and should be readier to press early for institutional care. By
contrast, resources spent on "supporting the supporters" may be

capable of greatly enhancing their capacity to cope. Prospective studies are needed here, but are difficult.

"STYLES" OF SUPPORT

I return to questions posed at the outset: how may professional workers be most effective in supporting others, and how may specialist staff best support the primary team? What I have in mind is not just the nature of levels of resources, but the "style" which seems most likely to give confidence.

Availability, unfussy and without delays, is essential; where there is a sense of crisis, response must be immediate. Urgency needs to be measured not just objectively, but on the subjective sense of crisis of those calling for help. Only urgent response to urgent referral will give confidence that the crisis is being taken seriously.

The care of demented old people can be as consuming and unremitting a task as that of small infants. The 'care needs' of both groups are similar, but the context is quite different. Children have parents who are usually willing carers — problems arise only when they are not. But for the demented there may be no-one. A demented relative is a misfortune; rearing a child is usually joyous, if strenuous, with anticipation of growth and development. Release from pressure of care for a demented relative is only through deterioration, by institutional care or death, bringing guilt, anger and depression. It is small wonder that families under these pressures may have a different view from that of dispassionate observers of what is a crisis.

The specialised service must go into patients' homes. Initial contact especially should be in the home rather than in a clinic, office, or worst of all by direct admission to hospital; for removal from home is a momentous step and often irreversible, pre-empting more appropriate solutions. If it is necessary to admit to hospital, this should be after home assessment, rather than in place of it.[2]

Collaboration thrives on close personal contact. This too is often best achieved in the patient's home, where problems can be jointly examined at their roots. By personal meetings over actual problems GPs and specialists can dispel fantasies about each other. The GP may better see the specialist's difficulties as a "rationer" of scarce services, while the specialist sees the scale of the burdens which the GP and the family are daily carrying; and each knows that the other knows. Such regular contact, and awareness of each other's style of working, are part of the case for sectorisation of services, bringing specialists into relation with a fixed and relatively small group of primary care colleagues.

Not all problems of the demented are surmountable; but that makes all the more necessary a realistic assessment of what is feasible, and acknowledgement of what is not. Willingness to work sensibly together is prime among our obligations to the demented and their supporters.

REFERENCES

1. J. Wattis, L. Wattis, and T. Arie, Psychogeriatrics: a national survey of a new branch of psychiatry, British Medical Journal 282:1529 (1981).
2. T. Arie and D. J. Jolley, Making Services Work: Organisation and Style of Psychogeriatric Services, in: "The Psychiatry of Late Life", R. Levy and F. Post, eds., Blackwell Scientific Publications, Oxford (1982).
3. L. Hemsi, Psychogeriatric Care in the Community, in: "The Psychiatry of Late Life", R. Levy and F. Post, eds., Blackwell Scientic Publications, Oxford (1982).
4. N.H.S. Health Advisory Service, "The Rising Tide", H.A.S., Sutton, Surrey (1982).
5. A. Norman, "Mental Illness in Old Age", Centre for Policy on Ageing, London (1982).
6. W.H.O., "Psychogeriatric Care in the Community": Public Health in Europe No.10, World Health Organization, Copenhagen (1979).
7. J. Williamson, Screening, Surveillance and Case-Finding, in: "Health Care of the Elderly", T. Arie, ed., Croom Helm, London and Johns Hopkins Press, Baltimore (1981).
8. A. Bowling and A. Cartwright, "Life After a Death", Tavistock Publications, London (1982).
9. T. Arie, Teaching Health Care of the Elderly in the Medical Course in Nottingham, Age and Ageing 12:19 Supplem. (1983).
10. N. Mace and P. V. Rabins, "The 36-Hour Day", Johns Hopkins Press, Baltimore (1982).
11. E. Grundy and T. Arie, Falling Rate of Provision of Residential Care for the Elderly, British Medical Journal 284:799 (1982).
12. Dept. of Health and Social Security, "Health Care and its Costs: The Development of the National Health Service in England", Her Majesty's Stationery Office, London (1983).
13. Scottish Home and Health Department and Scottish Education Department, "Changing Patterns of Care": Report on Services for the Elderly in Scotland, Her Majesty's Stationery Office, Edinburgh (1980).
14. K. Bergmann, E. M. Foster, A. W. Justice and V. Matthews, Management of the Demented Elderly Patient in the Community, British Journal of Psychiatry 132:441 (1978).

AFFECTIVE DISORDERS IN LATE LIFE: PHARMACOTHERAPY

Lissy F. Jarvik

Professor, Department of Psychiatry and
Biobehavioral Sciences,
University of California, Los Angeles
and
Chief, Psychogeriatric Unit
West Los Angeles Veterans Administration
Medical Center, Brentwood Division

THIS WORK WAS SUPPORTED IN PART BY NATIONAL INSTITUTE OF MENTAL
HEALTH RESEARCH GRANT MH-31357 AND VETERANS ADMINISTRATION MEDICAL
RESEARCH FUNDS. THE OPINIONS EXPRESSED ARE NOT THOSE OF THE
VETERANS ADMINISTRATION. THE DRUGS FOR THIS STUDY WERE SUPPLIED
BY PENNWALT CORPORATION.

The data were gathered by:

Psychiatrists
Ching Piao Chien
Robert Gerner
Richard Rosen

Research Assistant
Jeanne Aldrich

Psychologist
Joanne Steuer

Research Nurse
Shirley Linde

Data Management
Jim Mintz

Clearly, in the time available today I cannot do justice to
all of the currently fashionable treatments of depression in old
age, and certainly not the treatment of mania as well. Generally,
these treatments are similar to the treatments we favor for young
adults. Since I cannot do justice to all, I shall look at just one,
our own double-bind placebo-controlled study of doxepin and
imipramine.

Some of you may be familiar with preliminary reports of this 36-week study of outpatients who met the criteria for major depressive disorder, unipolar type (Jarvik et. al., 1982).

We analyzed data from 32 patients, ten each on doxepin and placebo, and twelve on imipramine. They ranged in age from 55 to 81 years, with a mean age of 67 years in each group.

On entrance into the study, the severity of depression, measured by Hamilton Depression Ratings (Hamilton, 1960), did not differ significantly for the three groups, but, at end point, had decreased substantially for both the doxepin and the imipramine groups (about 50%), not the placebo group (19%). The drug-placebo difference was statistically significant (p<0.03) despite the small number of patients involved. There was not much difference between the two active drugs, and no support for the contention that doxepin was less effective, dose for dose, than imipramine.

We asked two further questions:

(1) How soon can we tell whether a patient will go into remission? The textbooks say three weeks or so, but everything goes more slowly in old age, so be patient and keep increasing the dose for four, five, six weeks or more. That was not true in our study. In retrospect, we could have identified the ultimate remitters within the first week or two, even though the dose at that time was generally only 50 mg per day.

(2) What about side effects? Did remitters have fewer side effects than non-responders? Let us examine the major undesirable side effect in the elderly -- change in blood pressure: There was no significant change in either systolic or diastolic supine blood pressure with either doxepin or imipramine. Yet there was a definite increase in orthostatic hypotension on imipramine, but not on doxepin. On the average, orthostatic hypotension increased with increasing dose, as illustrated by patient #72 (Figure 1). However, there was wide individual variability as exemplified by another patient (#10) who remained on 50 mg a day throughout the study (Figure 2). Thus, we cannot expect clinical improvement in orthostatic hypotension by simply decreasing the dose.

Should we conclude, then, that we should exclude patients who show significant orthostatic hypotension before treatment? After all, they are the ones most likely to have trouble and, therefore, least likely to respond to the drug treatment. Not so. The patients with the larger pre-treatment orthostatic blood pressure drop seem to be the ones who go into remission (Jarvik et. al., in press).

390

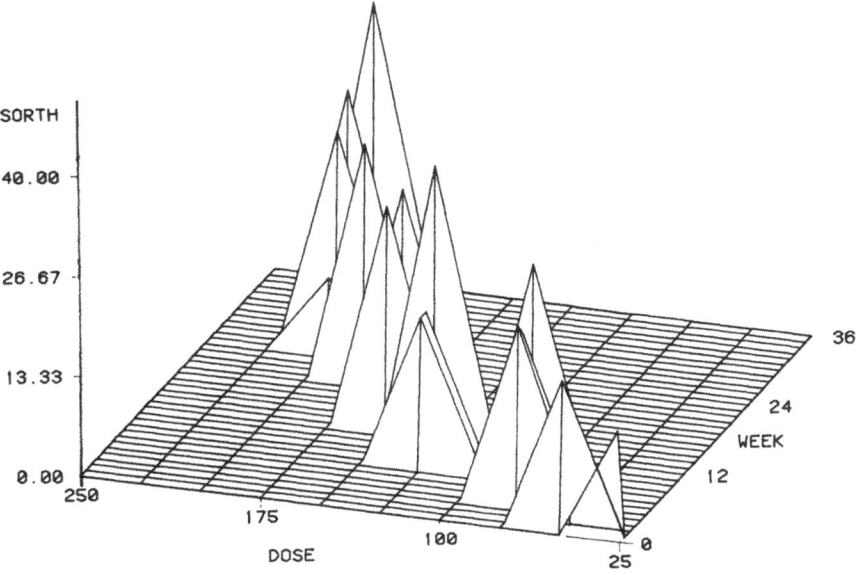

Figure 1

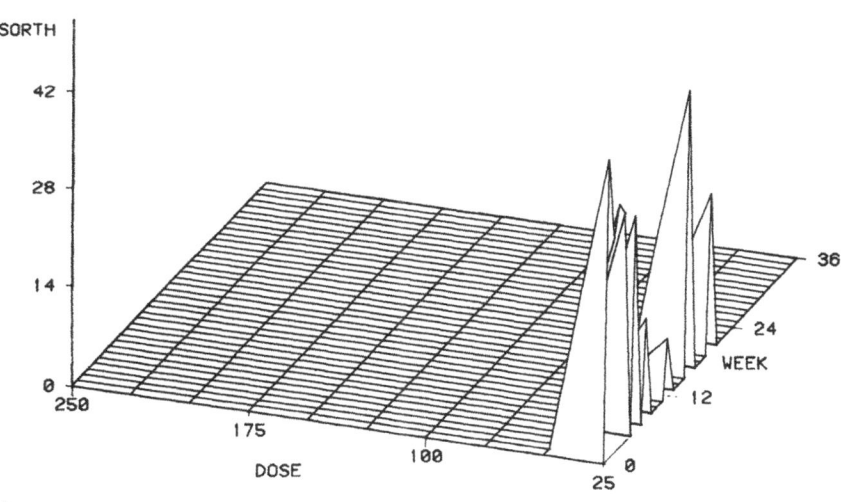

Figure 2

Thus, in the active drug groups, 91% of the patients with pre-treatment systolic orthostatic hypotension of 12 mm Hg or more improved or went into remission. Actually, 87% went into remission (Hamilton Depression score of 6 or less). By contrast, none of the patients with pre-treatment systolic orthostatic blood pressure drop of 10 mm Hg or less went into remission. In the placebo group, orthostatic hypotension did not distinguish remitters from non-responders.

Even though we attempted to include in our study only patients who were drug- and disease-free -- except for their depression -- we were not entirely successful in doing so. We wondered what would happen if we eliminated the patients with a history of cardiovascular disease -- nearly half the sample. Would we eliminate the predictive power of pre-treatment systolic orthostatic hypotension by cutting our data set nearly in half? No, indeed. If anything, we strengthened it. Now none were misclassified.

It was, of course, totally unexpected that those with high orthostatic drop would be the good responders to imipramine, a drug which produced orthostatic hypotension as a major undesirable side effect -- as well as to doxepin which did not differ from placebo in terms of producing orthostatic hypotension.

Of course, our result needs to be confirmed. If it is confirmed, we face the paradox that pre-treatment systolic orthostatic hypotension may become an indication rather than a contraindication to treatment with tricyclic antidepressants. If confirmed, we also need to identify the mechanism of action. At the moment, we have only speculation on that, no data. I do want to remind you, however, that our findings apply only to outpatients with a DSM-III diagnosis of major depressive disorder, who are between 55 and 80 years of age, not psychotic, not suicidal, not bipolar, and in relatively good physical health without major cardiovascular or other disease. They also apply only to the two tricyclic antidepressants which we studied -- doxepin and imipramine.

While we are awaiting confirmation and explanation of our findings, let me conclude this tale of one research project by reminding you that it merely confirms an observation made years ago by Voltaire:

"Doctors are men who prescribe medicines of which they
know little, to cure diseases of which they know less,
in human beings of whom they know nothing."

REFERENCES

Hamilton, M.: A Rating Scale for Depression. J. Neurol. Neuro-surg. Psychiatry, 23:56, 1960.

Jarvik, L. F., Mintz, J., Steuer, J., and Gerner, R.: Treating Geriatric Depression: A 26-Week Interim Analysis. Journal of the American Geriatrics Society, 30:713-717, 1982.

Jarvik, L. F., Read, S. L., Mintz, J., and Neshkes, R. E.: Pre-treatment Orthostatic Hypotension in Geriatric Depression: Predictor of Response to Imipramine and Doxepin. Journal of Clinical Psychopharmacology, in press.

PHARMACOTHERAPY OF THE ORGANIC BRAIN SYNDROME IN LATE LIFE

Thomas A. Ban and Theodore Hovaguimian

Vanderbilt University, Nashville, Tennessee, USA
Geriatric Institutions, University of Geneva, Switzerland
Division of Mental Health, World Health Organization
1211 Geneva 27-Switzerland

INTRODUCTION

Prerequisite for treatment of the two major dementias in the aged, i.e. Senile Dementia of Alzheimer Type (SDAT) and Multiinfarct Dementia (MID) is proper diagnosis.

The first attempt to systematize operational criteria for differential diagnosis of the 2 disorders was that of Mayer-Gross, Slater and Roth. Their findings were further substantiated by Roth and Myers (1975) who were able to separate the multi-infarct group by the following feature: abrupt onset, step-wise deterioration, fluctuating course, history of strokes, presence of significant hypertension and focal neurological signs.

On the basis of these features, Hachinsky et al. (1975) developed a rating scale for the differentiation of SDAT and MID patients. By correlating cerebral blood-flow and the "ischemic score" of the scale they revealed that patients with MID are distinctly different from patients with SDAT by having considerable more decreased blood-flow and oxigen consumption than other demented patients.

In recent years, our capability for differential diagnosis was considerably improved by the introduction of non-invasive technques for the measurement of regional cerebral blood-flow, computerized tomography and positron emission tomography (Royal College Committee on Geriatrics 1981).

In the treatment of MID cerebro-vaso-dilatators are frequently prescribed. Whether or not they can overcome the chronic state of hypoxia produced by the reduced cerebral flow has remained an open question. Sathananthan and Gershon (1975) argue that factors which cause vasodilation, such as autoregulation, lactosis and decrease in pH in and around the ischemic areas have already exerted their maximal vasodilating effect by the time of cerebro-vasodilators administration. Because of the differences in perfusion pressure, the healthy parts of the brain receive extra blood by the dilation of the healthyvessels (intra-cerebral steal syndrome) and may even shunt blood away from the ischemic areas under the influence of vaso-dilator drugs. But, even if the ischemic areas would obtain increased blood-flow, the increase in the blood supply might be in excess (luxury perfusion syndrome) of the metabolic demand. Furthermore, since the capillary network of the cerebral cortex develops an age-related increase in the mean capillary diameter and capillary length (per unit per brain volume), together with the increase in the mean capillary distance, Meyer-Ruge et al. 1978 have raised the possibility that the decrease in the cerebral blood-flow in the elderly is an attempt of adaptation to the changed autonomic parameters. Irrespec-tive of these considerations, there have been several cerebral vaso-dilators, such as papaverine, Cyclandalate, and Isoxsuprine used clinically during the past decade in patients with MID (Ban 1978). However, dihydroergotoxine has remained the most extensively employed among the various therapeutic agents.

Besides dihydroergotoxine, Vincamine has also been used and many other drugs have been tried (Witzmann and Blechacz 1977). Hall and Harcup (1969) observed some improvements with lypotrophic enzymes, a mixture of Citrogenase, aminoacidoxydase and tyrosinase.

Other attempts to treat the disorder included the administration of nicotin acid, beta-glucoronidase, cytochrome C and catalase (Altschul 1959; Hunter 1960; Kayatan 1960).

However, none of these various approaches to treatment have been verified by properly conducted clinical experiments.

SENILE DEMENTIA OF THE ALZHEIMER TYPE

During the past 20 years, numerous speculations, theories and hypotheses regarding the aetiology and nature of SDAT have been advanced and corresponding treatment modalities have been tried with limited success.

Collagene disease

In the late 1960's Chynoweth and Foley (1969) assumed that the Alzheimer disease belongs to the group of collagene diseases with autoimmune factors playing a role in its aetiology. With this assumption, they employed steroid hormones in the treatment of three presenile Alzheimer patients. As a result, they found that after intramuscular hydrocortisone administration all three patients improved. So far, their results have not been further substantiated in properly conducted clinical research.

Aluminium excess

While the notion that SDAT belongs to the collagene diseases has not been further pursued, in the early 1970's Crapper, Krishman and Dalton (1973) have made the observation that aluminium may be toxic to neurones and induces the formation of neurofibrillary tangles similar but not identical to those found in the brains of patients suffering from Alzheimer disease. On the basis of this observation, they raised the possible role of Aluminium in Alzheimer's dementia. nevertheless, while Crapper Krischman and Dalton (1973) found that brains of patients with Alzheimer's disease contain higher concentration of Aluminium than the brains of other psycho-geriatric patients, McDermott et al. (1977) maintain that Aluminium is not specific to Alzheimer's disease but rather increasing with age. If the aluminium hypothesis of SDAT would be substantiated by further evidence, chelating agents such as disodium edatate calcium with a similar binding constant to aluminium should be considered for treatment (Cole 1977). Whether this substance has a therapeutic effect and/or prophylactic action in SDAT remains to be seen.

Zinc deficiency

An alternative hypothesis suggests that, instead of an excess of aluminium, deficiency of Zinc might be the primum movens in Alzheimer's disease. Thus, Constantinidis and Tissot (1982) speculate that deficiency of Zinc might result in an alteration of the neuro-transmitter glutamate which in turn leads to gliosis and argyrophilic lesions. Nevertheless, to date no definite change in glutamate metabolism has been revealed (Pepeu 1982) and oral administration of zinc sulfate in Alzheimer's disease patients did not produce any clinical improvement.

Folate deficiency

While no definite change in glutamate and GABA metabolism in aging could be revealed (Pepeu 1982), a reduction in acetylcholine (Ach), dopamine (DA) and norepinephrine (NE) formation (Pradham 1980) with or without decreased 5-hydroxytryptamine (5 HT) levels (McGeer 1978) has been repeatedly confirmed in patients with SDAT. Since the rate limiting step in the synthesis of catecholamine (DA, NE) and endolamines (5 HT) is hydroxylation of the amino acids and since fola folate is the coenzyme of this process, the possibility has been raised that SDAT might be related to deficiencies in folic acid and vitamines B12 (Carney 1967; Hurdle and Williams 1966; Shulman 1967). Nevertheless in at least one clinical trial, folate administration has remained entirely ineffective (Shaw et al. 1971).

Increased MAO activity

Since folate deficiency could not explain the reduced activity in monoaminergic systems other possibilities were considered. A promising lead was created by the recognition of decreased activities of monoamine synthetizing enzymes, such as choline acetyl transferase, dopa decarboxylase and tyrosine hydroxylase, associated with increased activities of catabolizing enzymes, such as monoaminoxydase (MAO) and catechol-O-methyl-transferase (COMT) (Meyer et al. 1977; Pradhaus 1980; Terry and Davies 1980). Furthermore, it was also revealed that the increased MAO activity was restricted to the enzyme MAO-B (with beta-phenyl-ethylamine as substrate and was wirtually absent for the enzyme MAO-A (with 5 HT as substrate) (Adolfsson et al. 1978; Gottfries et al. 1979). Corresponding with these findings is the result of a clinical study in which the administration of 5-hydroxy-tryptophan (5 HTP) to patients with SDAT and MID has remained without therapeutic effects (Meyer et al. 1977).

Results of clinical trials with dihydroxyphenylalanine (1-DOPA) in patients with SDAT have yielded contradictory results (Kristensen, Olsen and Theilgaard 1977; Lewis, Ballinger and Presly 1978).

In view of the increased MAO activity in these patients, a rational approach to treatment would be a combination of 1-DOPA and a type B MAO inhibitor. No report on the therapeutic effect of such combination is available to date.

Reduced choline acetyl transferase

Among the various alteration in SDAT, most prevalent are the greatly reduced choline acetyl transferase concentrations in the neocortex and the selective loss of cholinergic neurones in the temporal lobes.

Considering the finding of reduced choline acetyl transferase, the enzyme responsible for the formation of acetyl choline, and that acetyl choline cannot be given because it is rapidly broken down and produces serious adverse effects, attempts were made to reduce the degradation of ACh by the administration of anticholinesterases, such as physostigmine. As a result, in one study, a dose dependent improvement has been reported following treatment with physostigmine in in patients with SDAT (Glen et al. 1979). In another study carried out in a smaller population significant improvement in picture recognition has been described using either physostigmine or the muscarine agonist of choline (Roth 1983). In addition to the results of these studies, there is also a report on a 42 year old patient with Alzheimer's disease; in this patient physostigmine significantly reduced the number of intention errors in the free recall and the cued-recall word lists, while it did not increase the amount of information recalled (Smith and Swash 1980).

Results of ACh precursor administration are considerably less rewarding. The clinical trials with choline chloride and choline bitartrate yielded conflicting findings (Drachman and Sahakian 1979); Smith et al. 1978). One possible reason for this is that there are some indications that choline has little role in the regulation of transmitter synthesis in the cerebral cortex. But even if it would have a role, there is substantial evidence to believe that there is too little available choline acetyl transferase to utilize choline for the synthesis of Ach in SDAT patients (Roth 1982). Another problem related to choline administration are side-effects, such as gastro-intestinal discomfort, exacerbation of urinary incontinence. Considering all these, it has been suggested that in further experiments lecithin, the precursor of choline or deanol, a substance which increases ACh concentrations should be used (College Committee on Geriatrics, 1981). In view of the insufficient availability of choline choline acetyl transferase for the synthesis of ACh, however, Peters and Levin (1979) suggest that ACh precursor administration should be combined with the administration of the anticholinesterase, physostigmine.

Impaired glucose oxydation

An additional dimension related to ACh synthesis was brought to attention by Bowen et al. 1979 who found selective reduction of all glycolytic enzymes involved in hexose-mucophosphate metabolism in SDAT patients. Since there is a reduction in ACh synthesis when glucose oxydation and/or utilization is impaired, the possibility of treatment with "cerebral activators", substances which improve cerebral glucose utilization has been raised. Included among these substances are meclofenoxate, naftidrofyril and pyritinol (Ban 1980). Although evidence for their usefulness in the treatment of SDAT is still lacking.

CONCLUSIONS

Pharmacological treatments to chronic brain syndromes in the aged have been reviewed with special reference to SDAT.

Although the various treatment modalities employed have yielded limited success, they contributed to the understanding of some of the pathomechanisms involved in SDAT.

ACKNOWLEDGEMENT

The authors are grateful to Miss B. Naulleau, Nazareth College, Rochester N.Y., for her help in the bibliographical research.

REFERENCES

Adolfsson, R., et al., 1978, Reduced levels of catecholamines in the brain and increased activity of monoamine oxidase platelets in Alzheimer's disease: Therapeutic implications, in "Aging, Vol. 7," R. Katzman, R.D. Terry, and K.L. Bick, eds., Raven Press, New York.

Altschul, R., 1959, Einfluss von Cytochrom C und Hämatoporphyrin auf Serumcholesterin, Z. Kreislaufforsch, 48:844-848

Ban, T.A., 1980, Psychopharmacology for the aged," S. Karger, Basel, München, Paris, London, New York, Sydney.

Ban, T.A., 1978, The treatment of depressed geriatric patients, Am. J. Psychother., 32:93-104.

Bowen, D.M., et al., 1979, Accelerated aging or selective neuronal loss as an important cause of dementia, Lancet, i:11-14.

Carney, M.W.P., 1967, Serum folate values in 423 psychiatric patients, Br. Med. J., 4:512-516.

Chynoweth, R., and Foley, J., 1969, Pre-senile dementia responding to steroid therapy, Br. J. Psychiat., 115:703-708.

Cole, J.O., 1977, Psychopharmacology update. Psychopharmacology and senile dementia, McLean Hosp., 2:210-221.

Constantinidis, J., and Tissot, R., 1982, Degenerative encephalopathies in old age: neurotransmitters and zinc metabolism, in "Aging, Vol.18," R.D. Terry, C.L. Bolis and G. Toffano, eds., Raven Press, New York.

Crapper, D.R., Kirshon, S.S., and Dalton, A.J., 1973, Brain aluminum distribution in Alzheimer's disease and experimental neurofibrillary degeneration, Science, 180:511-513.

Drachman, D.A., and Sahakian, B.J., 1979, Effects of cholinergic agents on human learning and memory, in "Nutrition and the brain, Vol.5," A. Barbeau, J.H. Growdon, and R.J. Wurtman, eds., Raven Press, New York.

Glen, A.I.M., and Whalley, L.J., 1979, Alzheimer's disease, in "Early recognition of potentially reversible deficits," Churchill Livingstone, Edinburgh.

Gottfries, C.G., et al., 1979, Monomines and their metabolites and monoamine oxidase activity related to age and to some dementia disorders, in "Drugs and the elderly. Perspectives in geriatric clinical pharmacology. Proceedings of a symposium held in Ninewells hospital, U. of Dundee, 13-14 September 1977," J. Crooks and I.H. Stevenson, eds., Macmillan, London.

Hachinsky, V.C., et al., 1975, Cerebral blood flow in dementia, Arch. Neurol., 32:632.

Hall, M.R.P. and Harcup, M., 1969, A trial of lipotropic enzymes in atheromatous (arteriosclerotic) dementia, Angiology,205:287-300.

Hunter, J.D., 1960, Nicotinic acid therapy in patients with coronary disease, N.Z. Med. J.,59:280-285.

Hurdle, A.D.F. and Williams, T.C.P., 1966, Folic acid deficiency in elderly patients admitted to hospital, Br. Med. J., ii:202-205.

Kayatan, S., 1960, Arteriosclerosis and β-glucuronidase, Lancet, ii:667-668.

Kristensen, V., Olsen, M., and Theilgaard, A., 1977, Levodopa treatment of pre-senile dementia, Acta Psychiat. Scand.,55:41-51.

Lewis, C., Ballinger, B.R. and Presly, A., 1978, Trial of levodopa in senile dementia, Br. Med. J., 1:550.

Mayer-Gross, W., Slater, E. and Roth, M., 1954, "Clinical psychiatry," London and Baltimore.

McDermott, J.R., et al., 1977, Aluminum in Alzheimer's disease, Lancet,2:710-711.

Mcgeer, E., 1978, Aging and neurotransmitter in the human brain, in "Aging, Vol. 7," R. Katzman, R.D. Terry and K.L. Bick, eds., Raven Press, New York.

Meyer, J.S., et al., 1977, Neurotransmitter precursor aminoacids in the treatment of multi-infarct dementia and Alzheimer's disease, J. Am. Geriatric Soc., 25:289-298.

Meyer-Ruge, W., et al., 1978, Alteration of morpholological and neurochemical parameters of the brain due to normal aging, in "Senile dementia: biomedical approach," K. Nandy, ed., Elsevier/North-Holland, New York, Amsterdam

Pepeu, G., 1982, Pharmacological control of neuronal aging, in "Aging, Vol. 18," R.D. Terry, C.L. Bolis and G. Toffano, eds., Raven Press, New York.

Peters, B.H. and Levin, H.S., 1979, Effects of physostigmine and lecithin on memory in Alzheimer disease, Ann. Neurol.,6:219-221.

Pradham, S.N., 1980, Central neurotransmitters and aging, Life Science, 26:1643-1656.

Roth, M., 1983, Some strategies for tackling the problems of senile dementia and related disorders within the next decade, Unedited working paper for the W.H.O. scientific group on senile dementia, Paris.

Roth, M., 1982, Dementia in relation to aging in the central nervous system, in "Aging, Vol. 18," R.D. Terry, C.L. Bolis and G. Toffano, eds., Raven Press, New York.

Roth, M. and Myers, D.H., 1975, The diagnosis of dementia, Br. J. Psychiat., 125: (spec. 9) 87-99.

Royal College Committee on geriatrics, 1981, Organic mental impairment in the elderly: implications for research, education and the provision of services, J. Roy. Col. Phys. London, 15: No. 3.

Sathananthan, G.L. and Gershon, S., 1975, Cerebral vasodilators. A review, in "Aging, Vol. 2," Gershon and Ranskin, eds., Raven Press, New York.

Shaw, D.M., et al., 1971, Folate and amine metabolites in senile dementia: a combined trial and biochemical study, Psychol. Med., 1:166-171.

Shulman, R., 1967, A survey of vitamin B_{12} deficiency in an elderly psychiatric population, Br. J. Psychiatry, 113:241-251.

Smith, C.B. and Swash, M., 1980, Effects of cholinergic drugs on memory in Alzheimer's disease, in "Aging, Vol. 13," L. Amaducci, A.N. Davison and P. Antuono, eds., Raven Press, New York.

Smith, C.M., et al., 1978, Lancet, 2:318.

Terry, R.D. and Davies, P., 1980, Dementia of the Alzheimer type, Annu. Rev. Neurosci.,3:77-95.

Witzman, H.K. and Blechacz, W., 1977, On the role of vincamine in the therapy of cerebrovascular diseases and impairment of cerebral function, Arzneimittel-Forsch, 27:1238-1247.

METABOLIC/CIRCULATORY ASPECTS OF GERONTOPSYCHOPHARMACOTHERAPY

S. Hoyer

Dept. of Pathochemistry and General Neurochemistry,
University of Heidelberg, D-6900 Heidelberg / F.R.G.

This paper is primarily concerned with the effects of drugs which are said to influence blood flow and oxidative metabolism of the brain (so-called nootropic drugs) in primary dementias.

Before these drug effects are discussed in more detail, some general aspects of dementia should be mentioned.

The most common cerebral illness in middle and old age is dementia. This condition may be defined as a global deterioration of higher mental functions in their intellectual, cognitive and emotional aspects[1]. Dementia may lead both to reversible and to irreversible mental deficits. The prevalence of severe dementia in people aged 65 years and older had been estimated at about 4 % in the 65 year old group increasing to more than 25 % in people who are 85 years and older. Mild to moderate forms of dementia occur in about 11 % in people 65 years and older[2,3].

Dementia may be caused either by degenerative neuronal variations in brain tissue or by disturbances in microcirculation. Both abnormalities produce primary dementia, i.e. autochthonous brain diseases. Dementias due to extracerebral diseases or due to brain diseases which cannot be accounted for by degenerative or vascular brain processes should be strictly distinguished in patho-physiological and clinical terms. They should be designated as secondary dementias.

Dementia of Alzheimer type (DAT) predominated with 60 to 70 %. Microcirculation disturbances cause dementia of vascular type (DVT) (synonym: multiinfarct dementia, MID) in 20 to 30 %, while both degenerative and microcirculation variations are found in 15 to

20 %. Nosologically, "simple" senile dementia, and both Alzheimer's senile and presenile dementia may be regarded as variations of the same degenerative brain disease[4,5]. Morphologically, DAT and DVT differ significantly. DAT is characterized by an atrophy which is most marked in the anterior parts of the middle and superior temporal gyri and the hippocampus along with neuritic plaques and neurofibrillary tangles which appear as paired helical filaments. The more plaques and tangles the more severe the dementia. The presynaptic cholinergic system in the hippocampus is particularly affected.

In DVT, circumscribed cell loss with gliosis in cerebral grey and white matter as expression of microcirculation disturbances are found. The multiple small infarcts scattered over brain cortex and white matter primarily produce dementia symptoms. If they merge into larger ones, they may be responsible for secondary neurological deficits such as TIA or PRIND in the history along with the respective psychiatric symptoms.

In the beginning of the diseases, these two main types of primary dementias are found to be associated with obviously characteristic changes in oxidative brain metabolism.

In DAT, cerebral blood flow (CBF) and the cerebral metabolic rate of oxygen (CMR-oxygen) were found not to be decreased but rather to be slightly increased. However, CMR-glucose was markedly reduced so that an imbalance between oxygen and glucose is present. Furthermore, the normally existing association between CBF and the respective metabolic rates of substrates is abolished: a dissociation can be demonstrated between CBF and CMR-oxygen on the one hand and CMR-glucose on the other[6,7].

It should be recalled that the brain utilizes only glucose to gain energy under normal conditions. Glucose metabolism in the brain is found to be closely related with acetylcholine formation via pyruvate which derives from glucose and which is known as a precursor of acetyl-CoA. Acetyl-CoA is a substrate for acetylcholine formation[8,9].

Acetylcholine synthesis was found to be reduced by about 60 % in DAT along with a decreased activity of choline acetyltransferase (CAT) which decreased most as the number of neuritic plaques and neurofibrillary tangles rose[10,11,12]. Although the relationship between disturbed glucose metabolism and reduced acetylcholine synthesis has not been substantiated in patients suffering from DAT, one may tentatively assume a close relationship between glucose metabolism and acetylcholine formation analogous to that in normal tissue, but on a reduced and thus abnormal level. This hypothesis may be supported by some other findings. In brain cortex of DAT patients, a profound decrease up to 10 % of normal controls was found in phosphofructokinase activity along with decreased activities of other enzymes working in glycolysis[13,14]. It might thus be tentatively assumed that the decrease in the activity of the glycolytic flux-controlling enzyme phosphofructokinase would lead to a decrease in glycolytic flux, i.e. to a reduced glucose consumption and thus reduced pyruvate formation in the brain. The decrease in acetylcholine synthesis in the brains of DAT patients might therefore be related to the reduced cerebral glucose consumption as was measured in many patients suffering from DAT. The increased cerebral release of lactate, i.e. the enhanced lactate production in the brain along with normal or reduced CMR-glucose occasionally found in DAT patients, may be assumed to be related to a disturbance in the pyruvate dehydrogenase complex which also may lead to a diminished acetylcholine formation[15].

It thus becomes obvious that at least in the beginning of DAT, no disturbance in cerebral circulation is present. The predominant biological abnormality is found in cerebral glucose metabolism including the associated acetylcholine formation and pyruvate oxidation, i.e. glycolysis and pyruvate oxidation as measured in a reduced CMR-glucose are primarily involved.

As a consequence for therapy in DAT, it would appear meaningless to medicate the undisturbed cerebral circulation as was propagated for many years. Therapy should be directed towards improving the abnormal glucose metabolism and the reduced acetylcholine synthesis or acetylcholine concentration, respectively.

Several studies were performed using choline or lecithin as precursors of acetylcholine synthesis to enhance acetylcholine synthesis. Lecithin or choline were administered in high dosages, in some cases over weeks or months. These procedures failed to improve the mental deficit of DAT or EEG changes of this dementia type[16,17,18]. Another approach was to inhibit the catabolism of acetylcholine by means of physostigmine. An improvement of memory could be demonstrated. However, the disadvantage of the administration of this acetylcholinesterase inhibitor is evident. The effect is only short-lasting so that it would be necessary to administer the drug repeatedly each day to maintain the mental improvement. The therapeutic range is exceedingly narrow[19,20]. It may thus be assumed that this mode of treatment will not be appropriate in medical practice. The situation may be similar for arecoline, a cholinergic agonist of short-lasting efficacy. On the other hand, an improvement of the predominantly reduced CMR-glucose and of the deranged cognitive capacities could be found in DAT after a three to four week treatment with either pyrithioxine or extractum sanguinum deproteinatum siccum (dried deproteinated blood)[21,22]. However, this therapy was not successful at all or only slightly successful in chronic DAT and in DVT. The underlying biological mechanism of action of these two drugs is as yet obscure and has to be elucidated.

As mentioned above, the underlying process of the formation of multiinfarcts may be related to disturbances in cerebral microcirculation. If this holds true, it might be expected that changes characteristic for ischemic/anoxia would dominate the metabolic derangement. The disturbed balance between normal cerebral oxygen consumption and abnormally increased cerebral glucose uptake indeed resembles metabolic changes which occur in acute anoxic damage, e.g. after hypoxic hypoxia[6,7,23]. In contrast to hypoxia, no augmentation of cerebral blood flow and CMR-lactate could be observed in DVT. In this dementia type, no distinct disturbance in any neurotransmitter system could be found.

The metabolic fate of the "surplus" of glucose taken up by the brain is as yet unknown. It may be speculated that this amount of glucose not oxidized by the brain may be falsely metabolized and/or abnormally stored in brain cells, i.e. in astrocytes near the vessels as glucose polymers comparable to the "glycogen" which was found after acute experimental ischemia or asphyxia[24,25]. If a similar storage of glucose polymers in brain cells occurs during the initial phase of DVT, this may lead to a disturbance of the glucose transport into the brain and to an impairment of the metabolic pathway of glucose in the brain. A decrease in CMR-glucose would have to be expected as a consequence in the further course of DVT. Such a fall in CMR-glucose along with reduced CBF and CMR-oxygen has indeed been measured in the course of DVT. As far as coupling between CBF, CMR-oxygen and CMR-glucose in DVT is concerned, it is maintained between CBF and CMR-oxygen also in this dementia type. However, a dissociation seems to be present between CBF and CMR-goxygen on the one hand and CMR-glucose on the other but in the opposite direction as has been mentioned for DAT[6,7].

As a consequence, therapy should be directed against the presumably ischemic/anoxic-induced metabolic changes. Such disturbances can be well defined pathophysiologically and in other fields by the results of experimental neurosciences. On the other hand, however, no direct information on drugs improving metabolism in ischemic/anoxic brain tissue lesions in patients are available. This also holds true for drugs which were found to improve decreased CBF and CMR-oxygen in DVT along with the psychiatric symptomatology. We studied the effects of centrophenoxin, pentifyllin and piracetam in DVT patients and found efficacy of these drugs mentioned after a three to four week treatment[21]. No effects could be observed in chronic states of DVT or in DAT.

That all drugs mentioned fail in chronic dementia states becomes clear when regarding the degree of derangement in blood flow and metabolism. Blood flow and oxidative metabolism of the brain had decreased progressively to approach a low functional level which may correspond to the reduced demands of the diseased brain. At this stage of advanced dementia, DAT and DVT are hardly distinguishable within clinical and in pathophysiological terms[6,7,26].

Increasing interest is attracted by another group of aged patients suffering from depression with late onset in old age. This affective disorder would seem to be different from monophasic or biphasic endogenous depression. Depression in old age often presents features which strongly suggest dementia for clinical reasons. However, dementia is mimicked and therefore this psychiatric disorder is often designated as pseudodementia[27]. In depression in old age, average CBF, CMR-oxygen and CMR-glucose were found to be reduced more or less pronounced even at the onset of the disease or during its exacerbation when in DAT and DVT CBF and CMR-oxygen show no deviations from normal. It is as yet completely unclear whether it is rational to treat this type of affective disorder exclusively with antidepressive agents which have more or less severe anticholinergic side effects. These drugs would be able to reduce acetylcholine production, which is strongly associated with DAT as was mentioned above. It still remains open to what degree thymoleptic or neuroleptic drugs may deteriorate or even initiate dementia iatrogenically.

It thus becomes clear that in DAT and DVT, the treatment of various metabolic derangements has high priority as against the treatment of circulation disorders. The therapeutic mechanisms of drug activity on either the disturbed glucose and acetylcholine metabolism in DAT or on the ischemic/anoxic lesions in DVT have to be elucidated in the near future to meet one of the most urgent demands in geriatric medicine: to reduce morbidity significantly and to improve the fate of dementia patients.

REFERENCES

1   W. Mayer-Gross, E. Slater and M. Roth, Clinical psychiatry, 3rd ed. Bailliere, Tindall and Carssell, London (1969)

2   K. Oesterreich and O. Wagner, Psychopathologie des Alterns und der Voralterung. - Historische Entwicklung der Begriffbildung, Z. Geront 15, 314 (1982)

3   R.D. Terry, Dementia. A brief and selective review, Arch.Neurol. 33,1 (1976)

4   B.E. Tomlinson, The structural and quantitative aspects of the dementias, in: Biochemistry of dementia, P.J. Roberts, ed., Wiley, Chichester (1980)

5. J. Constantinidis, Is Alzheimer's disease a major form of senile dementia? Clinical, anatomical and genetic data, in: Alzheimer's disease: Senile dementia and related disorders (Aging Vol. 7), R. Katzman, R.D. Terry, K.L. Bick, eds., Raven, New York (1978)

6   S. Hoyer, Blood flow and oxidative metabolism of the brain in different phases of dementia, in: Alzheimer's disease: Senile dementia and related disorders, (Aging Vol. 7), R. Katzman, R.D. Terry, K.L. Bick, eds., Raven, New York (1978)

7   S. Hoyer, Factors influencing cerebral blood flow, CMR-oxygen and CMR-glucose in dementia patients, in: Biochemistry of dementia, P.J. Roberts, ed., Wiley, Chichester (1980)

8   E.K. Perry, R.H. Perry, B.E. Tomlinson, G. Blessed, and P.H. Gibson, Coenzyme A acetylating enzymes in Alzheimer's disease: possible cholinergic "compartment" of pyruvate dehydrogenase, Neurosci.Lett.18, 105 (1980)

9   G.E. Gibson and J.P. Blass, Impaired synthesis of acetylcholine in brain accompanying hypoglycemia and mild hypoxia, J. Neurochem. 27,37 (1976)

10 N.R. Sims, D.M. Bowen, C.C.T. Smith, R.H.A. Flack, A.N. Davison, J.S. Snowden, and D. Neary, Glucose metabolism and acetylcholine synthesis in relation to neuronal activity in Alzheimer's disease, Lancet I, 333 (1980)

11 E.K. Perry, B.E. Tomlinson, G. Blessed, K. Bergmann, P.H. Gibson and R.H. Perry, Correlation of cholinergic abnormalities with senile plaques and mental test scores in senile dementia, Brit. J. Med. 2, 1457 (1978)

12 G.K. Wilcock, M.M. Esiri, D.M. Bowen and C.C.T. Smith Alzheimer's disease. Correlation of cortical choline acetyltransferase activity with the severity of dementia and histological abnormalities, J. Neurol. Sci. 57, 407 (1982)

13 D.M. Bowen, P. White, J.A. Spillane, M.J. Goodhardt, G. Curzon, P. Iwangoff, W. Meier-Ruge, and A.N. Davison, Accelerated ageing or selective neuronal loss as an important cause of dementia? Lancet I, 11 (1979)

14 P. Iwangoff, R. Armbruster, A. Enz, W. Meier-Ruge, and P. Sandoz Glycolytic enzymes from human autoptic brain cortex: normally aged and demented cases, in: Biochemistry of dementia, P.J. Roberts, ed., Wiley, Chichester (1980)

15 G.E. Gibson, R. Jope, and J.P. Blass, Reduced synthesis of acetylcholine accompanying impaired oxidation of pyruvic acid in rat brain minces, Biochem. J. 148, 17 (1975)

16 W.D. Boyd, J. Graham-White, G. Blackwood, I. Glen, and J. McQueen, Clinical effects of choline in Alzheimer senile dementia, Lancet II, 711 (1977)

17 N.L. Canter, M. Hallett, and J.H. Growdon, Lecithin does not affect EEG spectral analysis or P_{300} in Alzheimer disease, Neurology 32, 1260 (1982)

18 S. Gauthier, P. Etienne, D. Dastoor, B. Collier, and R. Ludwick, Lack of effect of a 3-months treatment with lecithin in Alzheimer's disease, Neurology 31, 89 (1981)

19 J.E. Christie, A. Shering, J. Ferguson, and A.I.M. Glen, Physostigmine and arecoline: Effects of intravenous infusions in Alzheimer presenile dementia, Br. J. Psychiat. 138, 46 (1981)

20 K.L. Davis and R.C. Mohs, Enhancement of memory processes in Alheimer's disease with multiple-dose intravenous physostigmine Am.J. Psychiat. 139, 1421 (1982)

21 S. Hoyer, G. Krüger, K. Oesterreich, and F. Weinhardt, Effects of drugs on cerebral blood flow and oxidative metabolism in patients with dementia, in: Cerebral vascular disease, J.S. Meyer, H. Lechner, M. Reivich, eds., Excerpta Medica, Amsterdam Oxford (1977)

22 S. Hoyer, K. Oesterreich, and K.D. Stoll, Effects of pyritinol-HCL on blood flow and oxidative metabolism of the brain in patients with dementia, Arzneim. Forsch./Drug Res. 27, 671 (1977)

23 J. Hamer, K. Wiedemann, H. Berlet, F. Weinhardt, and S. Hoyer, Cerebral glucose and energy metabolism, cerebral oxygen consumption and blood flow in arterial hypoxemia, Acta Neurochir. 44, 151 − (1978)

24 J. Klatzo, E. Fargas-Bergeton, L. Guth, J. Miguel, and Y. Olsson Some morphological and biochemical aspects of abnormal glycogen accumulation in the glia, in: Proceed. VIth Int. Congr. Neuropathol., Masson, Paris (1970)

25 M.J. Mossakoswki, D.M. Long, R.E. Myers, H. Rodriguez de Curet, and J. Klatzo, Early histochemical changes in perinatal asphyia, J. Neuropathol. Exp. Neurol. 27, 500 (1968)

26 W.D. Obrist, Noninvasive studies of cerebral blood flow in aging and dementia, in: Alzheimer's disease: Senile dementia and related disorders (Aging Vol. 7), R. Katzman, R.D. Terry, K.L. Bick, eds., Raven, New York (1978)

27 C.E. Wells, Pseudodementia, Am.J.Psychiat. 136, 895 (1979)

NEUROPHYSIOLOGICAL ASPECTS OF GERONTOPSYCHOPHARMACOTHERAPY

Bernd Saletu

Section of Pharmacopsychiatry
Psychiatric University Clinic
A-1090 Vienna, Austria

INTRODUCTION

Gerontopsychopharmacological agents are drugs with specific effects on the central nervous system (CNS) suggesting that they would be of particular value in the therapy of behavioral and mental disorders frequently occuring in the elderlies. However, as geronto-psychopharmacotherapy includes also the utilization of classical psychotropic drugs such as anxiolytics, antidepressants and neuroleptics (which were originally developed for a younger population), several synonyma have been suggested for these drugs such as nootropics, cerebral protectors, geriatrics, cerebral insufficiency improvers, antihypoxidotics, etc. Although most of these agents have found their way into gerontopsychopharmacotherapy based on some defined pharmacological action (for instance vaso-dilation, actions on brain metabolism, antithrombotic effects), they have one thing common: they act against cerebral hypoxidosis. Under "hypoxydosis" we understand since Strughold (1944) an impairment of the cerebral biological oxidation, which may be due to hypoxic, nutritive, histotoxic, ischemic or metabolic causes. The present paper describes changes in human brain function after the administration of anti-hypoxidotic drugs as measured objectively and quantitatively by computer-assisted spectral-analyzed EEG. The latter in combination with certain statistical procedures (called "quantitative pharmaco-EEG") has been proven to be of great value in the classification of psychotropic drugs and in the determination of their bio-availability at the target organ -- the human brain (Saletu, 1976, 1981). These findings will be viewed in the light of the neurophysiological

411

knowledge about normal and pathological aging.

I. Quantitative EEG changes after geronto-psychopharmacological
    agents ("pharmaco-EEG profiles")

        In the last 6 years we have studied systematically encephalo-
tropic and psychotropic effects of antohypoxidotics/nootropics by
pharmaco-EEG and psychometric methods (Saletu, 1981). In the double-
blind, placebo-controlled studies usually 10 elderly healthy volunteers above the age of 60 were included. They received randomized
(Latin square design) in weekly intervals single oral doses of the
potential antihypoxidotic drugs (a low, a medium and a high dosis),
a clinically widely used reference compound as well as placebo. A
3-minute vigilance-controlled EEG (V-EEG), a 4-minute resting EEG
(R-EEG), and behavioral and clinical measures were recorded at the
hours 0, 1, 2, 4, 6 and 8 after oral or parenteral drug administration. The EEG was analyzed off-line on an Intertechnique Plurimat
S computer system utilizing power spectral density programs. These
analyses in combination with statistical procedures demonstrated
that several antihypoxidotics induced statistically significant and
systematic changes in human brain function as compared with placebo,
characterized by a decrease of delta and theta activity and an increase of alpha and/or beta activity (Fig. 1).

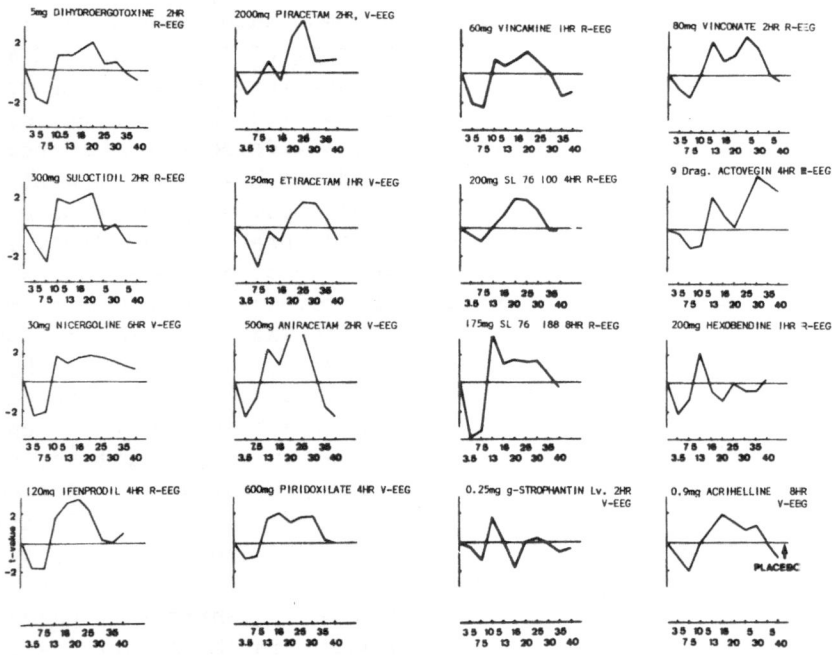

Fig. 1. Pharmaco EEG profiles of several antihypoxidotic/nootropics
    as compared with placebo. A common decrease in delta and theta
    and an increase in alpha and/or beta acitvity can be seen as com-
    pared with placebo, indicating improvement in vigilance.

Among these drugs were representative compounds of different chemical subclasses such as dihydroergotoxine and nicergoline of the ergotalkaloids; vincamine, vinconate, SL 76 100 and SL 76 188 of the vincamine alkaloids and analogues; ifenprodil, tinofedrin and suloctidil of the phenylethanolamines; piracetam, etiracetam and aniracetam of the pyrrolidine derivatives structurally related to GABA; etofylline of the xanthine derivatives; ouabain (g-strophantine) of the cardiac glykosides and acrihelline of the cardiac steroides; CRL 40028 - a benzhydrylsulfinyl-acetonehydroxamid acid and its main metabolite CRL 40476 - a benzhydrylsulfinylacetamid. Further drugs inducing such CNS changes were piridoxilate - a glyoxylic acid - substituted pyridoxine, Actovegin[R] - a standardized deproteinized hemoderivate; hexobendine, the xantinederivate etofylline and its combination Instenon forte[R]. Not only are the aforementioned drugs of different chemical provenance, but they do belong also to different subclasses regarding their mode of action. Metabolically active antihypoxidotics include dihydroergotoxine, nicergoline, vincamine, vinconate, SL 76 100, SL 76 188, piracetam, etiracetam, aniracetam, piridoxilate, Actovegin and suloctidil. Nicergoline and suloctidil have an additional antithrombotic effect, suloctidil is also rheologically active. To the vasoactive compounds one may count nicergoline, vincamine, hexobendine, Instenon forte[R], ifenprodil, suloctidil and etofyllin. Indirect antihypoxidotics are the cardiosteroids-and glycosides as they are providing more blood to the brain, although a direct mode of action is discussed.

II. Clinical/neurophysiological correlations and the concept of vigilance

The above described decrease of slow activity and increase of alpha and/or slow beta activity after antihypoxidotics represent changes in the CNS which are just oppositional to alterations seen in normally and pathologically aging subjects (Fig. 2). It is a rather well documented fact that the human EEG shows progressive slowing of the background activity with advancing age. Utilizing computer assisted quantitative analysis of the EEG this slowing can be objectivated by an increase of relative power in the delta and theta activity as well as by a decrease of the dominant frequency of the alpha activity (Fig. 3). Further age-related changes are a decrease of alpha activity and alpha adjacent beta activity as well as an increase of fast beta activities. Senile EEG features are accentuated in senile dementia-Alzheimer types, whereas the presenile cases show the most marked abnormalities (Obrist, 1980). The increase of delta and theta activity and decrease of alpha activity in normal and pathological aging are due to deficits in the vigilance-regulatory systems.

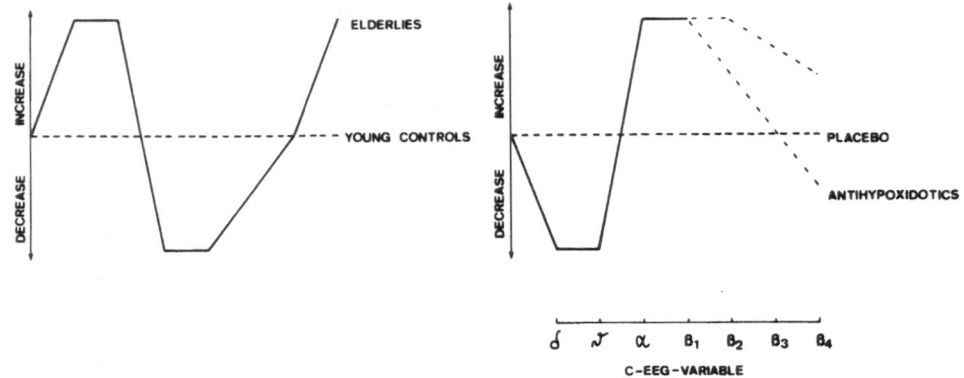

Fig. 2. Schematic quantitative EEG changes in the elderly and after
antihypoxidotic/nootropics. Certain antihypoxidotics induce
EEG alterations characterized by a decrease of delta and
theta and increase of alpha and slow beta activity. These
alterations are oppositional to age-related changes and indicative of vigilance-improving properties of the drugs.

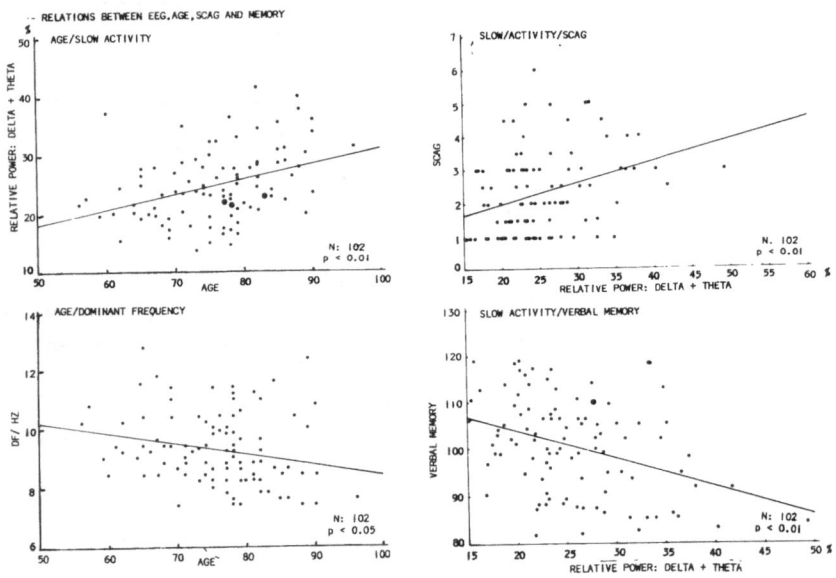

Fig. 3. Regression and correlation between quantitative EEG changes,
age, SCAG score and mnestic functioning (as evaluated by
means of the Grunberger verbal memory test). Slow activity
increases, while dominant frequency decreases with increasing age. The greater the relative power in the delta and
theta band, the higher the SCAG score and the worse the
mnestic performance.

According to Head (1923) vigilance is defined as the dynamic state of the neuronal network determining the availability and grade of organization of man's adaptability. Indeed, a deterioration of adaptive behavior with progressing age has been known by clinicians for quite some time. A correlation between slowing of the EEG and deterioration in clinical symtomatology and mental performance has been shown recently by us utilizing the SCAG score (completed by the psychiatrist) or the Grünberger Verbal Memory Test (completed by the by the patients themselves)(Fig. 3). The greater the relative power in delta and theta activity, the worse the SCAG score reflecting the clinical status of the patient and his mnestic performance (GVG score). Following up on the question whether differences between patients with good and bad memory are due to differences in vigilance at the time of acquisition or at the time of recall, we found that in both instances vigilance was better in the good performers.

III. Improvement of vigilance as therapeutic principle

If antihypoxidotics improve human behavioral measures by improving vigilance, one should be able to demonstrate such relationships after the administration of antihypoxidotic drugs. Indeed, we found for instance after etiracetam a significant regression and correlation between changes in delta activity in the EEG and "wakefulness" as evaluated by means of a semantic differential polarity profile in elderlies: the more increase in "wakefulness", the more decrease in relative power in the delta band. However, since vigilance as defined by Head reflects more than just mere "wakefulness" or "Vigility", one would expect that changes in neurophysiological measures are linked also to changes in other psychometric variables. This could be demonstrated after aniracetam administration, where we found that an increase in dominant frequency, decrease in delta activity and increase in slow beta activity was associated with an improvement in motor activity, complex reaction, reaction time, mood, affectivity, attention variability, tapping and an increase in CFF (Saletu, 1981). This association was not only found in acute studies, where it is most likely very difficult to demonstrate, but also after chronic administration of antihypoxidotics such as nicergoline.

Further evidence for our hypothesis came to the fore from therapeutic trials with antihypoxidotics in man, utilizing the experimentally induced hypoxidosis as well as the organic brain syndrom of the alcoholic patient. Hypoxic hypoxidosis was induced by a fixed gas combination of 11.3% oxygen and 88.7%nitrogen, which was inhaled under normobaric conditions by healthy subjects for a period of 23 minutes (Saletu and Grünberger, 1983). Oxygen tension decreased significantly from 98 mm/Hg to 40 mm/Hg within 14 minutes and remained stable thereafter. EEG spectral analysis EEG showed under hypoxia an increase in delta activity, decrease of alpha and slow beta activity as well as an increase in fast beta activity, which was attenuated significantly by aniracetam. These protective qualities could also be substantiated at the behavioral level as psychometric changes during hypoxia were dose-dependently mitigated. Another clinical approach lies in the utilization of the organic brain syndrom (OBS) of the alcoholic patient (Saletu et al., 1978). Antihypoxidotics such as methyl-thiomethyl-pyridine (EMD 21657) or pyridoxilate, which was predicted by pharmaco EEG and psychometric trials to have antihypoxidotic/nootropic properties, produced during a 6 weeks treatment period a marked improvement in the organic brain syndrom of the patients, which was significantly superior to the changes after placebo and were accompanied by a significant decrease of delta activity in the spectral analyzed EEG. A correlation between changes in the OBS score during piriloxilate therapy and those in delta activity was + 0.686 (p < 0.01).

REFERENCES

Head, H., 1923, The conception of nervous and mental energy. II. Vigilance: a physiological state of the nervous system. Br. J. Psycho., 14:125.

Obrist, W., 1980, Cerebral blood flow and EEG changes associated with aging and dementia, in: "Handbook of Geriatric Psychiatry", E.W. Busse, D.G. Blazer eds., Van Nostrand Reinhold, New York.

Saletu, B., 1976, Psychopharmaka, Gehirntätikeit und Schlaf, Karger, Basel.

Saletu, B., 1981, Application of quantitative EEG in measuring encephalotropic and pharmacodynamic properties of antihypoxidotic/nootropic drugs, in: "Drugs and Methods in C.V.D.", S.I.R. eds., Pergamon Press, France.

Saletu, B., Grünberger, J., 1983, Cerebral hypoxic hypoxidosis: Neurophysiological, psychometric and pharmacotherapeutic aspects, Adv.biol. Psychiat., vol. 13, Karger, Basel.

Saletu, B., Grünberger, J., Saletu, M., Mader, R., Volavka, J., 1978, Improvement of the alcoholic OBS with EMD 21657-a derivative of a pyritinol-metabolite: Double blind clinical, quantitative EEG and psychometric studies, Int.Pharmaco-psychiat., 13:177.

Strughold, W., 1944, Hypoxydose, Klin. Wschr., 23:221.

PARADOXICAL RELATIONSHIPS BETWEEN SERVICES, NEEDS AND OUTCOMES

Barry J. Gurland

Ctr. for Geriatrics and Gerontology, Columbia University
and New York State Office of Mental Health
100 Haven Avenue - Tower 3-29F
New York, N.Y.   10032

The United States - United Kingdom Cross-National project is a long standing collaboration between teams in New York and London. This project has completed several psychogeriatric studies using a cross-nationally reliable assessment technique, the Comprehensive Assessment and Referral Evaluation (CARE), which covers over 20 dimensions of psychiatric, medical and social problems. In this paper we single out the dimension of depression in order to demonstrate the paradoxical relationships that can exist between service delivery (in this instance treatment with antidepressants), public health indicators of the need for services (in this instance, depression) and outcomes reflecting the efficacy of treatment.

We have elsewhere (Gurland et al., in press) noted that rates of depression may vary between representative samples of the community elderly by as much as threefold. In three of the US-UK Project Geriatric studies we were able to examine the relationship between use of specific antidepressive treatment and variation in rates of depression. The US-UK Cross-National Geriatric studies under consideration are as follows:

Geriatric Community Study: Examination of a representative sample of 445 elderly subjects living in the community in New York and 396 in London. A one year follow-up was conducted. Services received and family support were also studied.

Geriatric Hospital Study: Examination of 50 consecutive geropsychiatric admissions in New York and 50 in London. A three month follow-up was carried out.

<u>Geriatric Institutional Study</u>: Examination of 162 and 159 geriatric residents randomly selected from all long term care facilities in respectively New York and London. Organization and costs of institutions were also studied.

In the Community Study (Gurland et al., 1983) we used a criterion-based operational diagnosis of 'pervasive depression' to refer to cases that had a clinically significant level of depression. Of these depressives (58 in New York and 49 in London), 3% received antidepressives in New York and 14% in London. Thus, the depressed elderly in London received antidepressives nearly five times as frequently as the New York elderly. Yet, rates of pervasive depression were much the same in the two cities (13.0% and 12.4% in New York and London respectively). Moreover, at 1 year follow-up, the outcomes were only equivocally favorable to London: Chronicity of depression (i.e. present at baseline and follow-up) in New York was twice as common as in London (15.1% vs. 7.6%) and mean scores of depression improved in London (5.1 to 3.2) but did not in New York (4.6 to 4.9). However, mortality of pervasive depressives was higher in London (10.2%) than in New York (6.9%).

In the Hospital Study (Copeland et al., 1975; Gurland et al., 1976) we found that antidepressants or EST were used during the first month of hospitalization about three times more frequently in London (14 out of 20 cases) than in New York (4 out of 16 cases) among patients receiving a research diagnosis of Affective Disorder. Yet the dimension of depression showed significantly greater improvement in New York than in London. A shorter duration of hospitalization in New York compared with London possibly returned the patient sooner to a supportive community environment and to an active life, thus alleviating depression.

Finally, in the Institutional Study (Cross et al., 1983), we found that antidepressants were given at about the same frequency (16% in New York and 12% in London) in the two cities to non-demented residents (50 in New York and 90 in London). Nevertheless, rates of depression (defined as a threshold score corresponding to a diagnosis of clinical depression) among these non-demented residents were distinctly higher in London (55%) than in New York (39%); especially with respect to severely disabled residents (over twice as frequent). Possibly, the more intense nursing - rehabilitative efforts that were noted in New York compared with London were effective at relieving depression.

CONCLUSION

The overall impression we gain from these cross-national comparisons of the use of a specific psychiatric treatment (i.e. antidepressants) is that there is at best weak evidence of an impact on indicators of psychiatric health among the elderly population. It is a far cry from showing a treatment to be effective under carefully selected and controlled conditions to assuming a substantial impact when that treatment is used under routine conditions and the population rather than the individual is the target of concern. There is perhaps not enough emphasis on this latter, public health aspect, of psychogeriatrics.

PROBLEMS OF PATIENTS AND RELATIVES AT REFERRAL: A Preliminary
Report of the Characteristics of Elderly Patients/Clients Referred
to Social Service Departments - Geriatric Medicine and Psychiatric
Services

David Jolley and David Wilkin

Research Section, Psychogeriatric Unit
Withington Hospital, Manchester

INTRODUCTION

    Whilst increasing life expectation has resulted in a gradual
increase in the proportion of old people throughout the world, this
has developed furthest in those countries where the benefits of
industrialisation came first. Arising, as it does, within the fabric
of well established towns, cities and counties, this freshly emphatic
source of need encounters a pattern of services that have evolved
slowly to take account of local expectations and draw upon a design
that was appropriate when relatively few people survived into the
senium. This is most apparent in the structure of services that are
called upon when immediate of 'primary' responses from family, family
medical practitioner and voluntary or informal carers are finding
matters too difficult or too complicated. Psychiatric services,
having been 'set apart' in the mental hospital system, have changed
considerably during the past forty years to seek siting within local
general hospitals and to provide for people who remain within their
own homes. Yet this transformation is very variably developed within
the different parts of the United Kingdom. The majority of
Psychiatric hospital beds are still sited in mental hospitals and
this is most certainly so for those occupied by and available to old
people. A drive to produce psychiatric services that are sensitive
and relevant to the needs of elderly people and to facilitate
collaboration with other services that are concerned with the Health
and Welfare of the Elderly, has seen the spread of specialist
'Psychogeriatric' services to many Health Districts (1,2,3). What
is being achieved within this variegated and changing kaleidoscope
and perhaps more importantly what needs are being left without a
relevant response, is not easily discovered. Routine national
returns of Health Service activity have not identified work with

the mentally disturbed elderly as a separate category. Descriptions
of the individual services or components of services are informative
and interesting in establishing essential similarities and
differences between them and certainly register a wealth of
enthusiasm and achievement. Yet the few systematic analyses that
have been undertaken have understandably looked at patients who have
been admitted to hospital (4). Understandable because this approach
is relatively easy to administer and indeed the original argument
for the creation of 'Psychogeriatric' units drew heavily upon data
concerned with the effects of misplacement of mentally, physically
and socially disabled old people at the time of admission to hospital
beds (5). Doubts have been expressed about the relevance of
Psychogeriatric Units in the spectrum of services when the
characteristics of their new admissions are compared with those of
local geriatric units. Yet the majority of work with the elderly
goes on in their own homes. It is the essence of the emerging
styles of service that 'secondary tier' resources interact with
primary care agencies and with each other and only a proportion of
referrals result in 'admissions' that take the patient/client away
from home. Thus we have attempted to describe and analyse the
contributions of those secondary tier services that constitute the
major elements of Health and Welfare services to the elderly - Local
Authority Social Services, Geriatric Medicine and Psychiatry. Within
the framework of a description of facilities and formal planning
and collaborative machinery, we have chosen to monitor their
activities by describing and following a sample series of patients/
clients from the time of their referral to these agencies. This
paper outlines the circumstances and the characteristics of patients/
clients at the time of referral.

METHOD

Parallel studies have been undertaken in Manchester in the North
West of England and Southampton in the South (6,7). In the
'Manchester' study the situation prevailing in the community served
by Salford Area Health Authority has been compared with that in the
community served by South Manchester Health District of the
Manchester Area Health Authority. In terms of services for the
elderly the former demonstrates the accepted pattern of Geriatric
Hospital which is separate from the General Hospital. The General
Hospital includes a small Psychiatric Unit but the bulk of
Psychiatric Services and certainly those for the elderly are based
on a larger mental hospital which is sited apart from the Geriatric
and General Hospitals and is indeed outside Salford. At the time
of the study no specialist team was identified within the Psychiatric
Service to provide for the elderly. In contrast Geriatric and
Psychiatric Services are provided from the main General Hospital
which is sited within South Manchester and the Psychiatric Service
includes a specialist 'Psychogeriatric' team.

Both Salford and Manchester include a range of environments through inner city, high-rise, owner-occupier, private rental to corporation housing estates. Areas were chosen, Eccles and Worsley in Salford and 'Area 5' of South Manchester that were roughly matched to include equal numbers of privately owned homes and homes occupied by tenancy from the corporation with a smaller balance of private rentals. Both areas are fairly described as representative of the suburban environment common to many towns and cities in the United Kingdom.

A sample of new referrals to Social Services, Geriatric Medicine, Psychiatry and Psychogeriatrics (South Manchester only) was taken to achieve a take up rate of roughly two patients from each service during each week of a six month period, October - March 1979 - 1980 (Salford), 1980 - 1981 (South Manchester). In practice this meant taking all Social Service, Psychiatric and Psychogeriatric referrals and one in two Geriatric referrals. As most patients/clients were at home at the time of referral (and most remained there subsequently) it was necessary to gain agreement not only from the professionals to whom they had been referred, but also from their General (Family) Medical Practitioner as well as the client/patient himself before making an assessment visit. Controlled time-tabling meant that initial assessment was made 2 weeks on from the day that the referral had been made. Thus the sample actually seen excluded people who themselves declined to be included or whose professional advisers felt an approach would be inadvisable (64 Salford, 59 South Manchester) or who died within the 2 weeks from the time of referral (22 Salford, 19 South Manchester).

Those patients accepted into the sample were visited and assessed by the project research psychiatrist (Dr. Ian Stout) using a standardised interview and examination schedule. In addition Dr. Stout made contact with the person's General Medical Practitioner to obtain further information and a research Social Scientist approached the person identified as providing most care or support to the elderly person and assessed this person's status, needs and views using a standardised interview schedule. Patients and carers have been followed up six months after the initial interview and reassessed using modified versons of the standardised interview and examination schedules and the pattern of help made available to them reviewed in detail when the original presentation had included problems arising from a dementing condition. Particular attention has been focussed on collaboration between services in meeting the needs of these patients and their informal carers.

The present paper, therefore, represents a preliminary report describing the characteristics of the sample of clients/patients at first referral.

FINDINGS

Total Referrals in the Sample;

	Geriatric	Psycho.G.	Psychiatry	Social Service	Total
Salford	37	////	44	43	124
S.Manchester	40	41	7	43	131

Source of referral.

Cross referrals between the agencies under study were excluded from the sample of new referrals, though referrals between these agencies that occurred during the six month follow up of the cohort represent an important element of the collaboration between services that we sought to monitor.   In both areas the specialist medical services accepted almost exclusively from other medical practitioners, 80% of their referrals were from General Practitioners.   Yet both Social Service departments received 80% of their referrals from non-medical, non-nursing sources - usually family, friends or neighbours.

Place of Residence at First Assessment (2 weeks post referral)

	Salford			South Manchester			
	Geriatric	Psychiatry	S.S.	Geriatric	Psycho.G.	Psychiatry	S.S.
Alone	30	27	42	25	32	43	56
With Spouse	19	27	12	23	10	29	19
With Others	0	4	0	13	7	0	14
Relatives H.	16	7	7	8	12	0	7
Sheltered H.	8	7	26	10	5	0	2
Part III	5	18	5	3	10	0	0
Private H.	0	0	0	5	7	0	0
Geriatric W.	14	0	7	13	0	0	0
P.G.W.	-	-	-	0	2	0	0
Psych.W	0	9	0	0	7	29	0
Other Hosp.	8	0	2	3	7	0	2
	100%	100%	100%	100%	100%	100%	100%

The point is amply made that most patients/clients were in private households.   Those patients noted to be within Part III accommodation (Local Authority Homes) had been residents for six months or more and were not receiving active social work involvement prior to referral to the medical specialties and were, therefore, not excluded from the sample.   Only 2 clients of Social Services (Salford) had been moved into Homes as an immediate response to the referral and referral to Geriatric Services in both areas had led to only 20% of patients occupying a hospital bed.   Similarly very few beds were being used by Psychiatric or Psychogeriatric Services.

424

Age at referral;

Age range.	Salford			South Manchester			
	Geriatric.	Psychiatry.	S.S.	Geriatric.	Psycho.G.	Psychiatry.	S.S.
65-74yrs	19	55	30	20	29	100%	24
75-84yrs	62	30	51	58	47	0	57
85yrs+	19	15	19	22	24	0	19
Total	100%	100%	100%	100%	100%	100%	100%

The greater part of the work of Health and Welfare of the Elderly services is concentrated in the '75 years plus' age group. Clearly the Psychogeriatric Service, where it exists has concentrated on this clientele, leaving other psychiatrists free to see some young old people and bringing itself very closely into line with Social Services and Geriatric medicine.

Sex distribution;

Similarly the Psychogeriatric service with M:F ratio of 1:4 fell more closely into line with Social Services and Geriatric Medicine whilst the 'comprehensive' Psychiatric service in Salford saw relatively fewer women M:F, 2:3.

Marital status;

The 'not now married' (mainly single or widowed) predominate in all services, but the Psychiatric services in both areas attracted a 40% married clientele whilst the Psychogeriatric (14%) service again aligned itself with Social Services (14% Salford, 21% Manchester) as reaching out to those now alone in the world even more emphatically than Geriatric Medicine (27% Salford, 28% Manchester).

Problems identified at first assessment;

Problem	Salford			South Manchester			
	Geriatric.	Psychiatry.	S.S.	Geriatric.	Psycho.G.	Psychiatry.	S.S.
Psychiatric	51	84	51	43	88	100	51
Physical	100	71	93	100	68	29	84
Social	60	57	74	53	71	43	63

Thus problems related to psychiatric, physical and social pathologies are common throughout the spectrum of referrals to all these services. Within the area delivering a specialist Psychogeriatric service physical and social pathologies are concentrated within its clientele to the (relative) protection of the General Psychiatric service. This seems likely to be a helpful device for facilitating the collaborative effort and cross fertilisation of ideas and expertise that is clearly necessary if the clients/patients of all services are to receive the optimal management of their multi dimensional problems.

Psychiatric diagnoses at first assessment;

%	Salford			South Manchester			
	Geriatric	Psychiatry	S.S.	Geriatric	Psycho.G.	Psychiatry	S.S.
Dementia	16	27	16	5	34	0	9
Depression	5	30	14	13	15	71	2
Other	35	46	23	26	39	14	40
NIL	47	16	45	58	18	14	45

The presence of a Psychogeriatric service appears to have sheltered Geriatric, Social Services and most certainly General Psychiatric services from problems arising from obvious dementing conditions. This would appear to be a useful device for facilitating further management by concentrating expertise and providing a focus for collaboration in the management of this difficult diagnostic group. Yet it remains true that a range of psychiatric pathology presents to non-psychiatric services giving rise to a need for training opportunities for the professionals working within them and means for collaboration in the management of difficult cases.

Severity of intellectual impairment at first assessment;

Error Score	Salford			South Manchester			
	Geriatric	Psychiatry	S.S.	Geriatric	Psycho.G.	Psychiatry	S.S.
0	45	42	61	73	33	71	69
1-3	24	26	18	22	29	29	28
4-6	10	5	16	2	16	0	0
7-12	20	26	5	0	20	0	3
Total	100%	100%	100%	100%	100%	100%	100%

Reporting the error scores on a standardised test of personal orientation emphasises the point that in the area with a reasonably developed Psychogeriatric Service, people with severe intellectual impairment are virtually all referred to that service for initial assessment and advice by the primary services when they feel in need of help. In Salford, without such a service, not only does it seem that severe intellectual impairment is more common at this point of referral (suggesting that the primary services and family have held on to a later stage in the process in more cases) but the pattern of referral is almost random for those most severely impaired people which constitue 30% of the case loads of both

Psychiatric and Geriatric services and 20% of the cases referred to Social Services!

Comment

Our efforts to move back the point of initial assessment to referral to the specialist Health and Welfare of the Elderly agencies rather than admission have been rewarded by identifying a large proportion of mixed pathology among these patients/clients. In addition it does seem clear that where a Psychogeriatric Service is established it attracts a client group with characteristics that make it ideally suited to work closely with Geriatric medicine and Social Service departments in catering for the very elderly with multiple and severe pathologies. General Psychiatry is released to devote its attentions to fitter younger patients. Primary level agencies practise referral of the most severely impaired intellectually to the most appropriate assessment resource and it seems likely they do this relatively easily so that within the spectrum of referrals to the secondary tier services, the most grossly deteriorated are less significant.

Further reports from this project which was sponsored by D.H.S.S., will describe the effects of these alternative patterns of service provision upon the experience of clients/patients and their carers both informal and professional after the initial referral.

REFERENCES

1. Jolley D., and Arie T. (1978) Organisation of Psychogeriatric Services, British Journal of Psychiatry. 129,418-23.
2. Arie T., and Jolley D. (1982) Making Services Work; organisation and style of Psychogeriatric services. In 'The Psychiatry of Late Life', edit. Levy and Post. Blackwell Scientific Publications Oxford.
3. Wattis J., Wattis L., and Arie T. (1981) Psychogeriatrics: A national survey of a new branch of Psychiatry. British Medical Journal, 282, 1529-33.
4. Copeland J. et al. (1975) Evaluation of a psychogeriatric service. British Journal of Psychiatry, 126, 21-24.
5. Kidd V.B., (1963) Misplacement of the elderly in hospital. British Medical Journal, 2, 1491-93.
6. Coleman P. et al. (1982) Collaboration between services for the elderly mentally infirm. University of Southampton research report.
7. Wilkin D. et al. (1983) Research Report No. 7. University Hospital of South Manchester Psychogeriatric Unit Research Section.

THE BOUNDARY BETWEEN PSYCHIATRY AND GERONTOPSYCHIATRY

G.H.M.M. ten Horn

Department of Social Psychiatry, State University
Postbox 30.001, 9700 RB Groningen
The Netherlands

INTRODUCTION

Mental health planning in the Netherlands distinguishes between services for childeren and adolescents(up to the age of 18 years), adults(from 18 to 65 years) and the elderly. Up to the present our various ideas about mental health care for the elderly have had the following two elements in common:
1. The population aged 65 years or more with regard to mental health problems can be considered as more or less homogeneous; and
2. The major issue is that of dementia.

In the Netherlands, retirement at the age of 65 years which became statutory in 1957, has so rapidly changed into a fact of life that it has almost become a biological inevitability, with considerable influence on mental health planning. Since recent economic pressures are bringing forward retirement age — which also influences the planning of health services — we are increasingly forced to reconsider the reality and significance of psychological and biological differences between people aged 65 years or more and those at the new retirement age of 62 or 61 years. If the mental health problems of people aged 55 to 64 years are not much different from those of people aged 65 to 74 years, while those of people aged 75 years or more are it can be argued that the target population of the mental health services for the elderly should not from now on include younger elderly following their earlier retirement. Instead, mental health services for adults might be better equiped to take over care of, for example, people up to the age of 70 or 75 years. In the Netherlands — where the age limit of 65 is the major criterion for assigning patients to a particular service — the mental health services for the elderly are mostly staffed by (social) psychiatric nurses and physicians who are trained to deal with the physical handicaps of elderly people and to deal with dementia, but who have little or no (psycho)therapeutic(psychiatric) training. It seemed that a study with a psychiatric case register could be helpful to gain insight and provide a basis for more rational planning.

THE REGISTER-AREA AND ITS SERVICES

On the 31st of December 1973 the Department of Social Psychiatry of the University of Groningen started a psychiatric case register, which covers a largely urban municipality of approximately 43.000 in the north of the Netherlands. The register has the Camberwell Register(Wing and Hailey, 1972) as its model:
1. It is based on a defined population;
2. It collects, longitudinal, information on all contacts of anyone from the area with all different psychiatric services (within and outside the study-area) serving the register-area; and
3. It orders the data patient-wise into a full record of all contacts the patient makes.

The mental health services involved in the register which serve the elderly are a psychogeriatric nursing home (104 beds), a unit for the elderly patients (with or without dementia) in a mental hospital (120 beds), a day hospital (9 places) and an out-patient team for the elderly, which is part of the so called Regional Institute for Ambulatory Mental Health Care ('RIAGG'). In the period studied the team consisted of one full-time social psychiatric nurse and two part-time physicians available to the elderly of the register-town but also of part of the province to which the register-town belongs. It delivers mainly care at a patient's home and is involved in the screening of patients before there eventual admission, although the service is administratively indepent from the in-patient services. For adult-patients uptill the age of 65 years there is a wide range of out-patient services within easy reach, including out-patient services of the mental hospitals and of the psychiatric departments of general hospitals, services for the addicted, an institute for psychotherapy and a social psychiatric service. Latter two are part of the already mentioned Regional Institute for Ambulatory Mental Health Care, since 1982 (Giel en ten Horn, 1982)

THE COHORTS

We collected four cohorts*of all elderly people in care of any of the (out-,day- or in-patient) mental health services covered by the register, during the first three months of 1975, 1977, 1979 and

---

*four cohorts of patients aged 65 years or more and only on cohort (1981) of patients aged 55 years or more.

1981. Included in this study are thus elderly patients, old en new, who were in (day-)hospital or with at least one face to face contact during (part of) the period of the first three months of the years studied. Each cohort was followed for a period of one year and patients could participate in more than one cohort if they were in care during more than one selection period. At the Third European Symposium on Social Psychiatry in Helsinki, september 1982, we presented the changes over a period of seven years, 1975 to 1982 (Giel, Brook and ten Horn, 1982). The findings form this cohort analysis showed that numbers and rates of patients aged 65 years or more were increasing up to 1979 after which they dropped again to the level of 1977*, which was 24 per 1000 of the population aged 65 or more. The majority of rates for females were higher than for males and the same counted for not married (single, divorced or widowed) versus married people.

Table 1 shows that the rates** for males as well as females and for married as well as not married persons in the age of 65-74 years are remarkably similar to those at age of 55-64 years. Above the age of 75 years rates appear to go up in each category and the differences between married and non married people get less, between males and females more, marked in the most elderly.

If the target population of the mental health services for the elderly should be going to include younger elderly of 55-64 years because of the earlier retirement, the clientele will increase with almost fifty per cent. On the other hand, if the target population of the mental health services for the elderly should be restricted to people aged 75 years or more the clientele will decrease with about thirty per cent, which leaves room for the growing numbers of elderly people.

Table 1. Three months period prevalence rates per 1000 population by sex, age and marital state

Age groups:	Rates: Males	Females	Married	Not married	Numbers* Males	Females	Married	Not Married
55-64	12,6	14,0	7,3	33,0	26	30	26	30
65-74	10,2	16,0	7,2	25,2	49	101	52	99
75-84	27,4	28,3	27,9	35,4	64	144	70	139
85 or more	54,0	74,9	70,3	67,0	34	88	23	99
Total	16,2	22,3	10,8	36,0	173	363	171	367

*age group 55-64 years based on the cohort of 1981; to compare the numbers of this age group with other groups they have to be multiplied by four

* Three months period prevalence rates of patients 65 years or more per 1000 population 65+: 1975:20,4(nr=90); 1976:23,9(nr=113); 1979: 29,9(nr=150); 1981:24,4(nr=127)

** Since inspection of the four cohorts revealed only minimal differences over the years we, lumped them together. The three months period prevalence rates were calculated by dividing the sum of the four cohorts by the sum of the four census populations at the 1st of January 1975, 1977, 1979 and 1981 and multiply the quotient by 1000.

431

To discover if the mental health problems of people aged 55 to 64 years are much different from those of elderly people we studied the types of mental disorders of the different age groups. As can be seen from table 2 the rates of the age group of 65-74 years are still remarkably similar to those at the age of 55-64 years. Although the rate of dementia is already rising, its breakthrough as a diagnostic category of great importance occurs at the age of 75-84 years and is still rising at 85 years or more. The rate of addiction drops with growing age, while the categories of psychosis and neurosis are still important at higher age.

If the target population of the mental health services for the elderly should be going to include younger elderly of 55-64 years, the distribution of the different diagnoses will change to 42% dementia and 58% other diagnoses compared with 59% resp. 41% of the 65-plus population at the moment. On the other hand, if the target population of the mental health services for the elderly should be restricted to people aged 75 years or more the distribution would be 75% dementia and 25% other diagnoses.

Table 2. Three months period prevalence rates of mental disorder, per 1000 population of the same age

Diagnosis:	Rates: Age groups:				Numbers[*] Age groups:			
	55-64	65-74	75-84	85+	55-64	65-74	75-84	85+
Dementia	0,7	3,4	23,3	54,3	3	38	150	98
Psychosis	3,1	2,2	0,8	1,7	14	24	5	3
Addiction	2,0	1,1	0,3	0,0	9	12	2	0
Neurosis and pers.disorders	4,2	2,3	2,6	2,8	19	26	17	5
Other diagnosis	1,3	2,9	3,7	6,6	6	32	24	12
Not known	1,1	1,7	1,7	2,2	5	19	11	4
Total	12,5	13,6	32,4	67,6	56	151	209	122

[*]age group 55-64 years based on the cohort of 1981: to compare the number of this age group with other groups they have to be multiplied by four.

Table 3. Type of care during year following first contact in first quarter of 1975, 1977, 1979, 1981, per diagnosis

Age groups:(N)	DEMENTIA					OTHER DIAGNOSIS					TOTAL				
	% Out-pt.	% In-pt.	(% Out + In pt)	Cont. per pt.	Days* per pt.	% Out-pt.	% In-pt.	(% Out + In pt)	Cont. per pt.	Days* per pt.	% Out-pt.	% In-pt.	(% Out + In pt)	Cont. per pt,	Days* per pt.
55-64 (3)	-	100	(-)	-	157	64	53	(17)	4,5	227	61	55	(16)	4,5	220
65-74 (38)	45	68	(13)	5,1	313	76	45	(21)	5,4	253	68	51	(19)	5,3	273
75-84 (150)	36	80	(15)	4,5	309	77	30	(8)	3,8	272	47	66	(13)	4,2	304
85 or more(98)	41	74	(15)	2,9	278	66	35	(12)	3,6	223	46	69	(15)	3,1	271
Total (289)	39	77	(15)	4,0	295	73	43	(16)	4,7	246	54	61	(15)	4,4	279

*per patient receiving out-patient resp. in-patient care.

Table 3 shows that the percentages of patients receiving out-patient respectively in-patient care of the age group of 65-74 years are very similar to those of the age group of 55-64 years and different from those of the elderly groups. Similar differences are found in the number of contacts per patient in out-patient care and the number of days per admitted patient: the younger groups had a higher number of contacts and a lower number of admission days.

People with dementia were less often out-patients (and with a lower average number of contacts) and more often in hospital (and with a higher length of admission) than people with another diagnosis.

Within the group of patients with dementia the eldest patients had fewest contacts and least in-patient days. Within the group of patients with another diagnosis the age group of 65-74 years was very similar to those of 55-64 years concerning the out-patient care, while the length of admission varied per age group.

If the target population of the mental health services for the elderly should be going to include younger elderly of 55-64 years, they would have to deliver 54% more out-patient contacts and 32% more in-patient days. On the other hand, a restriction to the age of 75 years or more would imply a decrease of out-patient contacts with 48% and a decrease of in-patient days with 25%.

If the mental health services for the elderly would restrict their target population to patients with dementia, leaving others to adult-psychiatry, it would imply a decrease of out-patient contacts with 61% and a drecrease of in-patient days with 24%.

STATE OF CARE AT THE END OF ONE YEAR

Table 4 presents the outcome at the end of one year according to diagnosis and age. Again the results suggest more similarity between age groups of 55-64 years and 65-74 years than between the latter and patients aged 75 years or more. People aged 75 years or more had more often died and were more often still in hospital, they were less often out-patients or not any longer in care.

Compared with patients with another diagnosis those with dementia had much more often died, were much more still in hospital and a lot less out-patient or not any longer in care.

Table 4. State of care at the end of one year as a percentage of the cases in each diagnostic-age group*.

Age groups:	DEMENTIA				OTHER DIAGNOSIS				TOTAL			
	Died	Not in care	Out-patient	In-** patient	Died	Not in care	Out-patient	In-** patient	Died	Not in care	Out-patient	In-patient
55-64	33	33	–	33	–	43	17	40	2	43	16	39
65-74	18	21	8	53	4	36	28	32	7	32	23	37
75-84	19	15	3	64	10	51	15	24	16	25	6	53
85 or more	24	20	5	50	17	46	12	25	23	25	7	45
Total	21	18	4	57	6	42	21	31	14	29	12	45

*for numbers in each diagnistic age group see table 2

**including those in in-and out-patient care

If the target population of the mental health services for the elderly should be going to include younger elderly of 55-64 years, they
would have at the end of one follow-up year percentage wise less
deaths(10 vs 15%), almost the same in hospital(44 vs 46%) and in out-
patient care(13 vs 12%) and more outside mental health services(32 vs
27%). On the other hand if they would be restricted to patients of
75 years or more the percentage of deaths at the end of a year would
go up(from 15 to 19%), also the number in hospital(from 46 to 50%)
while the number in out-patient care would drop(12 to 6%).
If the mental health services for the elderly would restrict their
target population to patients with dementia, leaving the others to
adult-psychiatry, it would imply at the end of one year an increase
in deaths(15 to 21%) and admitted patients(46 to 57%) and a decrease
of out-patients(12 to 4%).

DISCUSSION

     This study aimed at identifying similarities or differences in
the mental health problems and care of the middle aged and the elderly
which could guide us in planning(see also ten Horn,1980). Since recent
economic pressures are bringing forward retirement age it is important
to question whether the mental health services for the elderly should
also include the middle aged, at a time when demographic studies indicate tremendous increases in the population of the elderly. This
growth is strongest in the most elderly population which stands the
greatest chance of needing mental health care(Kramer,1980; Mann,1980).
Taking into account the number of cases there are strong arguments
for having psycho-geriatric services deal only with people aged 75
years or more, leaving the others to adult psychiatry. The results
from our study suggest more similarty between the age groups of 55-
64 and 65-74 years, concerning the rates of people contacting the
mental health services and the type of cases, than between the latter
and patients aged 75 years or more. If the psycho-geriatric services
would have to deal only with people aged 75 years or more it would
give them more room for dealing with the growing numbers in that age
group and for strengthening alternatives to in-patient care.
If the qualitative aspects of mental health care are to prevail it
might be concluded to do away altogether with the age criterion and
with the division between adult- and geronto-psychiatry. The relative
importance of other mental disorders than dementia in the elderly is
still considerable while the mental health services are not very
strong on the more intensive, therapeutic, forms of out-patient care.
It might be preferred to leave these patients to adult psychiatry.
Certainly this choice would require more attention to be paid to the
mental health problems of middle aged and elderly people than has
been done up till now in the services for adults.

REFERENCES

Giel, R., and Horn ten, G.H.M.M.(1982), Patterns of Mental Health Care in a Dutch Register Area, Social Psychiatry, 17, 117-123.

Giel, R., Brook, F.G., and Horn ten, G.H.M.M.(1982), Patterns of Mental Health Care for the Elderly: a Cohort Study in a Dutch Register Area, presented at the Third European Symposium on Social Psychiatry, Helsinky to be published in Acta Psychiatrica Finnica.

Horn ten, G.H.M.M.(1980), The use of a mental health case register for evaluation of mental health policy, in: Evaluation and Mental Health Care, Commission of the European Communities, 149-163.

Kramer, M.(1980), The rising pandemic of mental disorders and associated chronic diseases and disabilities, Acta Psychiatrica Scandinavica, 62, suppl.285, 382-396.

Mann, A.H.(1980), The Anglo-American geriatric studies, Acta Psychiatrica Scandinavica, 62, suppl.285, 279-284.

Wing, J.K., Hailey, A.(1972), Evaluating a community psychiatric service: Camberwell register 1964-1971. University Oxford Press, Oxford.

EVALUATION OF EFFECTIVENESS OF A PSYCHO-GERIATRIC

SECTOR ORGANIZATION

Jean Wertheimer

Service Universitaire de Psycho-gériatrie
1008 PRILLY (Switzerland)

As a foreword it seems necessary to note that the health organization in Switzerland is cantonal and not federal. This country is composed of 23 cantons or states and has no Health and Welfare Ministry. This system has the distinct advantage of promoting regional solutions to gerontological problems. Lausanne is the capital of the state of Vaud, and its population numbered 528'747 inhabitants in 1980 of which 15 % are over 65 years old. Ten years ago, this proportion was 12.6 %. The number of people 80 years and older in 1980 was equal to 3.1 % of the general population and to 20.65 % of the population 65 years and older.

Health Care Organization

The geographical situation of this canton is constituted from west to east by the Jura, the Plateau (where the most densely populated regions are found) and the Prealpes. Approximately half the cantons total population (250'000 inhabitants) live in Lausanne and its suburbs. Health care is supervised by the Department of the Interior and Public Health. Concerning the organization of physical care, the region is divided into 8 health districts which are organized locally but are under the strict supervision of the cantonal authorities. As concerns psychiatry, the canton is divided into 4 sectors (I: Center - II: West - III: East - IV: North). In sectors II, III, and IV where the population numbers 80'000 in each sector, the psycho-geriatric assessment and care is done by the adult psychiatric teams in the hospitals and ambulatory care centers (out-patient psycho-social centers). Sector I however, with the high urban concentration in Lausanne, provides separate services for adult and geriatric psychiatry.

The superposition of districts and sectors on the same territory is justified by the need of efficient planning. It does not constitute, in itself, an obstacle to the smooth fonctioning of the somatic and psychiatric structures. However, as concerns geriatric care, close coordination is especially imperative since the construction of homes for the elderly is the affair of the district, whereas the organization of psychiatric care concerns the sector.

The cantonal authorities instituted in 1967 a commission of gerontology whose role is that of consultant. It assembles the representatives of private and public organizations concerned with the problems of the elderly. Its duties are, among others, to evaluate needs, dictate guiding principles for the general organization of care, and to direct construction of medico-social establishments. A nomenclature has been introduced to distinguish between cases of type A (acute), B (intensive rehabilitation), C (chronic) and D (permanent care or nursing home).

One of the major efforts of the authorities in terms of gerontological care was to encourage the creation of a network of medico-social establishments disposing of C and D beds. Between 1966 and 1980 the number of C beds rose from 600 to 3130 (one per 166 inhabitants) and that of D beds from 1750 to 2216 (one per 235 inhabitants). Psycho-geriatric beds (118 in the central sector) are included in the C beds.

Simultaneously, an intensive effort was made to develop home-care programs. Housework help and meals on wheels are well organized, as well as nursing care and physical therapy. Psycho-geriatric care is made in the peripheral sectors by nurses trained in psychiatry and associated with psycho-social centers, and in the central sector by the Psycho-Geriatric Out-Patient Center (PGC) which is dependent upon the University Department of Psycho-Geriatrics (UDPG).

The UDPG is composed of two 150-beds hospitals, one located in the Lausanne region (Prilly), the other (Gimel) in the countryside about 30 kilometers from Lausanne. Gimel has a particular past history in that it served for 50 years as an asylum to which chronic patients were transferred from the Lausanne University Psychiatric Clinic. Entirely transformed into a modern psycho-geriatric hospital, its function changed in 1977. Whereas before it served as a "catch-all" for the overflowing University Clinic, it now works in parallel with Prilly and receives only emergency cases.

The PGC is located in the center of Lausanne. In a 12-room apartment works a team of 3 full-time doctors, 5 part-time doctors (who share their time with the psycho-geriatric hospital), 7 psychiatric nurses, 2 social workers, an ergotherapist and two secretaries. Professional activity consists of visits and out-patient consultations. Aside from out-patient care, the PGC personnel is often called as consultants in approximately 20 medico-social establishments. Finally, the UDPG has two day-hospitals of 12 places each, and whose activity is described elsewhere.(1)

Evaluation of Efficiency

A few statistics illustrate the activity of the UDPG and the importance for its function of the increasing number of available C beds, of the favorable influence of the activity of two hospitals working in parallel and following the same politic towards admissions, and finally of the development of home support and care.

At the Psycho-Geriatric Hospital in Prilly, the number of admissions was 152 per year in 1967 and has more than doubled in 1982 (319), the increasing efficiency being felt as soon as 1975. The discharges have also increased, and considering the various modes, one notes that the proportion of patients returning home during the same period (15.02 % in 1967 and 31.26 % in 1981) and those placed in other establishments (23.8 % in 1967 and 41.5 % in 1981) have increased considerably. Simultaneously, we note a net decrease in deaths which accounted for 35.5 % for the "discharges" in 1967 and 22 % in 1981. We also point out that the cases have become serious overall; for example the proportion of urinary incontinents was 33 % of the hospitalized population in 1966 and was 64 % in 1981. Between 1967 and 1981 the discharge diagnoses have changed, going from 63 % to 49 % for chronic psycho-organic syndromes and 29 % to 42 % for functional illnesses (thymic dysregulations, neurotics, delirious states). There appears to be a contradiction between, on the one hand, an increase of the dependency of the hospitalized population and on the other hand, a greater mobility of admissions and discharges and an increase in functional disorders. The apparent paradox can be easily explained. The creation of new C beds in medico-social establishments facilitates placing patients who do not need extensive care, and this is felt by the hospital population where patients who could be qualified as "unsuitable for placement" are concentrated. The development of home support and care programs delays hospitalization which, when inevitable is particularly difficult. Also, the existence of PGC favors the post-hospitalization out-patient care of those patients with functional disorders whose hospital stay can thus be shortened. In a psycho-geriatric hospital there are, necessarily, two types of beds, those occupied by chronic patients and those who constitute the flow of admissions and discharges (according to a gross estimation 57 % of the beds at Prilly are occupied by patients who have an extended hospital stay). One must see in this situation the advantages of a coordinated system which tends to preserve an optimal autonomy, and the disadvantage of the same system which tends to accumulate the most difficult cases in the hospitals. Efficiency is increased however, although the average occupation quotient of the 2 UDPG establishments has never been below 90 %.

In the psycho-geriatric hospital in Gimel, the change in organization naturally spurred an increase in admissions and discharges: 63 admissions and 31 discharges in 1975 and 153 admissions and 158 discharges in 1981. Patient mobility increased considerably, and we note a net increase in the number of patients returning to their own home or being placed in various establishments, and a simultaneous decrease in deaths.

It is interesting to note that since its creation, the PGC has had a fairly constant number of new cases per year, the number being around 300. However, the number of visits to private homes and medico-social establishments increases each year. In 1971 it was 2390 and ten years later 7166. We can conclude that as concerns out-patient care, undertaking serious cases requires frequent visits. This is clearly seen, though less spectacularly, in the number of consultations which was 1865 in 1971 and 3419 in 1981.

Conclusion

The description of the structure and the function of the University Service of Psycho-Geriatrics in Lausanne has no other aim but that of depicting a local solution to relevant problems concerning psycho-geriatric pathology in a population marked, as are all industrialized nations, by demographic ageing. This example seems to prove that the efficiency of such services is dependent upon the hospital and extra-hospital accomplishments made in the region and their role in the community. It is evident that the psycho-geriatric hospitals would function best when the team formed by these services works towards the prevention of hospitalization and follow-up care after discharge. Finally, the existence of specialized services insures a better knowledge of the community and suitable handling of the aged who suffer psychically. Psycho-geriatrics thus confirms itself as a whole.

References

Wertheimer J., Le-Dinh T. (1983) The Place of Day-Hospitals in a Psychogeriatric Sectorial Organization. Symposium Day Hospital Care for the Elderly. VIIth World Congress of Psychiatry. Vienna

Wertheimer J. (1981). Un service coordonné de psychogériatrie. Le Service universitaire de psycho-gériatrie de Lausanne. Hôpital Suisse 7:16

Wertheimer J., Le-Dinh T. Organisation sectorielle psycho-gériatrique: Le service universitaire de psycho-gériatrie de Lausanne. Psychologie Médicale. In the Press.

GEROPSYCHIATRY - STATUS AND SERVICES IN INDIA

A.Venkoba Rao and T.Madhavan

Institute of Psychiatry
Madurai Medical College &
Government Rajaji Hospital
Madurai-625020, India

The increase in life expectancy has been a spectacular achievement of our century but this has not been without fresh challenges.

Geropsychiatry has not yet been successful in claiming its priority in the health care system in the Indian subcontinent. Even the priority of the general Psychiatric care was not recognised until recently. There are no organised services for the aged in the country except for few voluntary ones. This lack of attention from the providers of care stems from the twin notions that old age is a period where any investment is attended by poor or no returns. The second is that the bulk of the population in the country is formed by adolescents who naturally claim health priorities. Those aged sixty and above form 7% of the India's population (683.8 millions) and they are estimated to number 41 millions: about the population of Spain. This figure is likely to rise to 60 millions by the year 2000 A.D. The morbidity rate for mental illness for this group has been estimated at 89/1000 population leading to a figure of 3.65 millions in the country - about the size of the country like New Zealand or even India's major city like Madras. (Venkoba Rao & Madhavan, 1982).

This presentation which deals with the status of Gero Psychiatry and its services in India is largely based on the findings from three sources in our Institute of Psychiatry namely Gero Psychiatry clinic, Community Mental Health Centre and Gero Psychiatric survey carried out by us in a semi urban area near Madurai. (Venkoba Rao & Madhavan, 1982). The Gero Psychiatric survey offers certain data. In a population of 15,668 (M:7,868 F:7,800) there were 686 (4.4%) aged 60 and above. 48.84% of them suffered from physical morbidity. The prevalence of psychiatric morbidity was 89/1000. 57% of Psychiatric group suffered from physical morbidity and 85% from sensory handicaps. Depressive illness contributed to 67% of the total psychiatric morbidity the rest by OBS (10%). Schizophrenia (5%), Neurosis (5%), Alcoholism (8%) and Possession status (5%), Freedom from physical illness, handicap and sensory deficit was noticed in 6.6% of the psychiatrically morbid group. This highlights the fact of concurrent presence of mental and physical morbidity in the aged and any form of services to the aged mentally ill must take this into account. Our experience has been that an elderly patient needs to have a minimum of 3 diagnoses.

We have been running a special Clinic for patients aged sixty and above for over 8 years. The Clinic functions once a week. Three beds are allotted for in patient care. The services comprise psychiatric, General medical, Geriatric, referrals, social and family care. In addition, supports of social and religious types are offered. Some States like Tamil Nadu offer monetary benefits, food and clothing to all those above 60 years.

The statistics of attendance at the Clinic during the last 7 years indicate that Gero Psychiatric patients contribute to 1.5 - 2.8% of the total General Psychiatry cases.

The Diagnostic categories encountered in the Gero Psychiatric Clinic are as follows: OBS: 33.4%, Affective Disorders 45.5%, Neuroses 8.5%, Alcoholism 1.3%, Schizophrenia 3.2%, Paraphrenia 3.9%, others 0.4%, Nil Psychiatry: 3.7.

Organic Brain Syndrome   Out of the total 457 cases,
153, (33.4%) suffered from OBS at the Gero Psychiatric
Clinic. Eighty two suffered from dementia, whereas
66 presented with acute OBS. In an indepth study of
150 successive elderly attending the out-patient
department, one third (48) suffered from OBS.

DEPRESSION:

        Depression is a major area of Psychopathology
in the Gero Psychiatric territory. The occurrence of
the depression in the elderly varied from 28.5% in the
Geropsychiatric Clinic to 67% of the total psychiatric
morbidity in a Semi urban area near Madurai (Venkoba
Rao, Virudhagirinathan and Malathi,1972; Venkoba
Rao, 1981; Venkoba Rao, Madhavan, 1982). The prevalence of depression is estimated at 60 per 1000 of
the geriatric population in the community. The
depressive illness in the community is invisible due
to factors like community tolerance, mistaking the
withdrawal features of the old person to the process
of ageing itself, failure to perceive the depression
as an illness by the family members and the society.
Wig and Murthy (1981) drew attention to the failure
of perception of depressive illness in the rural
population. The cases of Organic Syndrome, by virtue
of their symptoms of memory disturbance, wandering
incontinence, nocturnal delirium, may force them being
shifted to the hospital. The frequency of affective
disorders and OBS in our Gero Psychiatric Clinic
(34%; 43%) and the community (9.8%; 67%) offers a
striking contrast.

Social Factors

        According to our community survey findings
while 54.8% of the "normal" persons were socially well
integrated, only 26.2% of the psychiatrically morbid
fell in this group. Conversely 29.5% among the
psychiatrically morbid and 8.8% among the 'normal'
were not integrated. This runs counter to the theory
of "Disengagement" of Cumming and Henry (1961). We
have observed that social isolation does not affect
the elderly in the Indian setting (Venkoba Rao, et al
1972). Our present hypothesis is that it is lack of
social integration rather than social isolation that
is of importance. Living in the family, either joint
or extended does not guarantee, social integration

where the old ones are like "lonely islands". On the other hand living alone does not signify social isolation. Measures to enhance integration like guidance, counselling to the family members, financial support to the elderly, advising placements in the accepting family, visits by social worker are called for.

The recent Vienna Meet on the elderly declared that the family care was the best for the elderly. In our study 12% of the healthy and 16% of the psychiatrically morbid were living alone whereas nearly 50% were either in the joint or extended family and the remaining 30% in the nuclear type. Thus family setting continues to be available for the elderly and the advantage may be taken of this to augment the care to the elderly. A comprehensive health care comprising general medical and psychiatric in addition to the social and other supports will enthuse the family to keep their elderly with in its fold. This lessens the burden imposed on the family.

In a developing country like India, Gero Psychiatric care to be meaningful is to be the part of a comprehensive primary health care. The Programme needs to be incorporated into the existing health care system while drawing on the currently available resources from family, social, vocational, recreational and religious sectors and health education. The Primary Health Centre (PHC) each serving 100,000 population, forms the basic unit of the State Health services each with medical officers, health visitors, multipurpose workers. Training is offered to the PHC personnel in the method of detection of common illness, management with drugs and to enlist community support towards domiciliary care. There are on the whole 5,380 PHCs and 38,110 mini centres in the country. The aim of the Government is to create a PHC for every 10,000 population. The pattern of functioning at PHC level is from Multipurpose Health Worker - Health Visitor - Medical Officer - Referrel to hospital. We have chosen a primary health centre near Madurai with a catchment population of 97,070 with an expected aged individuals of 6,800. The main centre has 17 mini centres with a staff of 37, including medical and paramedical. The work is in progress and it is too early for evaluation. However services offered in the Gero Psychiatric Clinic for the last 7 years indicate a favourable trend when parameters like drop outs, mortality, and outcome are employed. The outcome study in which 73 out of 150 consecutive cases were so far followed up, revealed the following findings. In general complete recovery and partial recovery occurred in 58% and 24% of affective disorders, with 18% registering relapses. On the other hand in the OBS group there was a mortality rate of 41% and an unchanged or a worsening course in 18% each. There was 23% complete recovery in this group, which was however noticeable in acute confusional states. The contrast in the outcome of affective disorder group and the dementia group confirms the observation of Roth and others in their classical work.

The Geriatric health education including the Gero Psychiatric, is to be undertaken not at the Geriatric stage of one's life. It should be the part of health education to convey the message that the old age is the inevitable feature of the youth and the education is likely to be successful in the sense that the youth can take care of the elderly ones besides preparing itself for old age.

REFERENCES:

1. Cumming E and Henry W.E. (1961)
   Growing old, the process of disengagement, Basic Books, New York.

2. Venkoba Rao, A., Virudhagirinathan, B.S., Malathi, R (1972) Mental Illness in patients aged fifty and over - A Psychiatric Psychological and Sociological Study.
   Indian Journal of Psychiatry, 14, 319

3. Venkoba Rao, A (1981) Mental Health and ageing in India. Indian Journal of Psychiatry, 23, 11

4. Venkoba Rao, A and Madhavan T (1982) A Gero Psychiatric morbidity Survey in a semi urban area near Madurai.
   Indian Journal of Psychiatry, 24, 258.

5. Wig N.N. & Murthy R.S. (1981) Rehabilitation of
    depressed patients in a developing country <u>In</u>:
    <u>Rehabilitation of patients with depression and</u>
    <u>Schizophrenia</u>
    Eds:J.K. Wing, P.Kielholz W.M. Zinn. Huber
    Publishers, Bern Stuttgart, Vienna, 82.

FAMILY THERAPY IN SERIOUS AND TERMINAL ILLNESS

Claus Bahne Bahnson

Clinical Professor of Family Medicine and Psychiatry
University of California, San Francisco
Medical School, Fresno Campus

The seriously ill or terminal patient cannot be approached as an isolated individual without considerations for the many existing bonds between the patient, his family, his social group, and the medical institution and its staff members. Illness and death do not take place in a vacuum, but are intimately intertwined with social, family, and intraindividual dynamic processes.

Two basic concepts underlie our approach to the understanding and treatment of the terminally ill patient and his family. The psychosomatic holistic concept of disease and death, supported by hundreds of clinical studies, has taught us that a psychodynamic element interacts with several other factors in the production and course of illness and in the timing of death. Secondly, the historical approach suggests that the occurrence of, and response to, terminal illness are not random or solely genetically or environmentally determined events, but that both the production of an illness and the individual's response to the illness are anchored in his total life pattern and family dynamics, starting with childhood experiences, and followed by successive transitions called forth by new developmental phases.

Seen within the context of the family, untimely serious or terminal illness always is a family affair, both with regard to the etiology of the illness and to the responses and reactions to the illness. Premature or untimely serious and terminal illness in a family member most often reflects a failure in the emotional integration of the family forcing the patient to turn to self-relatedness and somatization. Illness expresses a defensive regressiveness to "somatic loneliness" and autogenesis from the more advanced projective emotional involvement with others and biologic or sublimated

449

heterogenesis. This concept is important to consider, because from this viewpoint the family is a co-creator of the very illness in one of the family members that then becomes a stressful problem with which the family has to cope. The illness of a family member is a "family symptom", and the family's reaction to this "symptom" must be understood within the dynamic context of it's meaning for the family. Therefore, we cannot treat the family and its reactions to the "symptom" of serious or terminal illness in a member without understanding the context within which it has been produced. We shall here only mention, but not discuss, the fact that the family and the patient also are part of larger social and institutional systems that interact, sometimes in very unfortunate ways, for the dynamic family system and the intrapsychic dynamic system of the patient. Particularly the interaction between the family and the medical treatment systems are complex and often destructive and may leave the patient suspended between two incompatible networks of belonging and demands. Thus, the targets for therapeutic intervention are not limited to the patient and the immediate family only, but also to the other involved "treatment families" of the patient and the many conflicts arising between these systems.

Previously I have emphasized that not only the present family, or family of procreation, but also the family of orientation, or childhood family, is of crucial importance for determining the latent proclivity of the adult patient to regress to somatization within the family of procreation. Therefore, the family therapist must consider this wider historical context also where the choice is not to seek a complete anamnesis. The patient will automatically bring information about relevant aspects of the historical context through current attitudes, defensive postures, or spontaneous associations.

Serious illness in a family member often develops when the family, via the nexus of the patient, has arrived at a blind alley or an existential crossroad, from which there seems to be no way out in either direction; perhaps because the pull from opposite directions immobilize action; perhaps because ambivalence is not resolveable; or perhaps because a movement forward is wrought in anxiety due to fear of hostility or betrayal. When the patient regresses into "somatic loneliness" in such life situations, old frustrated wishes and hopes from childhood and youth seem to re-emerge without immediate possibilities for satisfaction. Here it is the therapeutic task to prevent a re-repression of the old wishes and to attempt a new reintegration of the old desires in the present context of the patient and the family. Serious illness must nearly always be seen as a last alarm reaction on the part of the patient on behalf of both the self and the family, indicating that life under present circumstances is intolerable. It would therefore be both therapeutically cruel and blind to attempt a reconstitution, or "rehabilitation", of the patient by re-establishing exactly those family and life situations that constituted the precursors of the illness in the first place. The therapist must always attempt new solutions that integrate a larger proportion of the authentical needs within a new life constellation or context. To give up the old and to dare to look for new and untried solutions is usually associated with anxiety. The therapist must be available as an anaclitic agent for the family to temporarily allay this anxiety and make new resolutions possible, that may take the pressure off the patient's illness as a family solution, and may allow for an improvement or at least a diminuendo in the unrelenting destructive drive. We have seen cases in which, even late in a malignant illness, long periods of improvement, and in some cases complete remission, have taken place when patients and therapists have had the courage to attempt a completely new family - and thereby also individual - solution.

The reasons for using family therapy in the treatment of seriously and terminally ill patients are not only anchored in the joint and enmeshed roles of the patient and family in producing the illness, but also in the consideration that the serious illness of any family member relentlessly involves the lives and change the demands on all other family members. Irrespective of the functional role of the sick family member, the very fact that a part of the "family-body" is ailing, has a profound effect on all other parts or members of the "family-body". It is as if an attack on the undisturbed structure of the family all by itself carries the seed for profound anxiety in all family members irrespective of the practical implications. The disturbances in one part of the network are noticeable in all other parts of this net. The disease in one family member constitutes an immediate attack on the unconscious expectancy of maintenance of the archetypal family structure that serves as an unconscious ethological basis for life. This threat is more potent when it is directed towards a young adult family member carrying considerable responsibility, because this development threatens the survival of the system more acutely than when an old grandparent, or even a child, falls ill. In the case of the grandparents, the security of the family system over the future years is still intact; and in the case of a child, restitution always is possible, so that the system may survive. In all cases, whether for young or old family members, the serious or terminal illness also introduces anxiety because the family is confronted with the unknown, and because the myth of eternal survival of current structures has been shaken. Not only the uncertainty of the survival of a given family member, but also the uncertainty about any order and predictability in the family's life as a whole shatter the expectancies of constancy and safety.

One of the family therapist's great challenges is to help the family redefining and reconceptualizing a different future than previously, and perhaps unconsciously, expected, by letting all family members associate to possible new solutions, both when there is hope for an improvement and when the patient is terminal. In the prior case it is particularly important to involve the family and the patient together in structuring new solutions - never a reversion to the old - because the family's willingness to accomodate a new solution involving the patient may provide the crucial pivot for life encouragement for the patient, and thus be instrumental in bringing about an improvement. Where the destructive disassociation of the family has gone too far, and the disease has developed beyond the point of no return due to irreversible physiological changes, the therapist's job is to attempt to bring out into the open the many hidden agendas and issues associated with anger and guilt, that otherwise incapacitate the family because they bar all attempts at resolution.

When parents in active young families, where the children still live at home, fall ill, there are some typical reactions both on the part of the parents and the children that we need to pay attention to. When fathers fall ill both they and the families feel that they have failed as providers and guides, and there is ample guilt in the patient and covert anger in the rest of the family for this implied desertion of responsibility and care. Of course, the anger at the sick father cannot be expressed, is often thoroughly repressed and creats ample guilt in other family members. It is the family therapist's important purpose to gently and carefully uncover these feelings so that they can be dealt with in a more constructive way. Not uncovering such feelings, particularly among the children, often leads to psychosomatic and behavioral pathology in the youngsters, that then again may create more unconscious guilt in the sick father, starting a spiral of anger and guilt. Although parental roles today are less differentiated than some generations ago, it still seems that mother's terminal illness has other ramifications than father's. Here we see that the disturbance of the archetypal nurturance and security relationships with mother create deep anxieties in all family members about ever being able to be satisfied and cared for without the mother, and these frustrated dependency needs often have a stronger regressive pull for the family even than the sequelae of the loss of the father. The sick mother often feels tremendous guilt for not being available as the nurturant figure for her children and often verbalizes her need for seeing her children grow up, meaning that if she could care for them until adulthood, they might not be left without a source of nurturance later. Families with terminal mothers must learn to develop alternative resources for nurturance, since the mother not only must withdraw nurturance due to her own incapacitation during illness, but because she herself needs care from alternative family members so that the "mothering" within the family system now must be provided by other family members, best by figures on the parental level in the extended family, such as aunts and grandmothers, but basically by any workable constellation of other family members, including the father. In the

452

less traditional family the shifts are easier to bring about, but each family provides its own unique solution dependent upon the age of the children and the availability of extended family members. One important aspect is that the younger children need the stability of older nurturant family members in order to prevent a "parentification" and a load of responsibility incommensurate with their tender age. Whether conscious or not, young children often feel enraged that one of their parents is "deserting" them and is withdrawing the caring function. They often perceive it to be caused by their own inadequacy or hostility, and feel guilty and anxious over their imagined power to "create pain for their parents". Similarly, the parents feel guilty about depriving their offspring of a solid and protected childhood, and the healthy parental partner often feels rage against the terminally ill family member for deserting everybody and leaving all the burdens with the remaining parent. The fact that there is some truth to these difficult affects makes it even more important that the family therapist helps the family communicate these feelings to each other, so as to relieve the family system from the burden of repression and containment, that seems to reinforce the regressive somatization and thereby contributes to the exacerbation of disease. It is decidedly relieving for the family to be able to discuss even these difficult feelings during the illness of a family member, and clinically we see that both mood and course of illness take a more benign route after guided communication of these difficult issues.

When a child falls seriously or terminally ill additional problems arise in the family associated with the untimely and unexpected occurance of the inevitable. There is a natural sequence to the death of older members when younger members are growing up to fill the gap, but to have the roots cut away under your feet is disquieting and upsetting. Very much guilt is associated with serious illness in young children, particularly because on the unconscious level, this development suggests poor or insufficient parenting, and makes the parents feel that they have failed in some way they cannot easily define. Objectively, we do know that exacerbations in leukemia and Hodgkins disease in young people very often coincide with disintegration and strife in the family, so that to some degree these guilt feelings in the parents reflect reality. For the family therapist the goal is to work on the parental problems that may be associated with the exacerbation of the child's illness, and thereby take the pressure off the child as a mediator or "mentor" for the parents. Under no circumstances should the guilt be increased, but to the contrary, working in the family with issues not directly related to the child and its illness is paramount. We have seen that in some cases a resolution of the parents' conflict, associated with disintegration of the family system, can take the pressure off the sick child so that periods of remission may ensue. If the parents do no longer need the child as a mediator to keep the structure intact, and when the covert hostility as a part of the parents ambivalence about the child subsides, a tremendous weight is taken off the young family member, and a fresh reorganization can take place that often involves improvement in health status. Again, in the case of the young patient, it is important to understand that the therapeutic approach is exactly _not_ to force return of the child to the premorbid solution, be it effort in school, athletics, or other counterphobic forced activity. What should be arrived at in sensitive family sessions is a new role and purpose for the child's existence, defined much closer to the young person's needs, and framed within the current developmental stages of the youngster. Unfortunately, we often see very bad mental health in the handling of young somatic patients, in the sense that family, medical staff, and society at large pressures them to be able to perform "like other healthy children", a serious misunderstanding of what the child needs in this special situation, where the last thing the child yearns for is a return to the very status that contributed to unfolding the illness in the first place.

A common problem for both young and old terminal patients is that they very often, and with some right, feel deserted and shunned, although many individuals in their surroundings make a superficial effort at showing interest and care. "The leper" is never welcome, always reminds us all of our impending death, and appears as a phobic object. Since disintegration of the family system and isolation of the individual have a pathognomic effect on the production of disease, and since this isolation is reinforced when serious illness sets in, it is of particular importance for the family therapist to build contacts, rip down barriers, increase communication, facilitate cathartic expressiveness, and in all possible ways to counteract the emotional isolation of the terminally ill. To feel like a member of the family system again helps these patients tremendously, and they often find new roles for themselves, that not only help them regain their self respect and feeling of meaningfulness in the system, but which also represent a true helpfulness within the family system; for example, when a parent or grandparent can serve as advisor and confidant even when physically unable to be of practical help. Particularly for the classical father, the loss of control or power in the family is connected with high anxiety, and although power and control factors must be partially shifted around in the family when the father is ailing, there are probably many areas in which he can maintain a helpful consulting control to the benefit of all. This principle of course applies to mothers and other authority figures in the family as well, particularly in the new era where role differentiation is becoming less pronounced and sometimes completely reversed.

At a certain point in the progression of illness the question is no longer how to mobilize the patient and family psychosomatically against the disease, but where the goal turns towards the best possible resolution of the disengagement and the preparation for death. In treating families with terminal patients who are seen over longer periods of time with waxing and waning hopes for remission, we see that periods where support for integration and energizing is needed, alternate with periods of natural disengagement and the pain of object loss must hold the focus for the therapist. Sometimes these two elements can co-occur within very short time spans, when the patient and family the one minute talk and focus on strengthening conditions and in the next minute deal with the great Adieu. Several levels of reactions to the threat of death also can co-occur and the family therapist has to accept that no simple, logical approach takes priority in these situations. However, even when at the end of life, and even when having accepted the final fading within this universe, the family must be helped to support the patient and overcome their fear of the uncanny, so that the patient does not feel the classical despair expressed in the famous words: "Father, Father, why have you abandoned me...".

REFERENCES

1. Bahnson, C. B.: Psychophysiological complementarity in malignancies: past work and future vistas. In Bahnson, C. B., editor. Annals New York Acad. Sciences 164:319-374, 1969.
2. Bahnson, C. B.: Das Krebsproblem in Psychosomatischer Dimension. In Thure von Uexkull, editor. Lechrbuch der Psychosomatischen Medizin, Urban and Schwarzenberg, Munich, 685-698, 1979, 1981.
3. Bahnson, C. B.: Psychological Aspects of Cancer. In Y. H. Pilch, and T. K. Das Gupta, editors. Surgical Oncology. McGraw-Hill Book Co., New York, 231-253, 1984.
4. Bowen, M.: The use of family therapy in clinical practice. Comprehensive Psychiatry 7:345-374, 1966.
5. Eissler, K. R.: The Psychiatrist and the Dying Patient. New York, International Universities Press, 1955.
6. Freud S.: Beyond the Pleasure Principle (1920). London, Hogarth Press, 1955.
7. Jackson, D. D.: The question of family homeostasis. Psychiatry Quarterly Sup. 31: 79-90, 1957.
8. Simmel, G.: Tod und Unsterblichkeit in Lebensanschauung: Vier Metaphysische Kapitel. Munich, Dunker and Humbolt, 1918.

DAY-HOSPITAL CARE FOR THE ELDERLY

M. Bergener

Rheinische Landesklinik Köln
Wilhelm-Griesinger-Str. 23
D-5000 Köln 91 (Merheim)

INTRODUCTION

The entire population in Europe is going to increase by 17 % from 1970 up to the year 2000. The number of inhabitants being older than eighty will grow by 30 % or even by more than 60 % with regard to those being more than eighty years of age.

These data reflect the worldwide change in population structure by taking Europe as an example: We have to face an enourmous increase of people being older than eighty and a simultaneous decrease of the younger. The problems arising out of this development do in fact lead to consequences in every field of social life. In order to manage these problems an intensified interest of all kinds of scientific desciplines with regard to gerontology is required - this request is valid for biology and medicine as well as for psychology and sociology. The demand cannot be met without increased scientific commitment to gerontology. The exceptional position of gerontology and its particular status has recently been emphasized by the "World Assembly in Aging" (Vienna, 1982) which was initiated by the United Nations. The guidelines make plain how much is left to be done.

Still gerontology and also geronto-psychiatry representing a scientific sphere, largely placed outside medicine are generally ignored. Now as before, the outside attitude of many physicians towards old age diseases is determined by indifference and resignation. Up to the present negative stereotypes do establish an aversive attitude which has not been substantially altered yet thus causing disadvantages for the elderly. Without any radical reconsidering in this respect the withdrawal from obsolete and disorganized structures in medical care and its quantitative and qualitative deficits will not be accomplished. In fact these structures prevent the use of efficient methods of treatment and care in the medical and social fields.

Besides ambulant and mobile services to the patients the day-hospital care is regarded to be of particular importance.

In a regionally structured compound system consisting of different arrangements and services all medical and social aids are coordinated for every indivudual case. Moreover they ensure the coherence of their single effects. Therefore the function of day-hospital care is not limited to saving capacities in institutions of general medicine and psychiatry. The constant or at least temporary relief of primary groups being concerned seems to be even more essential. Any chronic diseases and long lasting need of care may often lead to serious and most severe stress for the patient's family thus presumably resulting in social decompensation and complete social isolation. This situation should be taken into account to a greater extent than it has been done before regarding the decision, as to the scope of help. In addition to profound diagnoses and therapy day-hospital care provides promissing rehabilitative alternatives after in-patient treatment. Therefore, it is out of question that whithin the scope of prophylactic as well as curative and rehabilitative actions, day-hospital care is assigned to pre-eminent tasks: an integral function, the key role in a system of extensive geriatric aids and respective medical care with different emphases.

The fact that the patients spend the evening, the night and the weekend at home does not mean less therapy but rather an extended type of therapy having a specific range of indication.

More than in case of full in-patient treatment factors deriving from the psycho-social environment largely influence therapeutic strategies thus counteracting any aversive and regressive trends.

Despite encouraging signs day-hospital care institutions have remained a chance mainly not taken advantage of in this country. In contrast to other European states it only gets accepted gradually in the Federal Republic of Germany. Neither positive experiences being made in different countries during decades nor the demands put forward in the psychiatry inquiry were able to change this situation. In England the day-hospital care movement already started in the fifties; immediately after World War II in the year 1947 the first day-hospital institutions were opened. One fifth of all patients are treated in these clinics. In the view of representatives of the British National Health Service the number of these patients has not yet reached the level which could actually have been achieved.

According to the British model, day-hospital care is provided for 65 patients within a standardized district of 100.000 inhabitants. However, in the Federal Republic of Germany massive barriers still delay a similar development. The question remains absolutely open whether at all or at least to what extent these barriers can be extinguished. Reforms in health services being overdue for a long time are blocked because of tendencies to preserve and defend conventional structures. In this respect "the bed in hospital" is regarded to be of particular importance. Another difficulty is caused by the present legislation establishing different cost regulations and responsibilites in the medical and social fields of activities. Day-hospital care is not only situated between in-patient and out-patient treatment. Moreover its functions substantially exceed the medical scope of duties and concentrate on preservation, support and restoration of physical, psychic and social competence. Thus, it terminates the still existing division between in-patient and out-patient treatment and their respective institutions. Even more decisive is the fact that they cross those boundaries between health service and social care, being caused by different laws.

Provided these dividing lines and the present dichotomy can be overcome, day-hospital care will not be anymore a chance largely not being made use of. Therefore basic reforms are required; this state of affairs has been discussed during the last years though without any results. Legislative initiatives seem to be a conditio sine qua non, in order to end the inadequate coordination of the incommensurability in the fields of medical and social care, to be found in essential spheres and under many different aspects. Repeated efforts to attain a kin of "joint activities" by all representatives have failed again and again.

In fact there are additional reasons which have been and still are responsible for problems in establishing day-hospital care elsewhere outside Great Britain.

For the patients as well as for their relatives and the physicians it is difficult to classify correctly day-hospitals which do not uphold conventional border lines between in-patient and out-patient treatment, but on the contrary, even try to overlap these boundaries. The terms commonly used for day-hospital care illustrate these difficulties thus leading not only laymen but also physicians to regard them as being somehow obscure and even absolutely superfluous. Day-hospitals are more than just insufficiently described and defined as "clinic without beds" or as a kind of medical care given to those patients who do not need an intensive in-hospital treatment and therefore may as well be treated by private physicians. Contrary to these views day-hospitals care most efficient instruments to ensure medical and psycho-social care.

The guide-lines correspond with the principles of multidimensional diagnosis, therapy and rehabilitation by employing interdisciplinary methods and strategies. Therefore, they are particularly qualified to represent the basic elements of geriatric aids. A multidimensional approach seems to be a promising way to treat multimorbidity in old age, by taking into account medical as well as psychologic and social aspects, at the same time though with changing prevalences.

A particular handicap in old age are different kinds of social isolation. Day-hospital treatment is able to counteract this development. Any relations being specific for primary groups are not endangered - on the contrary these relations are even supported and preserved.

Day-hospital care therefore represents integral elements within the entire therapeutic system. They do not directly compete with any other institutions. Day-hospital care is given to those patients who do not need full-time in-hospital treatment any more. Nevertheless, their complete medical and social rehabilitation is dependent on further medical, psychological and social help.

Day-hospitals for geriatric care could prove to be a model. Their efficiency may stimulate interdisciplinary cooperation, also in other medical and social fields within or outside national health and social services. In that case, it would be inevitable to modify the at present prevailing 'disease patterns'.

In the course of any illness the actual components the diesease consists of may change repeatedly. The interference of different determinations leads to a great variability in clinic symptomatology, as well as in the progress of the illness thus resulting in the demant for specific old-age diagnosis and therapy not limited to polypragmasy covering the symptoms.

No therapy whatsoever is able to reserve the process of aging itself.

Yet, geriatrics include effective treatment alternatives in order to cure geriatric diseased or at least contribute to soothe typical infirmities of old age. Day-hospital treatment is one of these alternatives and should be made available and utilized to a greater extent than it has been done before.

The development to convert every tenth and then, step by step every eighth "bed in hospital", being reserved for geriatric care into day-hospital capacity or provide them as such from the very start I would not regard as being an "abstract utopia", but as a quite justified requirement - a great opportunity and challenge for the eighties.

THE PLACE OF DAY-HOSPITALS IN A PSYCHOGERIATRIC

SECTORIAL ORGANIZATION

Jean Wertheimer

Service Universitaire de Psycho-gériatrie
1008 Prilly (Switzerland)

The University Department of Psycho-geriatrics in Lausanne (UDPG) exercises its function in a psychiatric sector composed of 250'000 inhabitants whose proportion of people 65 years old and older is 15 %.The Department is formed by two 150-bed hospitals, an out-patient policlinic called the Ambulatory Psycho-geriatric Center (PGC) and two day hospitals. This study aims to describe the role of the last two structures within the overall sectorial organization, that of the hospitals and the PGC being described elsewhere (1).

Within the concept of community medicine, the connections between ambulatory, intermediary and hospital care have, as a primary objective the promotion of optimal autonomy, adapting from individual to individual the mode of care. So, the UDPG offers the possibility of consultations, visits, day hospitalisation and short or long hospital stays. The transition from one structure to another is done quite smoothly.

Post-hospitalization

The two day hospitals are integrated, one into one of the psycho-geriatric hospitals (DH I), the other into the PGC (DH II). Day Hospital I has 12 places. It is run by a psychiatric nurse and patients can benefit from the hospital's infrastructure (ergotherapy, physiotherapy, animation and meals). Medical supervision is insured by one of the resident doctors in the psycho-geriatric hospital. Its principal action concerns the post-hospitalization phase. Its location in the hospital itself allows the hospitalized patients to be integrated into the group at the day hospital before returning home. The roles of the DH I are to take on the post-cure care, and to encourage a progressive return to greater autonomy, as well as to support on a long term basis chronic psychiatric patients (schizophrenics, depressives, alcoholics). This day hospital being located in a well-equipped hospital center, it also has a pre-hospitalization function for certain chronic psycho-organic cases that the families try to keep at home. These patients are integrated into the day hospital group or into a division in the hospital.

Before hospitalization

The Day Hospital II (DH II) occupies a 5-room apartment above the PGC. The team is composed of three psychiatric nurses, one nurses' aid and one ergotherapist. One resident doctor in the PGC detains the medical responsibility. There are also 12 places in the DH II. Meals are brought in from the psychiatric clinic (regeneration system). The action of DH II is primarily concerned with the pre-hospitalization phase, the patients coming for the most part from the PGC. Its roles are to treat acute or sub-acute situations (depression, psychotic decompensation, etc.) and to avoid hospitalization of these cases and also of chronic patients who can remain at home provided they have day care. A smaller number of the patients come from the psycho-geriatric hospitals, such that DH II also has a post-hospitalization role. In so far as it remains feasible, the patients come to the 2 day hospitals by their own means. If this is not possible, they are picked up and left off at home by a bus belonging to the UDPG.

Efficiency of Sectorial organization

The DH I has been in function for 10 years, the DH II for 7. Over the years, and especially since 1975 the community function of the UDPG has developed considerably and the canton has equipped itself with additional beds for chronic patients as well as with home care and support programs. It is therefore interesting to analyze the evolution of the patient population of these intermediary structures during this period.

Day Hospital I (DH I)

From 1973 to 1982, DH I has had 131 admissions, of which 99 were new cases and 32 readmissions. The low number of admissions coupled with the constant high occupation rate of 11, is a sign of prolonged hospital stays. To facilitate analysis, the ten-year span was divided into 2 periods, the first from 1973 to 1977, and the second from 1978 to 1982.

One notes first of all that the number of admissions has greatly increased during the second period (83 as compared to 48). New cases also increased but to a lesser extent, going from 42 to 57. One also notes that the number of readmissions also increased (20 as compared to 8) reflecting the ease with which a patient can be re-evaluated and cared for in the sectorial system.

Table 1

HJ 1	Admissions	New cases
1973-1977	48	42
1978-1982	83	57
	131	99

The source of admissions (table 2) undergoes slight modifications. The majority of the cases continue to come from the hospital, but there is an increase of those coming directly from home. This means that the number of psycho-organic patients has increased, which again shows the systems' adaptability, as a fair number spend their day in the ward rather than in the day hospital itself.

Table 2

HJ I   Origin of admissions (%)

(1973-1982)

	1973-1977	1978-1982
Home	33,5	42,0
Psychogeriatric H.	60,4	54,5
Others	6,0	3,5

Finally, one witnesses a distinct development in the proportion of patients returning home, the total number going from 15% to 43% (Table), as well as a simultaneous decrease in rehospitalizations in the psycho-geriatric hospitals. These statistics show the essential role of DH I which is to serve as a way-station between hospital and home.

Table 3

HJ I   Discharges Destination

	1973-1977			1978-1982	
	N	%		N	%
Home	6	15,5		34	43
Psychogeriatric H.	27	69,5		36	45,5
General Hospital (CHUV)	2	5		3	4
M.S.E.	-	-		4	5
Deceases	4	10		2	2,5

Day Hospital II (DH II)

From 1976 to 1982 DH II received 249 admissions. The average of 36 admissions per year has remained more or less constant, as has the number of discharges (34 as an average per year). The analysis of the source of these patients unfortunately could not be performed. However, that of the discharges (Table 4) shows an increase in the patients returning home up to 1980, followed by an impressive fall in their number, whereas hospitalizations in the psycho-geriatric hospital increase and patients placed in establishments for chronic illnesses decrease. These figures express without a doubt that the pre-hospitalization cases have become more serious and consist of a majority of psycho-organic syndromes, but also of psychotics and depressives.

Table 4

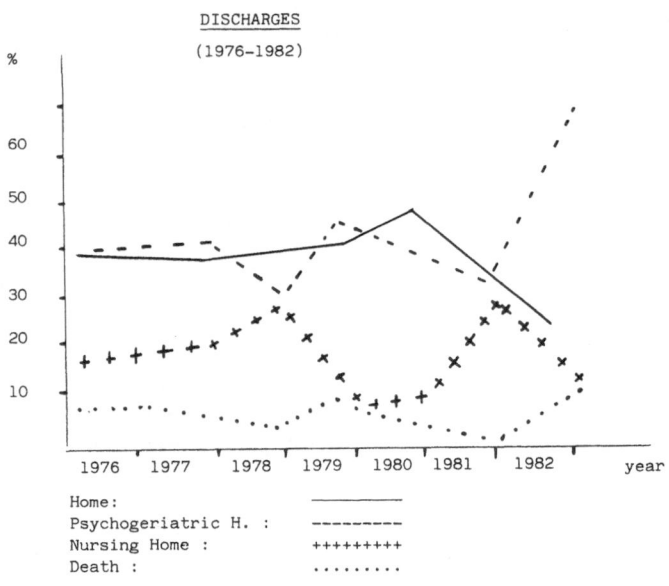

DISCHARGES
(1976-1982)

Home: _____
Psychogeriatric H. :   ---------
Nursing Home :   +++++++++
Death :   ....

Conclusion

The development of coordinated activity in a sectorial psycho-geriatric organization influences the day hospital structures concerned with the post-hospitalization phase by providing better patient mobility and an increase in the number of patients returning home. On the other hand, it influences those concerned with pre-hospitalization care by an increase in admissions to psycho-geriatric hospitals. This fact must stimulate the search for solutions to the problems concerning the care of chronic psycho-organic syndromes. In our experience, 12 places in DH II are insufficient. The number should be increased to at least 20, such that "functional" and "psycho-organic" sub-groups could be formed.This would limit the progressive invasion of psycho-organic syndromes on the structures provided for general psychiatry of the elderly.

References

Wertheimer J., (1981). Un service coordonné de psychogériatrie. Le service universitaire de psychogériatrie de Lausanne. Hôpital Suisse No. 7:16

Wertheimer J., Le-Dinh T., Organisation sectorielle psycho-géria-trique: Le service universitaire de psycho-gériatrie de Lausanne. Psychologie médicale. In the Press.

Wertheimer J., (1983). Evaluation of effectiveness of a Psycho-Geriatric Sector Organization. Symposium on Services to the Elderly: Evaluation of Effectiveness. VIIth World Congress of Psychiatry, Vienna

DAY CENTRES, DAY CARE AND DAY HOSPITAL IN THE UNITED STATES AND CANADA - OR HOW TO COMPARE APPLES, ORANGES, CARROTS AND SHOELACES

H. F. Reichenfeld

Ottawa, Canada

It is frequently argued that the cost of health services - the shoelaces which hold them together - will be significantly reduced by the adequate provision of domiciliary and ambulatory services and the concomitant reduction in demand for hospital and nursing home beds. The argument is fallacious and it has in fact been demonstrated that the provision of high quality ambulatory services has no significant effect on the utilisation of institutional facilities.[15] In fact the very opposite has been observed. As services expand, so demand for them grows and just as "Work expands so as to fill the time available for its completion".[9] "The demand for medical services will expand so as to occupy - nay, outstrip - the services offered".[12] It should come as no surprise that better services will be more expensive. In every other sphere of human activity it is accepted that high quality is associated with a higher price tag, and it would be unreasonable to expect that in the health care system alone the provision of better facilities should be accompanied by savings. So much for the shoelaces.

The role of specific ambulatory facilities will therefore be discussed from their functional aspect without consideration of the financial implications. There appears to be a great deal of semantic confusion about the terms "Day Care" and "Day Hospital" - are we talking about apples or oranges - and some authors use the terms terms synonymously.[1,4] In principle it is not difficult to differentiate between them.

A Day Hospital can be seen as the closest approach to the traditional medical model of a fully staffed facility under the direction of a specialist physician with facilities for adequate investigations and treatment of an identified target population.

467

Although there will be large variations between individual patients the investigative and treatment processes can be expected to take place within a finite time frame resulting in a regular turn-over of the patient population. If the goal of the Day Hospital is to provide effective treatment for a specified group of patients it follows that General Psychiatric, Geriatric and Psychogeriatric Day Hospitals will need to develop along divergent lines though maintaining a comparable overall philosophy. An appreciation of the different roles played by geriatric and psychogeriatric day hospital can be seen in the planning of the expansion of a well established centre for geriatric care which includes the establishment of both facilities as separate entities.[3]

In geriatric psychiatry the Day Hospital can be seen as part of a comprehensive network of psychogeriatric services with a number of quite specific goals. (Figure 1). They are:
1. To provide a treatment modality additional to out-patient and in-patient treatment for patients who need intensive therapeutic involvement but are able to maintain themselves in a community setting;
2. To provide an interim period of active therapy for discharged in-patients;
3. To provide a period of trial therapy in an ambulatory care setting in the presence of severe psychopathology;
4. To provide ongoing support for patients with a history of frequent in-patient admissions with the goal of avoiding the "revolving door syndrome".

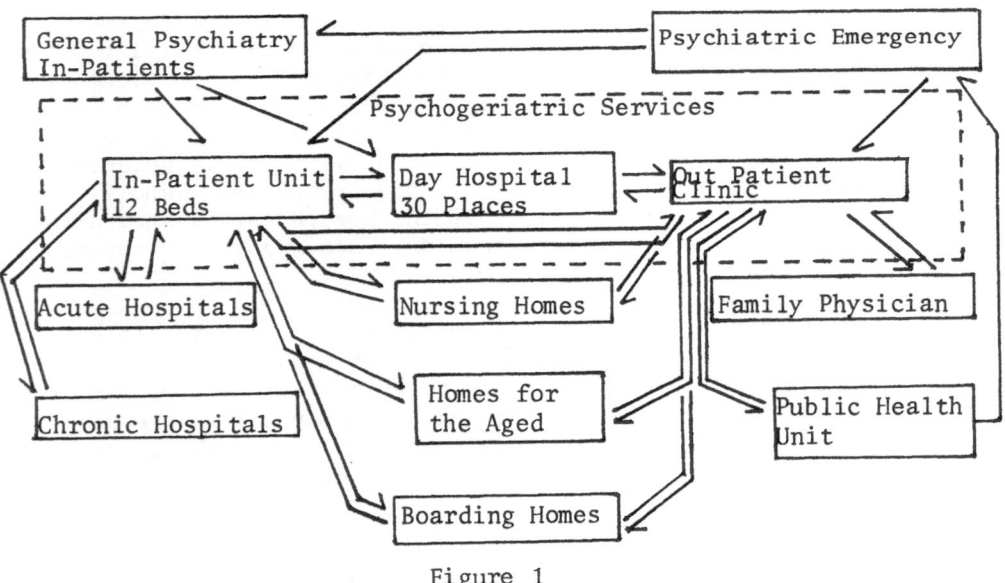

Figure 1

The effectiveness of the psychogeriatric day hospital has been specifically demonstrated in the treatment of elderly depressed patients. (Table 1) By focusing on this particular group of patients it has been shown that even with minimal though highly motivated and experienced staff half the patients discharged over a 1 year period were considered improved to the point that they were functioning adequately in the community without further psychiatric treatment. (Table 11)[13]

TABLE 1

DIAGNOSES

DEPRESSION	57
PSYCHOSIS AND SCHIZOPHRENIA	8
DEMENTIA	6
ALCOHOLISM	6
NEUROTIC DISORDERS AND ADJUSTMENT REACTIONS	6
	83

TABLE 11

OUTCOME

SUCCESS	
Discharged to own residence Living independently	31
PARTIAL SUCCESS	
Better adjustment in sheltered setting	14
FAILURE	
Not improved; admitted to In-Patient Unit	11
DROPPED OUT	6
TOTAL	61

In contradistinction to the day hospital with its expectation of
effective treatment and eventual discharge Day care can serve as the
classical paradigm for a long term service. This has been defined as
"one or more services provided on a sustained basis to enable individuals whose functional capabilities are chronically impaired to be maintained at their maximum levels of psychological, physical and social
well being".[2] It is directed at a population whose level of function-
in has placed them at the periphery of those who are in need of
institutional care. This need may have arisen from a variety of
causes or combinations of these. Foremost among them will be a
decline in cognitive or physical function associated with increasing
difficulty of the family to provide adequate support and/or supervision for the "identified" member. In view of the vital role of the
family in both recognising and accepting the need for long term care
their involvement in the process of accepting this specific modality
is difficult, lengthy but essential for the success of the program.

The Day Care program itself has been defined as providing the
"dynamic twins of supplementation and expectation".[8] By supplementation is meant the provision of services for identified needs which
the family is unable to meet, whilst expectation calls for a forth-
right approach towards realistic goals for both the applicant and the
family. Day Care may therefore provide such concrete services as
transportation to and from the centre, the creation of special rooms
and staff, but will also allow some flexibility in the program by
adapting the frequency and length of attendance to the needs of the
individual. Accurate assessment of the specific needs of the applicant and his family are obvious prerequisites and whilst the assessment process will frequently be somewhat lengthy this in itself will
contribute to the success of the program by producing a sense of belonging and group cohesiveness between applicant, family and staff
even before the program is formally entered.

Similarly, by making clear at the outset that acceptance into the
program will be accompanied by specific expectations active participation by both applicant and family is emphasized. Expectations will
apply to such concrete operations as insisting on proper attire and
conforming to the agreed schedule of attendance as well as appropriate
behaviour while attending the program. The latter will include participation in group activities as well as assisting in such operations
as serving coffee or welcoming new entrants.

In contrast to a psychogeriatric day hospital with its medical/
psychiatric/treatment orientation day care must be considered a social
service and is therefore most appropriately under the direction of
social workers. Medical or psychiatric input is limited to the provision of consultation services and clearing of the applicant for
fitness to attend or providing warnings about specific precautions
that may be necessary. Although it has been stated that "Day Care is
not designed primarily to serve cognitively impaired people"[10] in its

operation it has been found to be particularly helpful to this group of clients. Up to 15% of severely impaired members have been found to be tolerated, including disoriented individuals with tendencies to wander and showing severe agitation and an inability to form relationships with others. The usefulness of Day Care in cases of dementia should hardly be surprising. It is precisely the cognitively impaired individual who is most likely to benefit from a sustained service with continuity of care provided by the same team in a program which is sufficiently structured to counteract the inability of the individual to structure his own life yet flexible enought to allow for individual variations and changing needs over the course of time.

If the oranges and apples of psychogeriatric day hospital and day care cater to individuals showing a variety of psychiatric disorders of varying intensity and holding different prognoses day centres - the carrots in our comparison - basically deal with the healthy elderly. They therefore entail a great deal of autonomy for the user and as a result demonstrate even more diversity than other facilities. Though some of the earlier centres had developed as off-shoots of mental health services or retirement homes with a marked psychiatric orientation [5] the major emphasis is invariably centered on social activities, including the provision of meals, and maximum participation of the members in the running of the centre.

The Senior Centre has been defined as the "community focal point on aging where older persons as individuals or in groups come together for services and activities which enhance their dignity, support their independence and encourage their involvement in and with the community". [14,11] Though participant self government is one of its characteristics administrative relationship to an existing facility such as an old people's home has a great deal to be said for it. Sharing some activities will mitigate against the sense of isolation frequently experienced by residents of the home while the link between it and the centre will emphasize the principle of continuity of care. Another way of visualizing this principle consists of the concept of a Multi-Service Senior Centre (Figure 2) where some activities occur within the centre, others take place completely outside it with others still bridging the gap by being available both within and without.[14] Typical of the first are some health related services such as special clinics, screening programs and health education programs while referral to and information about community resources provide the link to other facilities. Day care and psychogeriatric day hospital would be included in these, again ensuring continuity of care. Other services bridging the gap will have a more definite social content, eg. advocacy, transportation and opportunities for employment whilst services geared to the specific needs of individuals will include the provision of meals both within the centre and in their home settings.

The utilisation and expansion of existing facilities to ensure a network of services for the provision of a continuity of care is a characteristic of the development in come Canadian centres, though these are in many cases only in the planning stage. In the U.S. fragmentation and lack of co-ordination among different providers

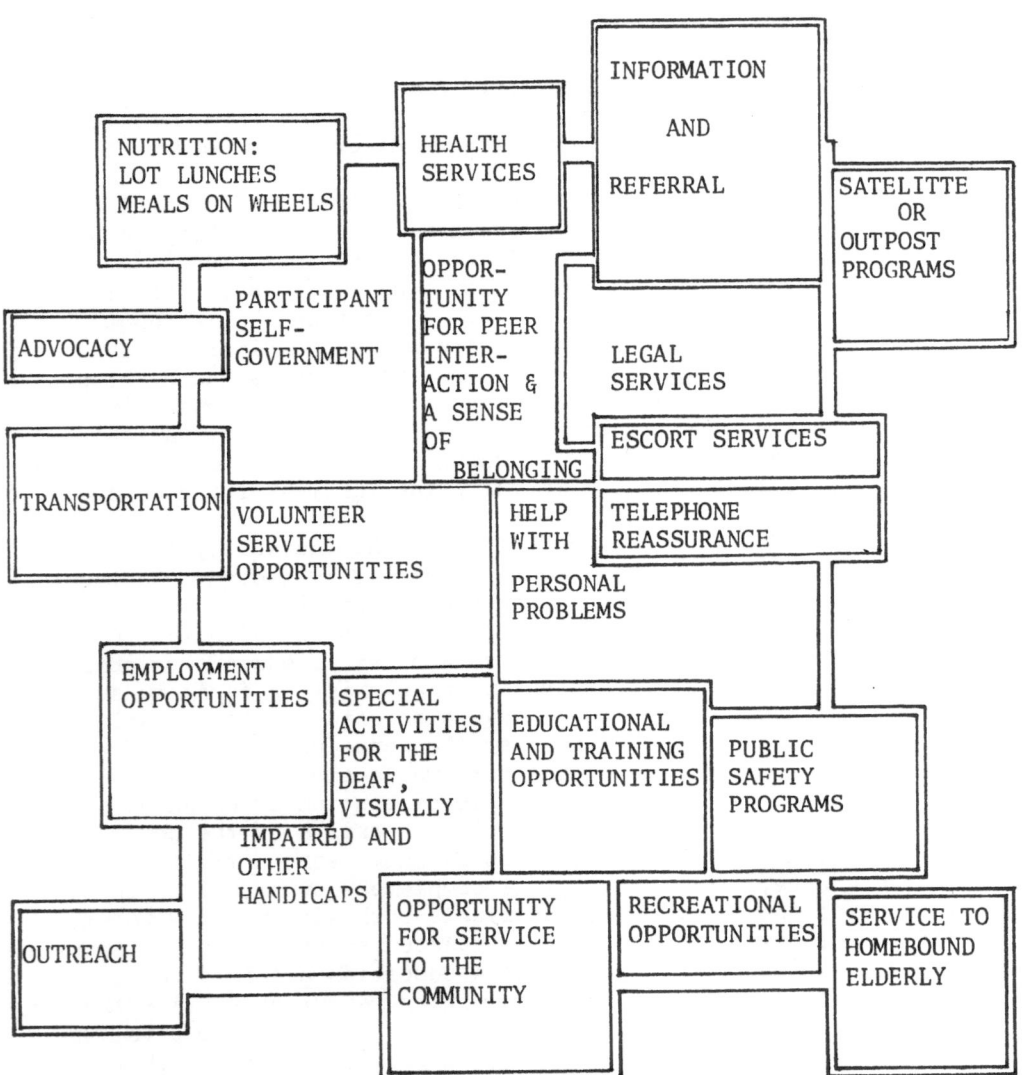

Figure 2   Multi-Service Senior Centre

have been identified as the greatest obstacles to obtaining appropriate care even when the level of community based services is adequate.[15]

A number of different solutions have been proposed. The Service Management Approach[6] consists of an ambitious attempt "to orchestrate the array of services into a co-ordinated, integrated treatment", and presupposes a client based comprehensive standardized assessment of current functioning leading to a written service plan, follow-up and reassessment. Quite appart from the difficulties which are usually encountered when different agencies try and collaborate on a unified approach this concept would exclude a large proportion of the most needy individuals, viz. those who are incapable of collaborating in the drawing up of an agreement on "problems identified, goals to be achieved and services to be pursued", in view of serious psychiatric disabilities.

Other approaches have considered the problem from the point of view of expanded home health care and its impact on the demand for institutional care, outcome, and cost.[15] Great difficulties in developing valid research instruments were encountered though it was generally concluded that expansion of home health care services would fail to bring about substantial savings. Increased availability inevitably leads to an increase in demand particularly from sections of the population currently not receiving any services though evidently in need of them. Further escalation of costs must ensue. This does not mean that cost effectiveness should not be considered in the development of services, but rather that the identification of specific target populations should be the first step in the expansion of ambulatory services. By defining the specific roles of day hospitals - geriatric and psychogeriatric - day care and day centres, and learning to differentiate between apples, oranges and carrots, it should be possible to devise the most appropriate services and treatment facilities for the ever growing number of elderly in our midst. At the same time it is necessary to have some estimate of the costs involved, otherwise the shoelaces that will hold these services together will either prove too short or break under the strain.

REFERENCES

1. Arie, T. - Day Care in Geriatric Psychiatry;Age and Ageing;8; Supplement;87-91;1979.
2. Brodie, E.M. - The Formal Support Network: Congregate Treatment Settings for Residents with Senescent Brain Dysfunction. In Miller, N.E. & Cohen, G.D. (eds) Clinical Aspects of Alzheimer's Disease & Senile Dementia. Aging Series Volume 15. Raven Press, New York, 1981.
3. Canadian Jewish News, 10 February, 1983.
4. Cooper, S. - A Day Hospital for Elderly Persons;The Canadian Nurse;41-43;February, 1970.
5. Glascote, R.M., Gudeman, J.E., & Miles, D.G. - Creative Mental Health Services for the Elderly;Joint Information Service of the American Psychiatric Association and the Mental Health Association;Washington, D.C., 1977.
6. Gottesman, L.E., Ishikazi, B. & Mac Bride, S.M. - Service

Management - Plan & Concept in Pennsylvania;Gerontologist; 19: 379-385, 1979.

7. Lorenze,E.J., Hamill, C.M., & Oliver, R.C. - The Day Hospital: An Alternative to Institutional Care. Journal Amer. Ger. Soc. 22: 316-320;1974.

8. Lyons, W., Day Care Programs: Problems and Prospects. Paper presented at the Annual Meeting of the National Conference of Jewish Communal Services;Washington, D.C., May, 1966.

9. Parkinson, C.N., Parkinson's Law or the Pursuit of Progress; p.4;John Murray;London, 1958.

10. Patashnik, M. - Providing Relief to Families of Impaired Day Care Members. Proceedings: Social Work Clinic Day - Baycrest Centre for Geriatric Care;52-54;1981.

11. Rapeljee, D.H. - Alternatives to Institutions;Proceedings of the 4th Annual Meeting of the Ontario Psychogeriatric Assocation, 109-112, Toronto, 1977.

12. Reichenfeld, H.F. - Letter to the Editor;The Lancet: 2: 1177; 1964.

13. Reichenfeld, H.F. - The Psychogeriatric Day Hospital - A Specific Treatment Modality in the Multidisciplinary Network. (To be published).

14. Stegmayer, H.E. - Personal Communication.

15. U.S. General Accounting Office. Report to the Chairman of the Committee on Labor & Human Resources, U.S. Senate GAO/1PE-83-1; December, 1982.

THE GERIATRIC DAY HOSPITAL IN FRANKFURT AM MAIN - HÖCHST: AN ALTERNATIVE

B. Kark, Hj. Werner, L. Waidner

Department of Internal Medicine

Städtisches Krankenhaus Frankfurt a.M.-Höchst

We report on our Day Hospital at Frankfurt - Höchst which openend 5 1/2 years ago and whose main concern is internal medicine. The stronghold of Geriatric Day Hospitals is in Britain, but they are prevalent in Switzerland and Scandinavia, too.

We set up the first such hospital in the Federal Republic, and others are following our path now. As it became obvious during our meeting on Day Hospitals two years ago, there is no common pattern for this type of hospital.

The actual type of geriatric day hospital and its establishment depend on the prevailing system of health care. In this country, the proposed day hospital has to be written into the official list of hospital beds first. Running costs are met by a daily charge. The actual rate is being fixed annually in negotiations with the health insurers (social security).

Other requirements include a densely populated catchment area with a suitable patient population and the attachment to a main hospital with full access to diagnostic and therapeutic facilities. In our case this is a hospital of the "maximum care" type. The Day Hospital was purpose-built to our own specifications to serve 60 elderly patients.

Staff includes two board certified internists, 5 nurses, 2 occupational therapists, 3 physiotherapists and a speech therapist.

The following services are provided:
Diagnosis and therapy as in any acute hospital; nursing care, occupational and physical therapy, and the services of a speech therapist. All sorts of medical appliances are available, too, of course. There is an additional voluntary service to help patients while they attend the hospital and after discharge.

The scope is not limited to strictly medical conditions since patients in this group tend to have multiple morbidity which covers all aspects of medicine. Constant cooperation with colleagues from other disciplines is mandatory. There is direct in-patient referral from family doctors in the area as well as referral from the various departments of the main hospital once the patient is able to get up. In earlier years, the majority of patients used to come from the main hospital. This ratio has been reversed now with 60% direct referrals from doctors in general practice and 40% of patients arriving from the hospital.

Any new case will receive a full diagnostic work-up unless this has been done during prior admission to the main hospital. Appropriate therapy will be instituted in due course which may mean referral to one of the other specialist departments such as for an operation.

Here are some frequently encountered conditions and their management:

(1) Heart disease: We offer long term E.C.G. monitoring, echocardiography, myocardial scintigraphy, right heart catheter, etc., so that a sensible choice of therapy can be made. We have an active group of elderly coronary patients who undertake specific group therapy with remarkable patient participation.

(2) Hypertension. We do not only provide thorough work-up but treat under conditions where the patients remain active. This, in our opinion, is superior to treatment where patients are kept in bed most of the time.

(3) We have full diagnostic facilities for occlusive arterial disease, i.e., Doppler sonography and angiography. Depending on findings, patients are recommen-

ded for an operation or put on full-scale conservative treatment. It is worth mentioning that patients like to use the treadmill simulator which allows self-assessment of progress.

(4) We use the full range of therapeutic support in stroke patients such as logopedics, occupational therapy and physiotherapy. Investigations are being completed as necessary.

(5) Diabetes is a frequent cause of referral. Both dietary counselling and planned exercise play an important role.

(6) The full diagnostic and therapeutic tools of the main hospital can again be aimed at disorders of sceletomuscular origin, and we make extensive use of the wide array of facilities of the orthopaedic department's physiotherapy section.

(7) Some malignant conditions are being investigated and treated as far as the framework of the day hospital allows.

(8) Some more benign forms of depression and dementia are being treated in the day hospital in cooperation with the neurology department.

We accept about 750 patients annually 60% of whom are women. The average length of stay is a little less than 20 days. The range is from 2 days where an operation is being arrranged to several weeks. 87% of patients can be discharged to their own homes.
The age distribution is as follows. 10% are from 50 to 59 years old, 80% are from 60 to 80 years, and a further 10% are older than 80 years. 40% of our patients have their own household, 56% live with spouse or relatives in the same home and only 3,3% were already cared for, single or with spouse, in an institution for the aged. Our average occupancy rate is about 90%. The waiting list is about one week, but urgent cases are being accepted directly.

In conclusion, here are the main features of our Day Hospital once again:
The main criterion is acute clinical illness; other cases will not attract payment for hospital treatment under our insurance system. This is in contrast to other countries where just caring support is made

available in geriatric day hospitals. For reasons inherent in our insurance system, we cannot provide therapy on a once or twice weekly basis as elsewhere.

The day hospital has to be attached to a main hospital for the sake of its diagnostic and therapeutic facilities and should have a densely populated catchment area so that enough patients can attend without too much travel. We have set a circle about 19 miles in diameter.

Our experience from 5 1/2 years tells us that a gap has been closed between in-patient and ambulatory treatment. Our success has led others to contemplate the setting up of day hospitals in many parts in the Federal Republic now.

TENTATIVE APPROACHES TO EVALUATING PSYCHOGERIATRIC DAY HOSPITAL TREATMENT

J. Husser and E.U. Kranshoff

Rheinische Landesklinik Köln
Wilhelm Griesingerstr 23
D-5000 Köln 91

During the last ten years there is an ongrowing number of psychogeriatric day hospitals being opened in West-Germany. But at the same time research work for defining the advantages of this treatment form compared with the traditional psychogeriatric wards evidently lacks. There are no definite criteria for the differential admission of a patient to a day hospital treatment or to a psychogeriatric ward as yet described. The often mentioned advantage of cheaper treatment in day hospitals is rather quickly changing into a disadvantage if the treatment period in the day hospital is longer than in the ward, thus resulting in the possibility of developing a new day hospital hospitalisation.

In our investigation we compared all first admissions of psychogeriatric patients of two open geriatric wards with the admissions to our psychogeriatric day hospital over a period of ten months. We investigated data of 84 patients, 20 from the day hospital and 64 from the two wards. Our data consist in informations about psycho-pathological status, physical and socio-demographic status, sex and age. The total of 12 variables were analysed by way of a cluster analysis technique.

Our research question was whether it is possible to describe factors which are relevant for the admission of a psychogeriatric patient either to an open ward or to day hospital treatment.

First a global description of our sample, divided into
the ward group and the day hospital group. (Table 1)

In the table you can see that in the age categories there
are more younger patients (65 - 69 years) in the day
hospital than in the wards. In the other age groups
there are no differences.

A smale difference,too, will be noticed in family status
where in the category of "widowed" ward patients are slightly
overrepresented. No difference was found concerning the
actual living situation, i.e. living alone or with others.

Concerning the psychiatric disturbances there is a trend
towards mild or moderate disturbances especially of the
psycho-organic and depressive and apathic syndromes in
the day hospital patients compared with the severe forms
of these syndromes in patients treated on the wards.

Concerning the global physical status patients with good
physical health primarily are treated in the day hospital,
patients with moderate or bad physical health on the wards.

As we were interested in variables forming clusters
which on one side could characterize day hospital patients and on the other side fully-stationarily treated
patients we performed a hierarchical cluster analysis.
Depending on statistical criteria a solution of seven
clusters was found to be optimal.

The results are presented in table 2. In three of the
seven clusters day hospital patients are overrepresented, i.e. they are represented twice as much as in
the total sample.

Two clusters showed no over - nor underrepresentation and two of the seven clusters showed an underrepresentation of day hospital patients.

In the three clusters with day hospital patients over-represented we find the following common variables which we think could be accepted as indicating day hospital treatment: these are "good somatic fitness", "moderate psycho-organic or mild depressive syndromes" and "no help reqiured in financial affairs".

Considering age groups none of the various age groups turned out to be more suitable for day hospital or fully stationary treatment respectively, the multivariate analysis thus contrasting the univariate analysis reported above.The next table (Table 3) presents the characterizing items of the two clusters in which day hospital patients are underrepresented: these are "moderate or bad somatic status", "severe depressive and mild or moderate paranoid symptoms" and "re-quiring much help in financial affairs".

The result seems trivial. It needs to be stressed, how-ever, that there is no influence of age, sex and living situation concerning the admission to one of the con-trasting treatments. From all of the investigated vari-ables the medical and the psychiatric indicators are the more important ones. From the whole field of social and demographic variables only the management of financial affairs had an influence, none of the various other supports in the daily living of old people not even the global rating of their living situation.

Table 1: Percentage Occurrence of Variables

Variable	Day Hospital (N=20) N	·/·	Open Wards (N=64) N	·/·
65-69 years	7	35	11	17
70-74 years	5	25	24	38
75-79 years	5	25	17	27
80+	3	15	12	19
male	5	25	12	19
female	15	75	52	81
unmarried	2	10	5	8
married	9	45	24	38
widowed	7	35	32	50
divorced/separated	2	10	3	5
living alone	9	45	28	44
living with family or others	11	55	36	56
deaths	8	40	17	27
dwelling: requiring no help	8	40	23	36
little help	4	20	13	20
much help	3	15	6	9
nothing alone	5	25	21	33
finance: requiring no help	9	45	25	39
little help	4	20	2	3
much help	2	10	9	14
nothing alone	5	25	19	30

Table 1: Percentage Occurrence of Variables (Continued)

Variable		Day Hospital (N=20) N	./.	Open Wards (N=64) N	./.
paranoid syndrome:	mild	2	10	5	8
	moderate	2	10	11	17
Psychosyndrome:	moderate	7	35	14	22
	severe	0	0	5	8
depressive syndrome:					
	moderate	15	75	39	61
	severe	0	0	9	14
apathic	moderate	12	60	19	30
	severe	2	10	16	25
physical health:	good	14	70	13	20
	moderate	5	25	36	56
	bad	1	5	15	23

Table 2: Clusters in which day hospital patients are overrepresented

Cluster IV	Cluster %	Total %
good physical health	100	32
70-74 years	100	35
no help in required in financial affairs	75	48
mild depr. syndrome	63	18
mild paranoid syndrome	25	8
N = 8		
Day Hospital: 210		
Open Wards: 66		

Cluster I	Cluster %	Total %
good physical health	100	32
75-79 years	90	26
no help required in financial affairs	70	48
N = 10		
Day Hospital: 208		
Open Wards: 69		

Cluster II	Cluster %	Total %
65-69 years	100	22
moderate psychoorganic syndrome	88	25
little help required in financial affairs	19	8
N = 16		
Day Hospital: 184		
Open Wards: 74		

good physical health

no or little help required in financial affairs

mild psychiatric symptomatology

Table 3: Clusters in which day hospital patients are <u>underrepresented</u>

Cluster VII	Cluster %	Total %
bad physical health	100	19
moderate para- noid syndrome	46	18
severe de- pressive syndrome	36	11
much help re- quired in fin- ancial affairs	27	14

N = 11
Day Hospital: 0
Open Wards : 119

Cluster III	Cluster %	Total %
70-74 years	100	35
moderate phy- sical health	93	49
severe apathy	33	22
mild paranoid syndrome	22	8

N = 15
Day Hospital: 28
Open Wards: 123

bad physical health

moderate or severe psychiatric symtomatology

much help required in financial affairs

DAY HOSPITAL CARE FOR THE ELDERLY IN THE NETHERLANDS

E.M.I. van Woerkom

Verpleeghuis Eikendonk
Eikendonklaan 2
5143 NG Waalwijk, The Netherlands

The subject of this paper is the development of daycare*in the
Netherlands. First I shall give you a short survey on ideas about
health care. In this survey I shall restrict myself to data which
relate to daycare. Next I shall further go into contents and
implications of this form of care: namely the indication policy,
the role of professional aid and relations and the conditions
for optimal realisation of the intended course of treatment.
Furthermore some recent Dutch publications will be mentioned.

At the moment the structure of health care in the Netherlands is
subject to change. Predictions about composition of the population
have led to an increase of the care for the elderly. Up until now
there was a rapid increase of nursing homes. Due to the economic
recession and a changed way of thinking about health care, when
it comes to the granting funds the out-patient care will be
emphasized. For example the number of hospital beds will be reduced
and consequently there will be more work for nursing homes, out-
patient care and such. The development of daycare fits in: daycare
has a preventive character and supports the out-patient treatment.
At the moment there are 327 nursing homes with 47.624 beds[1].
The standard for the somatic beds is 1.2% of the number of people
above 65 and the standard for psychogeriatric beds is 1.25%.
The standards for daycare are also laid down by the law. The number
of daycare centres has been established on 6% of the total of
nursing home beds; there are 0.72 °/oo somatic daycare places and
0.75 °/oo psychogeriatric daycare places.
Since 1977 there is a regulation on that puts the responsability
for daycare to the Health Insurance Fund. In 1977 25 nursing
homes were considered for financial aid; already in 1982 the total
was 139.

---

* In this article, daycare implies daytreatment

Table 1: Figures on daycare over the year 1982[1]

Daycare	Number	Available places	Treated patients	Average use of 1 place
Somatic	49	671	1.937	2.9
Psychogeriatric	33	445	1.035	2.3
Both categories	57	935	3.572	3.8
Total	139	2.051	6.544	

In recent years the number of daycare wards has increased as well as the number of people using these facilities.
A daycare centre at a nursing home has at least 5 places. With a total of 15 places a separate ward cen be built. A ward has somatic places, psychogeriatric or both (i.e. separated from each other).

After this presentation of figures and standards I shall go into the contents of this form of care.
What are the advantages of daycare? Daycare has medical, economic and social advantages. A great deal about these advantages has been published. These advantages can be found in the objectives which are pursued by the institutions. They can be summarized as follows:
1. delay or prevention of total admission; 2. relief of care at home and 3. care after release from hospital or nursing home.
All day centres support the main objective to keep the patient in his own surroundings for as long as possible. However, the day centres can differ mutually in a. the concrete realisation of these objectives and b. in the emphasis they put on their treatment philosophies.
In 1981 the National Health Institute [3] (N.H.I.) has done some research on daycare. This research was intended to see how daycare has worked out in the past 5 years. The centres do have some freedom, for example in indication policy, type of patients, objectives and whether they have contact with the out-patient care. The ideas of those who work in nursing homes with daycare and the demands from the outside world (patients, referring institutions) do ultimately result in a certain kind of care.

On account of the above there may exist differences between daycare centres. Jongeneel[4] found 4 different forms:
1. Most important is treatment, which will be limited in time. Staff members work individually; the nursing home doctor plays a central role.
2. Besides physical health, the psychological and social functioning are important; the care is a multi-disciplinary affair.
3. The nearest relations of the patient are involved in the

treatment, e.g. in joint talks on treatment.
4. Resocialisation of the patient is crucial. Recovery is not
the main objective, but the dealing with the handicap by
patient and his nearest relations.
The care involved from the first to the fourth form shows a
growing complexity.
There is no point in judging which is the best form (that depends
on all kinds of factors), even though it would be worthwhile
if each separate daycare centre makes a choice of policy in the
kind of form ånd in the quantity of differentiation with the
chosen form.

One of the differences between daycare centres is their indication
policy, i.e. a. the procedure around reference and indication and
b. the indication criteria that are being used.
How does the reference come about?
Patients are directed to a day centre by a general practioner
or by some referring institution (e.g. a Municipal Geriatric
Service). 3)
The N.H.I.[3] pleas for a multidisciplinary screening (by a doctor,
psychiatrist, psychologist, the nursing staff, a social worker
and eventually a neurologist). This screening is especially
necessary for psychogeriatric patients, because in this group
of patients mental, physical ånd social factors cause a complex
pattern of complaints. The screening takes place in one day
or during a longer observation period. After the screening a
discussion follows with the general practioner, the spokesman
of the referring institution, the nearest relations and the
daycare staff.
One can see the following advantages of such a screening:
1. to achieve the most appropriate admission
2. to accomplish a file with relevant background information
about the patient
3. to intensify contacts with out-patient care.

Which indication criteria are being used?
The Health Insurance Board states that the difference between
a daycare patient and a nursing home patient is that the environment of the daycare patient can satisfy the needs of the patient
during the time he is not in the daycare residence.
The Health Insurance Board [6] states that relief for environment
cannot be the only indication criterium. [4]
All daycare wards in hte N.H.I. research[4] put prevention of
an admission first; one ward states that patients can be
considered for treatment only if the perspective for improvement
exists. Some wards emphasize the releif for the home front;
this bridges the final admission. Most wards however, strongly
reject the idea of a daycentre like a 'crèche'. Crèche means
that a patient is offered the possibility to remain in an atten-
tive, professionally guided surroundings, in which a number

of stimulants are given to which the patient barely reacts. The
N.H.I. questions the fact that these patients should stay on
a day ward. Daycare for this reason is too expensive and the
possibility of overcrowding is greater.
In practice however, we can see an aggrevation of infirmity
of referred patients (among other things due to lack of provisions)
by which the amount of crèche patients is bound to increase in
the future.

Until now some research has been done on indication criteria and
reasons for admission.
A research of Monincx and van Oorsouw [7] shows that for 1/3 of the
research group relief of the home situation counts as a principal
reason for admission. Other often mentioned reasons were symptoms
of dementia and demand for reactivation. Relations mention the
following disturbing factors at the moment of admission: mental
deterioration, namely memory deficits, problems in the daily
care for oneself and restlessness during the night.
The research of van Woerkom[8] also shows that the reasons for
admission always had been the relief of the home environment in
combination with either reactivating or maintaining, respectively
improving the psychical level of the concerned. 1/3 of the cases
counted for crèche patients. Those who apply for daycare very
often mentioned the following symptoms which had been of crucial
significance to call for a similar aid: passivity, apathy and
depression. One hopes that (re)activation can be achieved through
daycare. Also disturbing factors were the following behavioral
aspects: wandering around, agitation, paranoia, meddlesomeness,
restlessness at night and the fact that it is impossible to
leave the patient on his own.
Monincx concludes that it is not clear which admission criteria
have been applied, in other words which degree of dementia is
acceptable. All abovementioned symptoms occur in the less infirmed
patients in nursing homes. Other factors, like the
situation of the family play a role in a. making their choice
between total admission or daycare and b. in the amount of time
a patient can stay at home.
In the past few years there have been publications about the role
of the family in the nursing process.
Jacobs en van de Schoot[9] come to the following conclusion:
the motivation of the family to carry on with the help depends
on their standard of values, the quality of the past and present
relationship between family and patient and especially the
positive and negative interactions at the moment. The condition
of the patient was not the most important factor; the psychological
and physical condition of the family however were crucial.
Daycare turns out to have a positive influence because the
family can take some distance from the nursing process.

I shall end this paper with some recommendations for the future. Some conditions have to be fulfilled for the realisation of the preventive character of daycare:

1. Information to out-patient care and relations about:
   a. the special function of a daycare centre and
   b. disturbances at old age.
   In this way an early diagnosis of psychological and physical detoriation will be possible.
2. Multidisciplinary screening before admission
3. On applying explicitation of the exact demand of help and expectations with regard to daycare; and next formulating of individual objectives.
4. To have a clear insight into those factors that are crucially important to family in order to continue their care.
5. Guidance to family by means of individual or group therapy.
6. Insight into the local or regional situation (presence or absence of provisions of other institutions) by which eventually it will be possible to influence the inflow of patients.

Up to now there has been too little systematic research on the problems I have dealt with in this paper. Only by scientific support the direct aid can be optimalised.

References:

1. J.J.G. Lorsheijd: Bedbezetting 1982, Nationaal Ziekenhuis Instituut, Utrecht (1983).
2. K. van Eekelen: Dagbehandeling in het verpleeghuis, Nijmegen (1975); E.M.I. van Woerkom: Dagbehandeling, de dagbehandelingspatient en zijn partner,Ned.Tijdschrift voor Gerontologie.
3. F. Jongeneel, J. Leenders: Tussen thuis en verpleeghuis, Nationaal Ziekenhuis Instituut, Utrecht (1982).
4. F. Jongeneel: Dagbehandeling in verpleeghuizen: een perspectief, Tijdschrift voor Gerontologie en Geriatrie 14 (1983)
5. Ziekenfondsraad: Advies inzake opneming dagbehandeling in verpleeghuis in het verstrekkingenpakket, Amstelveen (1976).
6. Nationale Ziekenhuis Raad: Nota dagbehandeling in verpleeghuizen, Utrecht (1981).
7. I. Monincx, J. van Oorsouw: Dagbehandeling Psychogeriatrie, verpleeghuis Rosendael, Utrecht (1983).
8. E.M.I. van Woerkom: Redenen voor aanvraag op een psychogeriatrische dagbehandeling, Verpleeghuis Eikendonk, Waalwijk (1983)
9. R. van Brummelen, P. Tjoa, M. Wardenaar: Onderzoek naar de gevoelens en ervaringen van ouderen met een dement funktionerende partner. Rijksuniversiteit Utrecht (1981). M. Jacobs, M. van de Schoot: Mantelzorgers van ouderen in dagbehandeling, Rijksuniversiteit Utrecht (1982)

PSYCHOINVOLUTE DISTURBANCES: THERAPEUTIC POSSIBILITIES

Roger Maximiliano Montenegro

Centre for Research in Medico-Psychological
Communication
Juncal 2425 - 8°B
(1425) Buenos Aires, Argentina

I wish to speak of a whole range of psychoemotional disorders of involution, few classified as syndromes and of major significance given that our elderly population, with increased means for prolonging life, is tending to grow exponentially and its disturbances with it.

We shall limit this broad range to disturbances ocurring during the ageing process, excluding those complaints where a history of morbidity could be noted before the involute period.

This distiction is of course artificial and open to some question; for instance it is by no means demonstrable at the moment that problems manifesting themselves for the first time in old age are in any clear way linked to the involution of the organism. Being a period of enormous change, old age may simply reveal what had been hidden or compensated for in earlier life. Similar doubts apply to those psychosis of late appearance where the gerontological changes (biological and psychometric) indicate nothing more than a physiological involution; in these cases it would be fanciful to blame the ageing process for the appearance of the psychosis.

We are going to consider the extensive group of psychoses, neuroses and other multiple behavioural disturbances occuring in this characteristic age group: "The involution", resulting from purely functional changes or reactive behaviour. We shall exclude the other large group of senile mental pathologies, understood as dementias, or general deterioration of mental faculties. We shall also exclude, somewhat arbitrarily, disturbances manifested before the involution.

Etiopathogenic considerations on involute disturbances

Using fairly flexible criteria we can identify the period of transition from maturity to the begining of ageing as between 45 and 65 years.

These limits will vary according to biological structure, predominant cultural models, family organization and existing personality. Equally they vary between individuals, and in the same individual, between each organ or function and in different moments.

The complexity and acuteness of these changes is such that the stage has been compared with the other age of enormous adjustment: Adolescence.

The most well-adjusted personalities will adapt satisfactorily to the change however complicated. Others with unresolved conflicts or lacking the capacity to deal with these intense experiences will manifest more or less pathological behaviour.

It is a stage of great losses needing both grieving and readjustment, that is to say a redistribution of the libido in relation to the losses transferring it to other internal and external objects, depending to a greater or lesser extent on the developement of the existing personality.

There is a strong genetic affinity between psychoses of involution and the group of schizoid and schizophrenic psychoses.

The old person and death

"Nothing is nearer to life that death as our time passes."

The image of death and the individual's idea of it is more important than the biological phenomenon itself. L. M. Goodman (in 1975) has shown that fear of death is less in individuals who have developed their creative potential more during their lives.

There is a relationship between the individual's view

of death and his life-style. The relative serenity or anxiety of old people is related to their degree of acceptance of death (in this respect the intense and common anxiety of the involution has been linked to the conscious or unconscious rejection of death).

The unbearable position of man in relation to death appears to stem from a narcissistic position. The subject is unable to make the smallest distinction between himself and the image of his world.

Social death

For many old people, social death comes before biological death. Louis Vincent Thomas has analysed it profoundly: "Old people like all condemned men awaiting execution, have lost all power; biologically finished, spent, socially useless (unproductive modest consumers) deprived of their functions (resting before eternal rest) usually living in precarious financial circumstances (especially if they belong to the least favoured classes of society) and in a cruel solitude."

The loss of a social identity based on productivity demands a reorganization of the personality but many old people have no alternative but to seek refuge in sickness and stagnation and, as a result, to enter an institution.

"The hospice (comments L.V. Thomas) is the result and most perfect instrument of social death in that it institutionalises the alienation of the old person while relieving the family of blame."

Semiology

We shall consider both involute psychoses and neuroses and other behavioural disturbances giving special attention to the pathology of grief, to suicide and to sexual behaviour in old age. Psychoses are identifiable in two broad areas: Involute melancholy and involute psychoses of delirium.

Involute melancholy was isolated by Kraepelin in 1896 who distinguished it from manic-depressive psychosis. It is the most common of these psychoses (70%), ocurring mainly in women (70%) between the ages of 50 and 55 after the menopause; it is characterised usually by feelings of lascitude, boredom, hypocondria or slight depression. After a while and reflecting the fundamental involute situation, and as a result of some emotional release factor the full range of symptoms is observed. There are recurring hysterical and hypocondriac symptoms as well as hallucinatory activity ideas of ruin, pessimism and ultimately self-destruction. The anxiety is so intense in its desperation that it may eventually lead to suicide attempts.

Involute psychoses of delirium generally appear as more or less systematic deliriums, hallucinatory or interpretative and of a paranoic turn. These cases have been given varying titles and correspond broadly to the involute paranoic state or senile paraphrenia of the C.I.E. (Code 297.1). They have also been called senile schizophrenia or late paraphrenia. They generally reflect a history of strong personality distrubances even without psychotic histories.

Neuroses. The most common are hystero-hypocondriac neuroses with varying symptoms of tyranny, refuge in sickness, conversions, romancing and deceit. Pruritus, pains and genito-urinary disturbances also occur. Acute regressive stages are common with disorientation and behavioural pseudo-demential disorders, without neurological symptoms.

Obsessive and phobic neuroses are more rare and they are accompanied by strong depressive tendencies and general anxiety (rituals and general phobic behaviour). Neurotic depressions also occur characterised by anxiety, hypocondria and depressive reactions.

Other behavioural disturbances comprise a range of changes in behaviour often seen in old people to varying degrees. These cases correspond to the "Adaptive Reactions in old age" (Code 307.4 of C.I.E.). According to current criteria these conducts are more linked to socio-cultural and psychological factors than to underlying biologico-involute processes. They are characterised as, rigidity, conservatism, agression towards the younger generation, incontinence and exaggerated worries about health, money, death etc. These symptoms, common among many old people but in an exaggerated form with depressions, anxieties, disturbances of sleep and varying functional disorders, are not identified clearly as clinical histories but are a frequent cause of consultation.

Pathological grief is also a common behavioural disturbance in old age. Equally suicide is not uncommon in the involution, caused by many factors not only loneliness or organic and mental illnesses. Recognising the danger of suicide is of major importance in psychiatry. The danger may increase for a number of reasons including hereditary predisposition, previous attempts, depressive bouts, and isolation or worries about money or health.

Disturbances of sexuality

Sexual relations reflect the subject's own models. Master and Johnson completed two illuminating studies on the sexuality of the aged of great use in understanding their disturbances. The elderly man and woman, they found can maintain an active sex life until their 80s. Studies of the changes accompanying ageing are few and have tended to relate changes in sexual behaviour simply to biological decline; but recent studies shed new light.

Many men become impotent because they do not understand normal changes in sexuality which ageing brings; a reduction in intercourse and in masturbation and nocturnal emissions. Possibly the most important factor is the early years of sexual formation of the individual; a regular sex life is the best means of maintaining sexual potency. Men who have been sexually active in a formative period are the ones who usually maintain an active sex life in old age. For women social and psychological factors are qualified by the changes and hormonal decline during the pre-menopause and menopause.But regular sexual activity is also important to maintain the women's sexual capacity. In this respect even women suffering from signs of vaginal steroid deficiency will maintain despite this high level of sexual activity. Many neurotic conditions of sexual and seductive exaltation both in the man and in the woman appear to be a result of defensive behaviour overcompensating for an impoverished reality.

Such senile behaviour was attributed to cerebro-biological changes ignoring the possibility of changes in libido and compensatory behaviour. It is possible for instance that the loss of awareness of new things and the concentration on old memories or hypocondria may in fact be due to the impoverishment of the libido and its narcissistic regressive displacement than to cerebral damage.

To end this clinical summary I would draw attention to the frequency with which in practice aspects of biological deficit can be overvalued, diagnosing many patients incorrectly as "senile dementia" or "cerebral arteriosclerosis", when a more serious examination would discard such simplistic diagnoses.

Therapeutic possibilities

Three possible levels of preventive action are presented by G. Kaplan viz: a) <u>Primary prevention</u> aiming to reduce the incidence of mental pathology in ageing by acting on socio-cultural factors in a variety of ways, seeking a better understanding of the problem and the social status of the old person, offering him chances to find a creative response to his problems; eg. by changing brusque unilateral and compulsory retirement to more gradual forms with adequate guidance and training for the future. b) <u>Secondary prevention</u> by adventurous diagnosis and treatment which would reduce the prevalence of disturbances and c) <u>Terciary prevention</u> or rehabilitation seeking to reduce the level of deterioration. The two latter levels suggest a series of basic premises: 1) Avoiding hospitalization and isolation 2) Maintaining an adequated social and family integration but avoiding mechanical imitations of the values of the consumer society 3) Maintaining a fine geriatric balance with correct evaluation of the subject's bio-physical state 4) Encouraging adequate doctor-patient relationships in the geriatric medicine 5) Recognising the importance of psycho-pharmacological therapy in psychiatric treatment.

Treatments cannot be mechanically applied; we need to seek the appropriate balance of social, institutional, psychotherapeutic and medicational approaches, based above all on technical training and a particular richness of humanity.

Psychotherapy should be the support, guide and illumination of the patient in his involute changes and his problems at work, at home and in society at large. We need to remember that therapy is complicated by the individual's rigidity and denial of his conflicts, defence mechanisms in the face of a disagreable reality.

The psychotherapy of the patient and the guidance and correction of the possible distortions in his domestic environment offer the chance of regaining a lost equilibrium and a tranquile and creative existence which we like to call health.

AUTHOR INDEX

Depression, 355, 443, 467
Development, 95
Developmental disability, 227
Diagnostic and therapeutic
    range, 475
Differentiation, 493
Distractibility, 41
Disturbance, 189
Dopamin receptor, 89
Dopamine, 311, 317
Dopaminergic system, 59
Dose prediction test, 377
Double mourning, 117
Down syndrome, 283, 311
Drug interactions, 377
DSM-III, 9, 289
Dysfunction, 41

Early adolescence, 17
EEG, 277
Epidemiology, 253
Epilepsy, 73
Expressive language, 221

Family conditions, 133
Family integration, 443
Family therapy, 221, 449
Frontal syndrome, 317
Functioning, 333

Geriatric community study, 417
Geriatric day hospital, 475
Geriatric hospital study, 417
Gerontocracy, 493
Gerontopsychiatry, 437, 457,
    461, 479, 487
Gerontopsychopharmacology, 403,
    411
Geropsychiatric clinic, 443
Glucose utilisation, 283

Handicap, 133
Handicapped children, 217
Higashimurayama plan, 235
Hyperactivity, 41
Hyperkinesis, 41, 59
Hypertension, 295
Hyperxydosis, 411

Hypothalamus, 311
Hypoxia, 411

Immigrant child, 141
Immigration, 27
Inattention, 41
Incoordination, 41
Indio-Chinese children, 109
Indonesia, 33
Infantile hyperkinetic syndrome,
    59
In-patient care, 429
Institutionalisation, 383
Insufficiency, 277
Insulin tolerance test, 89
Intracranial tumors, 305
Ischemic score, 277

Kanner's syndrome, 47

Language impairment, 47
L-Dopa, 59
Learning disabilities, 41
Leeds scales, 123
Lithium, 79, 83
Long term service, 467

Mamillary body, 311
Manic-depressive illness, 65, 79
Mediator, 203
Medical model, 467
Memory, 333, 411
Memory disorders, 339
Menengiomas aneurysms, 305
Mental health planning, 429
Mental health screening, 103
Mental health services, 241
Mental illness, 221, 247, 367
Mental retardation, 133, 177,
    195, 203, 221, 217, 227,
    235, 241, 247
Microsurgery, 305
Mild emotional disorders, 103
Mild mental retardation, 103
Mild motor dysfunction, 103
Minimal brain damage, 11, 41
Minor psychiatric illness, 117
Mother-baby relationship, 171

502

SUMMARY

CONTENTS OF

VOLUMES 1-8

VOLUME 1

CLINICAL PSYCHOPATHOLOGY

NOMENCLATURE AND CLASSIFICATION

VOLUME 2

BIOLOGICAL PSYCHIATRY

HIGHER NERVOUS ACTIVITY

BIOLOGICAL PSYCHIATRY
Biological Aspects - Organic Brain Syndromes
Biological Aspects - Functional Psychoses
Genetic Aspects of Psychiatry
New Prospects in the Treatment of Depression
Clinical and Research Aspects of Affective Disorders
Pathochemical Markers in Major Psychoses
Steroids in Psychiatry
Frontiers in Psychoneuroendocrinology
Positron Emission Tomography I + II
Laterality and Psychopathology
Serotonin and Disturbances of Mood
    (Sérotonine et troubles de l'humeur)
Psychobiology of Depression - Recent Findings and Theoretical Models
The Old Amine Theory and New Antidepressants
Biology of Mania
Lithium Transport Research: From Cellular Membrane to Clinical Practice
Clinical Applications of Plasma Levels in the Management of Schizophrenia
Dosing Neuroleptic Medication with the Help of Electric Registration of
    Extrapyramidal Fine Motoricity
      (Dosierung der Neuroleptika mit Hilfe der elektronischen Registrierung
      der extrapyramidalen Feinmotorik)
Movement Disorders and Tardive Dyskinesia
ECT: Background and Current Research
Psychic Changes in Patients with Cerebrovascular Diaseases I + II
Systems Science and Systems Therapy
Psychobiology of Anxiety
Psychobiology of Anorexia Nervosa
Physiological Basis of Anxiety
The Development of Human Stress Response: Research Findings and Clinical
Application
Stress and the Heart
HIGHER NERVOUS ACTIVITY
Physiological Investigations of Psychological Processes in Health
    and and Psychiatric Diseases
Orienting Reflexes in Psychophysiological Health and Disease

VOLUME 3

PHARMACOPSYCHIATRY

VOLUME 4

PSYCHOTHERAPY

PSYCHOSOMATIC MEDICINE

VOLUME 5

CHILD AND ADOLESCENT PSYCHIATRY

MENTAL RETARDATION

GERIATRIC PSYCHIATRY

VOLUME 8

HISTORY OF PSYCHIATRY

NATIONAL SCHOOLS

EDUCATION

TRANSCULTURAL PSYCHIATRY